the
Human Nervous System

AN ANATOMICAL VIEWPOINT

Second Edition

Murray L. Barr, M.D., F.R.S.C., F.R.S.

PROFESSOR OF ANATOMY, HEALTH SCIENCES CENTRE,
THE UNIVERSITY OF WESTERN ONTARIO;
CONSULTANT, CHILDREN'S PSYCHIATRIC RESEARCH INSTITUTE;
HONORARY CONSULTANT, VICTORIA HOSPITAL AND
ST. JOSEPH'S HOSPITAL, LONDON, ONTARIO, CANADA

Contents

Preface
TO THE
SECOND EDITION

The encouraging acceptance of this book, combined with an awareness of numerous changes that needed to be made, led to the publication of a Second Edition. In addition to changes in the text, many of them minor but some rather substantial, several of the illustrations have been either modified or replaced by new ones. The author is greatly indebted to users of the book who made helpful suggestions, and to Dr. Vernon B. Brooks, Professor of Physiology, University of Western Ontario, for advice with respect to CHAPTER 10: CEREBELLUM.

London, Ontario   M. L. B.

Preface

TO THE
FIRST EDITION

Because of the intricacies of neuronal connections and the necessity of being able to visualize structures three-dimensionally, the anatomy of the central nervous system offers a particular challenge to the student. It is only through an adequate understanding of the structure of the brain and spinal cord that concurrent studies along physiologic and clinical lines can progress. In particular, the interpretation of neurologic signs and symptoms must rest on a sound basis of neurologic anatomy. It is hoped that this textbook will provide such a basis for students in the health sciences and others studying the central nervous system of man. The book is written for those approaching the neurosciences for the first time; several excellent larger books on neurologic anatomy are available to the advanced student.

The material has been arranged in four sections. The first section deals mainly with neurohistology. The second and largest section is concerned with the regional anatomy of the central nervous system, beginning with the spinal cord and progressing to the highest levels of the brain. Although the sensory and motor systems are discussed regionally, experience in teaching has shown the necessity of reviewing these clinically important systems in their entirety, and this is done in the third section. The fourth section deals with the blood supply of the central nervous system, its meningeal coverings, and the cerebrospinal fluid.

Eponyms are used freely in neurology, in spite of attempts to eliminate them; they frequently offer welcome alternatives to the more formal, and sometimes formidable, anatomic terms. Some facts concerning individuals whose names are attached to structures are provided at the end of the book for students who are curious about the source of the eponyms. In addition, since many neurologic terms are derived from Greek and Latin, a glossary is included for those students who have not received instruction in the classics.

It is a pleasure to acknowledge the valued assistance of several persons. A special note of appreciation goes to Mrs. Margaret Corrin for the preparation of the drawings, all of which are her own work. Illustrations of this type are of particular importance in a textbook of neurologic anatomy. I also wish to thank Mrs. Aileen Densham, who carried out the secretarial work most efficiently. I am greatly indebted to Mr. J. E. Walker for the technical preparation of anatomic specimens for reproduction, to Mr. C. E. Jarvis for the photomicrographs, and to the staff of the Art Service Department of this Health Services Centre for their fine photography.

Several colleagues have given of their time to read drafts of all chapters and make valuable suggestions. They are Dr. H. W. K. Barr, of the Department of Clinical Neurological Sciences, and Drs. R. C. Buck, M. J. Hollenberg, and D. G. Montemurro, of the Department of Aanatomy. I am also grateful for the many helpful discussions on specific topics with Dr. J. P. Girvin, of the Departments of Clinical Neurological Sciences and Physiology, and with Dr. A. Kertesz, of the Department of Clinical Neurological Sciences. Finally, I wish to express my appreciation to the staff of Harper & Row for their patience, advice, and assistance.

London, Ontario   *M. L. B.*

the
Human Nervous System

AN ANATOMICAL VIEWPOINT

Introduction and
Neurohistology

1

An Introduction to the Major Regions of the Central Nervous System

It is helpful to refer to embryologic development when defining the principal regions or divisions of the central nervous system. The brain and spinal cord have their origin in the neural tube, which forms at the end of the third week of gestation by a midline invagination of the dorsal ectoderm. The nerve cells that eventually constitute the central nervous system, together with most of the interstitial or neuroglial cells, are therefore derivatives of the outer ectodermal layer of the embryo, like the epidermal cells covering the body surface.

Growth and differentiation are greatest in the rostral portion of the neural tube, from which the large and complex brain develops. Three swellings, the *primary brain vesicles*, appear toward the end of the fourth week; they are called the *rhombencephalon, mesencephalon,* and *prosencephalon* (Fig. 1–1A). The caudal and rostral primary vesicles each divide into two swellings during the fifth week, so that there are five *secondary brain vesicles;* these are called the *myelencephalon, met-*

encephalon, mesencephalon, diencephalon, and *telencephalon* (Fig. 1–1B). There is a pronounced flexure in the mesencephalic region.

DERIVATIVES OF THE BRAIN VESICLES

The various regions of the brain which develop from the foregoing vesicles acquire a distinctive structure, and some of the formal embryologic names are replaced by others for common usage (Table 1–1 and Fig. 1–2). The myelencephalon becomes the medulla oblongata, while the metencephalon develops into the pons and cerebellum. The mesencephalon of the mature brain is usually called the midbrain. The names diencephalon and telencephalon are retained, largely because of the diverse nature of their derivatives. A large mass of gray matter, the thalamus, develops in the diencephalon. Adjacent regions are known as the epithalamus, hypothalamus, and

3

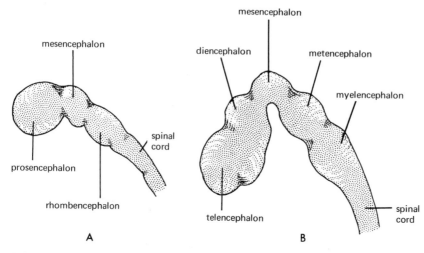

FIG. 1–1. A. Primary brain vesicles, fourth week of gestation. **B.** Secondary brain vesicles, sixth week of gestation.

subthalamus, each with distinctive structural and functional characteristics. The telencephalon undergoes the greatest development in the human brain, in respect both to other regions and to the telencephalon of other animals. It includes the olfactory system, the corpus striatum (a mass of gray matter with motor functions), an extensive surface layer of gray matter known as the cortex or pallium, and a medullary center of white matter.

The medulla, pons, and midbrain together make up the brain stem, to which the cerebellum is attached by three pairs of peduncles. The diencephalon and telencephalon constitute the cerebrum, of which the telencephalon is represented by the massive cerebral hemispheres. The lumen of the neural tube is converted into a lateral ventricle in each cerebral hemisphere, a third ventricle in the diencephalon, and a fourth ventricle bounded by the medulla, pons, and cerebellum. The third and fourth ventricles are connected by a narrow chan-

TABLE 1–1.   DEVELOPMENT OF THE MATURE BRAIN FROM THE BRAIN VESICLES

Primary brain vesicles	Secondary brain vesicles	Mature brain
Rhombencephalon	Myelencephalon	Medulla oblongata
	Metencephalon	Pons and cerebellum
Mesencephalon	Mesencephalon	Midbrain
Prosencephalon	Diencephalon	Thalamus, epithalamus, hypothalamus, and subthalamus
	Telencephalon	Cerebral hemispheres, consisting of the olfactory system, corpus striatum, cortex, and medullary center

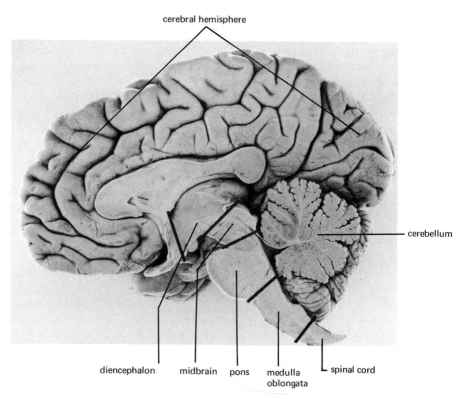

FIG. 1–2. Regions of the mature central system, as seen in sagittal section. ✕⅝

nel or aqueduct that traverses the midbrain.

SUMMARY OF MAIN REGIONS OF THE NERVOUS SYSTEM

Certain features of the main regions are noted in the following summary, by way of introduction and to provide a first acquaintance with some neurologic terms.

SPINAL CORD

The *spinal cord* is the least differentiated component of the neuraxis. The segmental nature of the spinal cord is reflected in a series of paired spinal nerves, each of which is attached to the cord by a dorsal sensory root and ventral motor root. The central gray matter, in which nerve cell bodies are located, has a roughly H-shaped outline in transverse section. White matter, which consists of nerve fibers running longitudinally, occupies the periphery of the cord. The spinal cord includes neuronal connections that provide for important spinal reflexes. There are also pathways conveying sensory data to the brain and other pathways conducting impulses from the brain to motor neurons in the spinal cord.

MEDULLA OBLONGATA

The fiber tracts of the spinal cord are continued in the *medulla,* which also contains clusters of nerve cells called nuclei. The most prominent of these, the inferior olivary nuclei, send fibers to the cerebellum through the inferior cerebellar peduncles, which attach the cerebellum to the medulla oblongata. Of the smaller nuclei, some are components of the following cranial nerves: hypoglossal (CN12), accessory (CN11), vagus (CN10), and glossopharyngeal (CN9). Nuclei of the vestibulocochlear nerve (CN8) are partly in the medulla and partly in the pons.

PONS

The *pons* consists of two distinct parts. The dorsal portion has features shared with the rest of the brain stem. It therefore includes sensory and motor tracts, together with nuclei of the facial (CN7), abducens (CN6), and trigeminal (CN5) nerves. (Trigeminal nuclei are also present in the medulla and midbrain.) The basal portion of the pons is special to this part of the brain stem. Its function is to provide for extensive connections between the cortex of a cerebral hemisphere and that of the contralateral cerebellar hemisphere. These connections are important for maximal efficiency of motor activities. A pair of middle cerebellar peduncles attaches the cerebellum to the pons.

MIDBRAIN

Like other parts of the brain stem, the *midbrain* contains sensory and motor pathways, together with nuclei for two cranial nerves, the trochlear (CN4) and the oculomotor (CN3). There is a dorsal region, the roof or tectum, which is concerned principally with the visual and auditory systems. The midbrain also includes two important motor nuclei, the red nucleus and the substantia nigra. The cerebellum is attached to the midbrain by the superior cerebellar peduncles.

CEREBELLUM

The *cerebellum* is especially large in the human brain. Receiving data from most of the sensory systems and the cerebral cortex, the cerebellum eventually influences motor neurons supplying the skeletal musculature. The function of the cerebellum is to influence muscle tonus in relation to equilibrium, locomotion and posture, and nonstereotyped movements based on individual experience. The cerebellum operates behind the scenes at a subconscious level.

DIENCEPHALON

The *diencephalon* forms the central core of the cerebrum. The largest component of the diencephalon, the *thalamus,* receives data from all sensory systems except the olfactory and in turn projects to sensory areas of the cerebral cortex. Part of the thalamus is involved in reverberating circuits with nonspecific cortical areas that are concerned with complex mental processes. Other regions of the thalamus participate in neural circuits related to emotions, and certain thalamic nuclei are incorporated in pathways from the cerebellum and corpus striatum to motor areas of the cerebral cortex. The *epithalamus* includes small tracts and a nucleus, together with the pineal gland, an endocrine organ. The *hypothalamus* is the principal autonomic center of the brain and as such has an important controlling influence over the sympathetic and parasympathetic systems. In addition, neurosecretory cells in the hypothalamus synthesize hormones that reach the blood stream by way of the neural lobe of the pituitary gland or influence the hormonal output of the anterior pituitary through a special portal system of blood vessels. The *subthalamus* includes sensory tracts proceeding to the thalamus, nerve fibers originating in the cerebellum and corpus striatum, and the subthalamic nucleus (a motor nucleus). The retina is a derivative of the diencephalon; the optic nerve (CN2) and visual system are therefore intimately related to this part of the brain.

TELENCEPHALON (Cerebral Hemispheres)

Within the *telencephalon,* the corpus striatum is a large mass of gray matter with motor functions, situated near the base of each hemisphere. The corpus striatum consists of caudate and lenticular nuclei, the latter being subdivided into a putamen and a globus pallidus. The medullary center of the hemisphere consists of 1) fibers connecting cortical areas of the same hemisphere, 2) fibers crossing the midline in a large commissure known as the corpus callosum to connect cortical areas of the two hemispheres, and 3) fibers passing in both directions between cortex and subcortical centers. Fibers of the last category converge to form a compact internal capsule in the region of the thalamus and corpus striatum.

Small areas of cerbral cortex have an ancient lineage (paleocortex); they are olfactory in function, forming part of the rhinencephalon or nosebrain, which dominates the cerebrum of lower vertebrates. Certain areas of cortex were once part of the rhinencephalon but acquired other roles in the evolution of the mammalian brain. These areas are referred to as archicortex; they are included in the limbic system, which is involved with emotions and the influence of emotions on visceral function through the autonomic nervous system. The development of cortex still further removed from olfactory influence (neocortex) was a most significant event in phylogeny. There is very little nonolfactory cortex in the brains of reptiles; the presence of substantial amounts of neocortex is a mammalian characteristic. Its extent and volume have increased during mammalian phylogeny, and the human brain is notable for having much more neocortex than the brain of any other animal. Nine-tenths of the cortex of the human cerebral hemispheres is neocortex, which provides areas for all modalities of sensation, exclusive of smell, and special motor areas. There are also extensive areas of association cortex in which the highest levels of neural function take place, including those inherent in intellectual activity. The unique place of the human species is an endowment conferred by an expanse of neocortex that is possessed by no other animal.

The weight of the mature brain varies according to age and body stature. The normal range in the adult male is 1100–1700 gm (average 1360 gm). The lower figures for the adult female (1050–1550 gm, average 1275 gm) reflect the smaller body stature of females in general, compared with males. There is no evidence of a relation between brain weight, within the normal limits, and a person's level of intelligence.

2

Cells of the Central Nervous System

There are two classes of cells in the central nervous system aside from the usual cells found in walls of blood vessels. *Nerve cells* or *neurons* are specialized for excitation (or inhibition) and nerve impulse conduction, and are therefore responsible for most of the functional characteristics of nervous tissue. The number of neurons in the human central nervous system has been estimated to be of the order of 14 billion. *Neuroglial cells,* also known as interstitial cells, have important ancillary functions. There are four kinds of neuroglia, namely, astrocytes, oligodendrocytes, microglial cells, and ependymal cells.

The central nervous system consists of gray matter and white matter. *Gray matter* contains the cell bodies of neurons, each with a nucleus. In sections prepared by a standard histologic stain such as hematoxylin and eosin, the cell bodies are separated by a complicated network of fibers known as the *neuropil,* which cannot be resolved into its components. With special staining methods or with electron microscopy, the neuropil is seen to consist of nerve cell processes and glial cells permeated by a capillary network. *White matter,* on the other hand, consists of relatively long processes of nerve cells, the majority being surrounded by myelin sheaths. Both the gray and the white matter include large numbers of neuroglial cells. In some parts of the brain, notably the brain stem, there are regions that contain both nerve cell bodies and numerous myelinated fibers and are therefore an admixture of gray matter and white matter.

The cytology of the nervous system is described in some detail in standard textbooks of histology. However, a subject so basic to the neurologic sciences can hardly be omitted from a students' textbook of neurologic anatomy. An account of the cellular components of the brain and spinal cord is therefore introduced at this point.

THE NEURON

The unique feature of neurons is that they are specialized for reception of stimuli, which may be either excitatory or inhibitory, and conduction of the nerve impulse. The part of the cell that includes the nucleus is called the *cell body* or *perikaryon*. *Dendrites* are typically short, branching processes which form a major part of the receptor area of the cell. Most neurons of the central nervous system have several dendrites and are therefore multipolar in shape. By reaching out in various directions, these processes improve the capacity of a neuron to receive stimuli from diverse sources. Each cell has a single *axon*. This process, which varies greatly in length from one type of neuron to another, conducts impulses away from the cell body, usually to other neurons. Axons of efferent neurons in the brain stem and spinal cord end on striated muscle fibers, or on nerve cells in peripheral ganglia in the case of autonomic neurons.

Each neuron is a morphologic and functional unit. This statement is implicit in the Neuron Theory, which is an extension of the Cell Theory to include nerve cells. The Neuron Theory, as opposed to the view that nerve cells form a continuous reticulum, was advanced by His on the basis of embryologic studies, by Forel on the basis of the response of nerve cells to injury, and by Ramón y Cajal from his observations with silver staining methods. The Neuron Theory was given wide distribution in a general review of the whole subject of the individuality of nerve cells by Waldeyer. Because of the special relationship between neurons at synapses (see below), wholly convincing evidence in support of the Neuron Theory had to await the introduction of electron microscopy. It is now clear that the plasma membranes of two neurons are separated at the synapse by an interval about 200 Å wide (Å = one ten-thousandth of a micron). The Neuron Theory is therefore more than a theory; it is a fact or law.

VARIETIES OF NEURONS

Although all nerve cells conform to the general principles outlined above, there is a wide range of structural diversity. The size of the perikaryon varies from 5 μ for the smallest cells in complex circuits to 135 μ for large motor neurons. Dendritic morphology, in particular the pattern of branching, varies greatly and is distinctive for neurons composing a specific cell group or nucleus. The axon of minute neurons is a fraction of a millimeter in length, exceedingly fine, and devoid of a myelin covering. The axon of large neurons, on the other hand, is several feet long in extreme cases, has a substantial diameter, and is typically enclosed in a sheath of myelin. Large and small neurons are known as Golgi type I and Golgi type II neurons, respectively. Intermediate grades, difficult to assign to type I and type II, occur in special locations. The following examples will serve to illustrate the range of variability among neurons of the central nervous system.

Examples of Large Neurons

Pyramidal cells of the cerebral cortex, Purkinje cells of the cerebellar cortex, and motor cells of the spinal cord are familiar examples of Golgi type I neurons. These cells and examples of small neurons are illustrated in Figure 2–1 as they might appear in sections stained by the Golgi bichromate–silver or bichromate–osmium method, or one of the many modifications of the Golgi technique.

The *pyramidal cell* derives its name from the shape of the cell body. An apical dentrite extends toward the surface of the

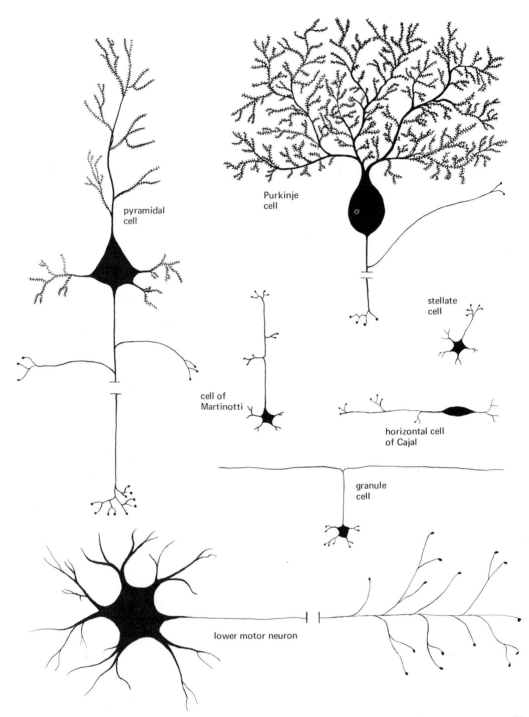

FIG. 2–1. Examples of neurons to illustrate variations in size, shape, and branching of processes. The axon of the lower motor neuron traverses cranial or spinal nerves and branches terminally within a muscle. The other neurons shown are confined to the central nervous system.

cortex, and there are several basal or horizontal dendrites. The dendrites branch extensively, and the smaller branches are beset with minute protuberances (dendritic spines or gemmules), with which axons of other neurons make synaptic contact. The axon of a pyramidal cell arises from the base of the perikaryon or occasionally from the root of a basal dendrite. It leaves the cortex and may continue for a considerable distance, even to lower levels of the spinal cord. The axon gives off collateral branches and these, together with the terminal branches, make synaptic contact with other neurons.

Purkinje cells form a single layer throughout the extensive cerebellar cortex. The cell body is flask-shaped, tapering into one or two dendrites which extend toward the cortical surface. The dendrites of these cells are remarkable in several respects. The branching is more profuse than in any other type of nerve cell, occurring in a plane at right angles to the cortical fold or folium. The branches bear many thousands of dendritic spines, providing for unusually abundant synaptic contacts with cells relaying data from outside the cerebellum. The axon arises from the base of the cell body, gives off one or more collateral branches, and then runs through the white matter to the central nuclei of the cerebellum.

Lower motor neurons are found in the ventral gray horns of the spinal cord and motor nuclei of cranial nerves. They are "lower motor neurons" in the sense that they come under the influence of "upper motor neurons" whose cell bodies are at higher levels, including the cerebral cortex. These large multipolar cells give off several dendrites which branch in the vicinity of the cell body. Large numbers of axon terminals (up to 2000 in spinal motor neurons) establish synaptic contact with the dendrites and the cell body. The axon leaves the central nervous system in a spinal or cranial nerve and terminates in motor end-plates on striated muscle fibers.

Examples of Small Neurons

Although Golgi type I neurons are impressive because of their large size, they are vastly outnumbered by Golgi type II cells. The latter are variously called intercalary, intercalated, or internuncial neurons (or simply interneurons) because they are typically interposed between other neurons to establish circuits that may be of great complexity. Such circuits are basic to the most complex neural functions, including the intellectual capabilities of man. These small cells are especially numerous in the cerebral cortex.

In the cerebral cortex and at certain other sites, many of the Golgi type II neurons take the form of *stellate cells,* so-called because their multipolar form gives a star-shaped profile (Fig. 2–1). Several short dendrites branch close to the cell body and establish contact with axon terminals. The thin axon, which is unmyelinated in Golgi type II cells, ends on one or more nerve cells in the immediate vicinity. *Cells of Martinotti* and *horizontal cells of Cajal* are additional examples of interneurons in the cerebral cortex. The cell of Martinotti is like a stellate cell, except that the axon is somewhat longer and directed toward the surface of the cortex. The horizontal cell of Cajal lies in the outer cortex with its long axis parallel to the cortical surface.

The *granule cell* of the cerebellar cortex is another example of a Golgi type II neuron. The small perikarya of these neurons are closely packed in the deepest of the three cortical layers. Several short dendrites establish contact with axons conveying impulses from outside the cerebellum. The axon is directed toward the surface of the cortex, bifurcates on reaching the outer layer containing Purkinje cell dendrites, and establishes synaptic contact with many Purkinje cells by running parallel with the cortical fold or folium.

The examples given above will serve to illustrate the morphologic diversity of nerve cells within the broad limits of a common pattern. In addition to size differences, there are variations in the number of dendrites, the pattern of dendritic branches, and other morphologic characteristics, according to the specific role of the neuron. It follows that the neurons of different cell aggregates or nuclei tend to be structurally similar within the nucleus. For example, neurons of distinctive morphology occur in the corpus striatum, thalamus, inferior olivary nucleus of the medulla, and many other gray centers of the brain.

CYTOLOGY OF THE NEURON

The intrinsic structure of the neuron, although basically like that of other cells, has some specialized characteristics. Knowledge of neurocytology has accumulated over many decades through the application of an assortment of staining methods for light microscopy and more recently through the use of electron microscopy. Hematoxylin and eosin stain, which is so useful for most tissues and organs, has less to offer with respect to nervous tissue, mainly because the processes of nerve and glial cells are not revealed. Many staining methods have been devised to demonstrate the processes of these cells and specialized components or organelles of the cytoplasm. Because of chemical differences between the various organelles, each requires a specific staining method. In order to visualize the nerve cell in its entirety, it is necessary to combine the results of several staining methods conceptually. This is true of most cell types, but the situation is made more difficult in the case of neurons by the cell processes, synaptic contacts, **and** myelin covering of axons.

Electron microscopy has the distinct advantage of showing the components of a cell without differential staining, depending instead on variations in scattering of electrons as they pass through the cell. The necessity of using ultrathin sections makes it difficult, although not impossible, to reconstruct the neuron three-dimensionally. In the end, a combination of light and electron microscopy gives a comprehensive view of neuronal structure. Figure 2–2 does not pretend to represent a typical neuron because the diversity among nerve cells makes the "typical neuron" an abstraction. The figure is intended to represent, in simplified and semidiagrammatic form, a large nerve cell as one conceives it when the results of several cytologic techniques are combined. The drawing also forms the basis for comments on the ultrastructure of the cellular components as shown with the electron microscope. It is assumed that most users of this book have become acquainted with cell ultrastructure through courses in biology or histology. Where this is not so, standard texts in those subjects may be consulted.

Cell Surface

The surface or limiting membrane of the neuron assumes special importance because of its role in the initiation and transmission of nerve impulses. There is a plasma membrane composed of lipid and protein molecules together with an external "cell coat" consisting of glycoprotein and sialic acid. The arrangement of the lipid and protein molecules is a subject of current research. Briefly stated, the participation of the cell surface with respect to the nerve impulse is as follows.

The cell membrane, considering the plasma membrane and the cell coat as a

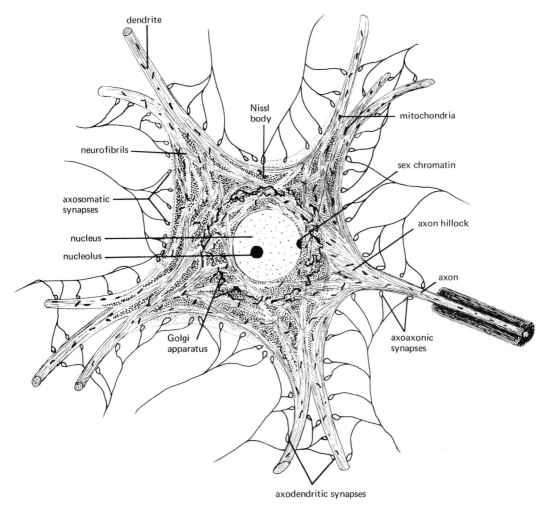

FIG. 2–2. Semidiagrammatic representation of the constituents of a nerve cell.

unit, is semipermeable in that it allows diffusion of some ions through it, but restricts others. In the resting state, the membrane is disproportionately permeable to K$^+$ ions. The latter diffuse from the cytoplasm, in which they are in high concentration, to the outer surface of the cell membrane. In this way, the outer surface acquires a positive resting potential of about 80 mV (millivolts). During excitation, when the membrane potential has been reduced by about 10–15 mV to threshold value, there is a sudden functional alteration in the membrane, characterized by a selective increase in permeability to Na$^+$ ions. These surge locally from the outer to the inner surface, the concentration of Na$^+$ ions being relatively high externally, causing a reversal of charge or *action potential.* Once generated, the action potential is self-propagated along the membrane by local circuits of electrical current. This is the *nerve impulse,* which can be recorded electrically from the outer surface of a nerve fiber as a wave of negative potential. The resting and active membrane potentials of excitable cells are dependent upon the semipermeable nature of the membrane noted above and the ion concentration differences which are maintained by active metabolic processes that make up the so-called "sodium pump."

Nucleus

The spherical nucleus is typically vesicular with finely particulate chromatin. The nucleus is usually situated centrally in the cell body; one exception is cells of the nucleus dorsalis or Clarke's column of the spinal cord, in which the nucleus is eccentric. There are a few binucleate nerve cells in sympathetic ganglia. The *nuclear membrane* or *envelope* has the usual double-layered ultrastructure with numerous small pores. Although the pores are closed by thin diaphragms, they enhance the permeability of the nuclear membrane for passage of certain chemicals from the nucleoplasm to the cytoplasm or in the reverse direction. There is usually a single prominent *nucleolus*. The large size of the nucleolus is related to its role in the synthesis of ribonucleic acid (RNA) and the transfer of RNA to the cytoplasm. The further role of RNA in protein synthesis has a special significance in nerve cells, particularly Golgi type I neurons, because an unusually large volume of proteins must be maintained in the long cell processes. In females, one of the two X chromosomes of the interphase nucleus is compact (heterochromatic), rather than elongated (euchromatic) like the remaining 45 chromosomes of the complement. The compact X chromosome is evident as a mass of *sex chromatin*, which is usually situated at the inner surface of the nuclear membrane. A small, spherical intranuclear structure of unknown significance, called the *accessory body of Cajal*, is

seen in sections stained by silver methods (Fig. 4–5). The nucleus and nucleolus of small neurons are correspondingly small, and the chromatin is likely to be in coarse clumps.

Cytoplasmic Organelles

Neurofibrils, Neurofilaments, and Microtubules. When certain silver stains are used the cytoplasm is seen by light microscopy to contain neurofibrils, sometimes grouped into bundles, running through the perikaryon and into the cell processes. In electron micrographs of nerve cells, the cytoplasm contains neurofilaments of the order of 75–100 Å in thickness; they are probably responsible for the neurofibrils of light microscopy, although this is uncertain. Electron microscopy also shows microtubules about 200–300 Å thick, similar to those of other types of cell. These appear to be involved in the rapid transport of essential metabolites from the perinuclear zone throughout the neuron. The neurofilaments and microtubules consist of helically organized protein threads.

Nissl Material. When nervous tissue is stained with basic dyes such as cresyl violet or thionine, clumps of basophilic material are seen in most nerve cells. These are known as Nissl bodies after Franz Nissl (1860–1919), a Heidelberg neurologist. The amount of Nissl material increases with the size of the neuron, and its arrangement varies from one type of nerve cell to another. For example, the clumps are coarse in motor neurons (Fig. 2–3), while the basophilic material is more finely distributed in sensory neurons. The Nissl substance extends into dendritic processes, but is lacking in both the axon hillock, i.e., the peripheral zone of the perikaryon where the axon emerges, and the axon itself. Nissl material is the same as the

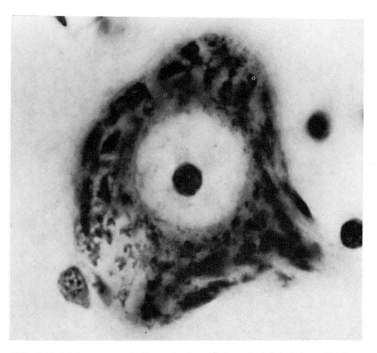

FIG. 2–3. Motor neuron in the spinal cord. Cresyl violet stain. ×1000

basophilic substance, sometimes called ergastoplasm or chromidial substance, in the cytoplasm of cells such as those composing the pancreatic acini.

The nature of the Nissl substance was made apparent by electron microscopy. Virtually all cells of the body contain an ultrastructural cytoplasmic constituent, known as the *granular endoplasmic reticulum,* in amounts ranging from scanty to abundant. This consists of a system of flattened cisternae or vesicles bearing ribosomal particles on their outer surfaces, and often with free ribosomes in the adjacent cytoplasmic matrix. The ribosomes contain RNA, and the granular or rough–surfaced endoplasmic reticulum is therefore basophilic. The clumps of Nissl substance consist of orderly arrays of granular endoplasmic reticulum with many free ribosomes (Fig. 2–4). The ribosomes participate in the synthesis of structural and enzymatic proteins, accounting for the abundance of Nissl material in large neurons having considerable cytoplasm to maintain in long processes. To be more specific it has been shown by several methods, including autoradiography following the administration of labeled amino acids, that the proteins of nerve cells are synthesized in the perikaryon, then flow along the neuronal processes, notably the axon, at a rate of about 1 mm a day. The axoplasmic flow away from the perikaryon replaces proteins that are degraded during cellular activity. This aspect of cell metabolism is even more important during growth of neurons and regeneration of peripheral nerve fibers. Axoplasmic flow is of cardinal significance in the phenomenon of neurosecretion by certain cells in the hypothalamus.

Mitochondria. These cytoplasmic organelles are scattered through the perikaryon,

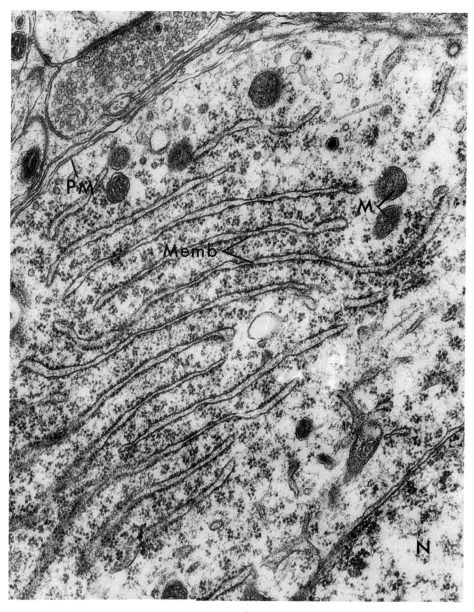

FIG. 2–4. Electron micrograph of a portion of a neuron in the preoptic nucleus of the rabbit's hypothalamus. The series of membranous profiles, together with the free ribosomes (polysomes) between the profiles, constitute the Nissl material of light microscopy. *M,* mitochondria; *Memb,* membranes of endoplasmic reticulum; *N,* nucleus; *PM,* plasma membrane. (Courtesy of Dr. R. Clattenburg) ×36,000

dendrites, and axon. They are spherical, rod-shaped, or filamentous, measuring from 0.2 to 1.0 μ in their greatest dimension and about 0.2 μ in diameter. With electron microscopy, the mitochondria show the characteristic peripheral double membrane and internal folds or cristae. Mitochondria are the repository of enzymes that are involved in several aspects of cell metabolism, including the respiratory and phosphorylating enzymes of the Krebs citric acid cycle. Mitochondria are therefore important in nerve cells, as in all cells, in the energy-producing reactions of cellular physiology.

Golgi Apparatus. The Golgi apparatus (complex) is a universal cytoplasmic organelle with special historic interest in relation to nerve cells, having been first demonstrated in these cells by the Italian histologist, Camillo Golgi (1843–1926). With a silver–osmium staining method for light microscopy, the Golgi apparatus appears as a dark, irregular network, which is often disposed around the nuclear envelope, midway between the latter and the cell surface. The Golgi apparatus appears in electron micrographs as clusters of closely apposed, flattened cisternae, arranged in stacks and surrounded by many small vesicles. This membranous system is continuous with agranular or smooth-surfaced endoplasmic reticulum, and the latter is continuous with granular endoplasmic reticulum. The three membranous systems are in a sense regional differentiations of a single, extensive cytoplasmic organelle. The function of the Golgi complex is imperfectly understood. In secretory cells, there is good evidence that the secretory products are "packaged" in the Golgi area, including incorporation of the carbohydrate moiety of the secretory product. In cells generally, the Golgi apparatus appears to be in dynamic relationship with vacuoles and other membranous components of the cytoplasm.

Centrosome. This cell organelle, which includes a pair of centrioles, has an important role in the dynamics of mitosis. A centrosome is present in the precursors of mature neurons during the developmental period, as is to be expected, and has been seen in nerve cells cultured in vitro. A centrosome is lacking, or poorly developed at best, in mature neurons. This raises the question of nerve cell multiplication. It is generally believed that there is little increase in the neuronal population after birth, although some increment in the number of small internuncial neurons during infancy is a distinct possibility. The size of the brain increases most during the latter part of fetal life. The increase in size of the brain and spinal cord during the postnatal growth period is due to a number of factors. These include further development of existing neurons, especially branching of dendrites and growth of axons, and completion of myelination of fiber systems.

Pigment Material

The perikaryon may contain nonliving material or cytoplasmic inclusions, of which the most important are pigment granules. *Lipofuscin* (lipochrome) pigment occurs as clumps of yellowish-brown granules. Traces of this pigment appear in neurons of the spinal cord and medulla at about the eighth year of life, and in cells of spinal and sympathetic ganglia at about the same time. The amount of the pigment increases with age. The significance of lipofuscin is unknown, except that it is related to the aging process and is found at other sites, including cardiac muscle fibers. Some types of neurons, of which Purkinje cells are an example, do not accumulate lipofuscin, even in old age.

The presence of dark *melanin* pigment in the cytoplasm is restricted to a few cell groups, the largest being the substantia nigra, a motor nucleus in the midbrain. The significance of melanin at this site is not known with certainty, although the melanin may be a by-product of a series of chemical reactions in which tyrosine and dihydroxy-phenylalanine (dopa) figure prominently. The pigment appears at the end of the first year, increases until puberty, and remains relatively constant thereafter. Fine, iron–containing granules are present in some nerve cells of the substantia nigra and in the globus pallidus, a component of the corpus striatum. The amount of this material is not age-dependent.

Processes of the Nerve Cell

Dendrites taper from the perikaryon and branch at acute angles in the environs of the cell body. The branching may be exceedingly profuse and intricate, the Purkinje cell of cerebellar cortex being outstanding in this respect. In some neurons, the smaller branches bear large numbers of minute projections, called dendritic *spines* or *gemmules,* which participate in synapses. The surface of the perikaryon may be included in the receptive area or "dendritic field" of the neuron. In motor neurons of the spinal cord, for example, large numbers of axon endings are in synaptic relationship with the cell body, as well as with the dendrites.

The single *axon* of a nerve cell tends to have a uniform diameter throughout its length. It is a short delicate process in the case of Golgi type II cells, branching terminally to establish synaptic contact with one or more adjacent neurons. In Golgi type I cells, the diameter of the axon increases in proportion to its length. Collateral branches may be given off at right angles to the main axon. The terminal branches are known as

telodendria; they typically end as swellings or synaptic end-bulbs. The cytoplasm of the axon is called *axoplasm* and the surface membrane is known as the *axolemma.* The axoplasm includes neurofilaments and microtubules, scattered mitochondria, and patches of smooth–surfaced or agranular endoplasmic reticulum.

Axons of Golgi type I neurons are surrounded as a rule by a myelin sheath, which begins near the origin of the axon and ends short of its terminal branching. Within the central nervous system the myelin is laid down by oligodendrocytes and consists essentially of closely apposed layers of their plasma membranes. The sheath therefore has a lipoprotein composition, and interruptions called nodes of Ranvier indicate where regions formed by different oligodendrocytes adjoin. The thickness of the myelin sheath tends to be directly proportional to the diameter and length of the axon. The greater the diameter of the nerve fiber, the faster is the conduction of the nerve impulse. (A nerve "fiber" in the central nervous system consists of the axon and the surrounding myelin sheath, or of the axon only in the case of unmyelinated fibers.) The formation and structure of the myelin sheath are discussed in the following chapter in the context of peripheral nerve fibers, in which these aspects of the myelin have been studied in greater detail.

Synapses

A neuron brings its influence to bear on other neurons at junctional points or synapses. "Synapse," meaning a conjunction or connection, was introduced by Sherrington in 1897. A nerve impuse can be propagated in any direction on the surface of a nerve cell. However, the direction followed under physiologic conditions is determined by a consistent polarity at the synapse, where transmission is from the axon of one neuron to the cell surface of another neuron.

Synapses assume a variety of forms, ranging from a simple apposition of axon and dendrite to rather complicated arrangements. In most instances, a synapse consists of an expansion of the end of an axonal branch in close apposition to the cell surface of another neuron (Fig. 2–5). The terminals are variously called *synaptic end-bulbs, end-bulbs of Held-Auerbach,* or *boutons terminaux.* Synaptic endings are always present on dendrites of cells in the central nervous system, the role of dendritic processes being to receive stimuli.

Depending on the type of neuron, there may also be synaptic terminals on the cell body, on the proximal portion of an axon before the myelin sheath begins, or even synaptic association between end-bulbs derived from different neurons. On the foregoing basis, synapses are said to be *axo-dendritic, axosomatic,* or *axoaxonic.* Depending on the role of the parent nerve cell and the nature of the chemical medi-

ator at the synapse, the influence of an end-bulb on the succeeding neuron is either excitation or inhibition. Axodendritic synapses are usually excitatory, while axosomatic synapses and the less frequent axoaxonic synapses are likely to be inhibitory.

When examined in electron micrographs (Figs. 2–6 and 2–7), the end-bulb usually contains a number of mitochondria; bundles of neurofilaments continue into some end-bulbs but not into others. The most characteristic constituent consists of large numbers of *synaptic vesicles,* which tend to accumulate near the synaptic surface. The vesicles vary from 200 to 650 Å in diameter, the majority being about 500 Å. They are thought to contain the chemical mediator of nervous activity across the synapse. Acetylcholine is known to be the mediator at synapses between preganglionic and postganglionic neurons of the autonomic system, at terminals of postganglionic parasympathetic fibers, and at motor end-plates on striated muscle fibers. Norepinephrine (noradrenaline) is the

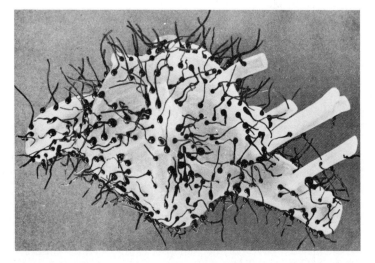

FIG. 2–5. Model of a nerve cell in the spinal cord, prepared from sections stained by Cajal's silver nitrate method. (From Haggar RA, Barr ML, J Comp Neurol 93:17–36, 1950)

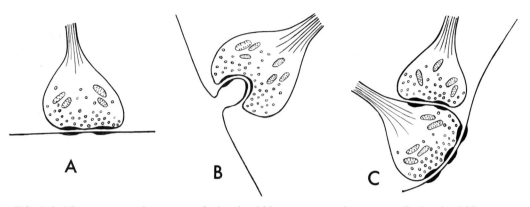

FIG. 2–6. Ultrastructure of synapses. **A.** Axodendritic or axosomatic synapse. **B.** Axodendritic synapse, in which an end-bulb is in synaptic relation with a dendritic spine. **C.** Axoaxonic synapse of the end-bulb to end-bulb type. See text for details.

transmitter agent at the terminals of post-ganglionic sympathetic fibers. Synapses are therefore classified as cholinergic or adrenergic. Establishing specific sites within the central nervous system at which acetylcholine, norepinephrine, or other substances act as neurotransmitters is an important aspect of current research.

The apposed surfaces of the end-bulb and the neuron on which it terminates are called the *presynaptic* and *postsynaptic membranes,* respectively. They are separated by a 200-Å-wide *synaptic cleft.* The pre- and postsynaptic membranes are thickened here and there, with a slight increase in density of the cytoplasm under the thickened areas of the postsynaptic membrane. These configurations bear some resemblance to the desmosomes that maintain cohesion between epithelial cells. If the synapse is excitatory, the chemical mediator released from the synaptic vesicles by a nerve impulse produces a functional alteration in the postsynaptic membrane, which may result in an action potential, as described above. If the synapse is inhibitory, release of the transmitter substance stabilizes the postsynaptic membrane and lessens the possibility that an

action potential will originate in the vicinity of the synapse. There are indications that distinctive differences in the size and shape of synaptic vesicles and in the ultrastructural details of the synaptic membranes may be correlated with the type of transmitter substance and with excitatory or inhibitory properties of the synapse.

NEUROGLIAL CELLS

Although neuroglial cells are not involved in the first instance with excitation, inhibition, and propagation of the nerve impulse, they have their own essential roles. It has also become evident that certain of these cells have an intimate relationship with nerve cells, leading to a high degree of interdependence. As noted above, the neuroglia are classified as astrocytes, oligodendrocytes, microglial cells, and ependymal cells (Fig. 2–8). The first two mentioned are sometimes combined under the heading of *macroglia.* All but the microglia differentiate from neural tube cells in the embryo and are therefore ectodermal in origin. Microglial cells are mesodermal derivatives.

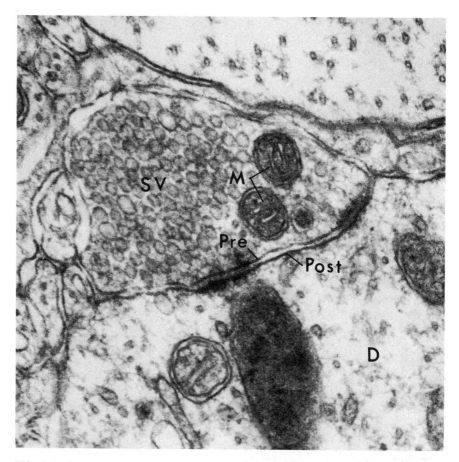

FIG. 2–7. Electron micrograph of a synapse in the suprachiasmatic nucleus of the rabbit's hypothalamus. *D*, dendrite; *M*, mitochondria; *Pre*, presynaptic membrane; *Post*, postsynaptic membrane; *SV*, synaptic vesicles in the end-bulb of an axon. (Courtesy of Dr. R. Clattenburg) ×82,000

ASTROCYTES (Astroglia)

Astrocytes are present in profusion throughout the gray and the white matter of the brain and spinal cord. Cytoplasmic processes reach out in all directions, and the name of these cells is derived from the conventional representation of a star. The nucleus is round or oval in profile, often indented, and in general larger than the nuclei of other neuroglial cells. The nucleus is moderately vesicular and the nucleolus is small, if visible at all. It is difficult to distinguish nuclei of astrocytes from those of small neurons in sections stained with basic dyes. The cytoplasm contains granules (gliosomes), which are resolved by electron microscopy into clumps of mitochondria or of lysosomes. The latter are membrane-bound vesicles, containing enzymes that digest macromolecular material, not only taken up by the cell, but also wornout protoplasm (autophagia). Electron micrographs also show numerous

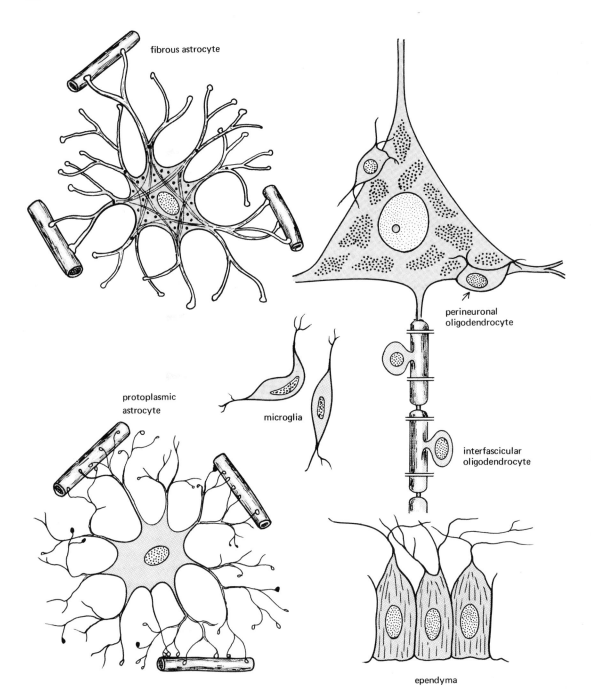

FIG. 2–8. Neuroglial cells of the central nervous system.

gliofilaments 75–100 Å in thickness; they are similar to the neurofilaments of nerve cells and the microfilaments of other cell types. Endoplasmic reticulum is scanty, but free ribosomes may be present.

Special staining methods, such as the gold-sublimate method of Cajal, are necessary to show the processes of astrocytes in light microscopy. Many of the processes end on capillaries or vessels of larger caliber as foot-plates or perivascular feet. Much of the capillary wall, perhaps 80 percent of its surface, is covered with astrocytic foot-plates, which are attached to the basement membrane surrounding the endothelial lining. The processes of astrocytes in the gray matter also end in close apposition to neurons at such intervals as are free of synapses. The processes of atrocytes near the surface of the brain and cord are attached as foot-plates to the pia mater, a thin meningeal layer that adheres to the surface, to form an *external limiting membrane*. The ventricles are lined by a single layer of ependymal cells giving off short processes from their deep aspect. There is a concentration of astrocytes beneath the ependyma, and their processes intertwine with those of ependymal cells to form an *internal limiting membrane.*

Astrocytes in the white matter tend to have rather coarse processes and contain bundles of gliofilaments visible as fibrils with the light microscope. This type of cell is called a *fibrous astrocyte.* The *protoplasmic astrocytes* found in gray matter have more delicately branching processes; the gliofilaments are not sufficiently numerous to be seen as fibrils with light microscopy. There are intermediate grades between typical fibrous and protoplasmic astrocytes, especially in transitional zones between white matter and gray matter.

The conventional view is that astrocytes, by virtue of the attachment of processes to blood vessels, constitute a structural and supporting framework for nerve cells and capillaries. However, they no doubt have an additional, more dynamic, role. It now seems likely that the transport of chemicals essential for the metabolic reactions of nerve cells occurs partly within astrocytes, some astrocytic processes being adherent to capillaries and others being adjacent to the surfaces of neurons. The above is a corollary of the narrow intercellular spaces of nervous tissue, which are of the order of 200 Å in width.

OLIGODENDROCYTES (Oligodendroglia)

The *oligodendrocytes* have, until recently, been the most underrated cells among the neuroglia because no satisfactory stain for their study by light microscopy had been developed. They could be seen only as cells rather smaller than astrocytes with spherical nuclei, scanty cytoplasm, and a few short processes (accounting for their name). They are situated adjacent to nerve cells in gray matter and in larger numbers among the nerve fibers of white matter.

As in certain other aspects of neurocytology, the morphology of oligodendrocytes has been placed on a sound basis by ultrastructural studies. This is especially true of the *interfascicular oligodendrocytes* of white matter, where they make up some 75 percent of neuroglial cells. The cytoplasm contains a considerable amount of endoplasmic reticulum and many ribosomes. But the most striking revelation is that the oligodendrocytes are responsible for the formation of myelin sheaths, in the same way as neurolemmal or Schwann cells form the myelin sheaths of peripheral nerve fibers. As noted above, the lipoprotein plasma membrane of an oligodendrocyte is wrapped abound the axon in numbers of layers that determine the thickness of the myelin sheath. The intervals between the territories of oligodendrocytes are identified as nodes of Ranvier. One oligodendrocyte forms internodal myelin for from 3 to

50 fibers, depending in part on the caliber of the fibers. A single oligodendrocyte also surrounds numerous axons when the fibers are unmyelinated, but the plasma membrane is not wrapped around the axons in layers to form myelin sheaths.

Other oligodendrocytes lie close to the cell bodies and dendritic processes of nerve cells. These *perineuronal oligodendrocytes* seem to have a symbiotic relationship with nerve cells in the central nervous system, similar to that of the satellite cells surrounding nerve cell bodies in peripheral ganglia. The close relationship between neurons and neuroglia is demonstrated in cultures of nervous tissue, in which neurons do not thrive and grow unless they are surrounded by neuroglial cells.

EPENDYMA

The *ependymal epithelium* lining the ventricular system of the brain and the central canal of the spinal cord is included among the neuroglia. The cells of this epithelium are arranged as a single layer in the adult and they are flattened endothelial-like to cuboidal-columnar in shape. Throughout most of the ventricular surface, the epithelium is characterized by a carpet of cilia projecting into the ventricle (Fig. 2–9). In other areas ciliated ependymal cells are interspersed among nonciliated cells. The deep surfaces of some ependymal cells give off processes that intertwine with those of astrocytes to form an internal limiting membrane. Suitable staining methods show

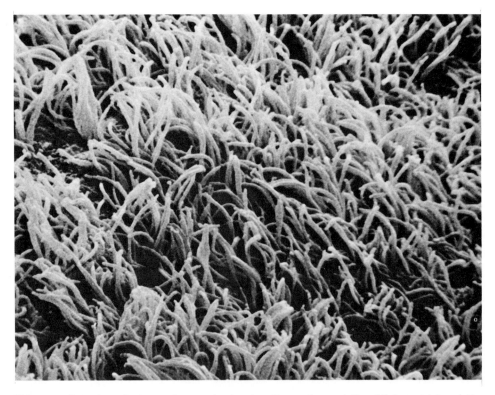

FIG. 2–9. Scanning electron micrograph showing the surface of the third ventricle of the rabbit. This illustration represents an area in which the ependymal lining is heavily ciliated. (Courtesy of Dr. J. E. Bruni and Dr. D. G. Montemurro) ×2,880

intracellular fibrils similar to those of fibrous astrocytes.

MICROGLIAL CELLS (Microglia)

There remain the *microglial cells,* which are scattered through the gray and the white matter in fewer numbers than the macroglial cells. The microglia can be stained by the silver-carbonate method of Rio Hortega. As mentioned above, these are the only neuroglial components that are not of ectodermal origin. Instead, they are mesodermal derivatives, invading the central nervous system late in fetal development, and hence known alternatively as *mesoglial cells.*

Microglial cells are small and have an irregular-shaped nucleus; the cytoplasm is scanty and there are several short, branching processes. No special function has been attributed to the microglia under normal conditions. However, when nervous tissue is damaged from any cause, the cells become rounded and enlarged, and display ameboid and phagocytic properties. Under these circumstances, the cells ingest and digest tissue debris. In view of their mesodermal origin and role as scavenger cells,

the microglial elements are regarded as belonging to the reticuloendothelial system of the body, with properties similar to those of histiocytes in connective tissue.

DEVELOPMENT OF NEURONS AND NEUROGLIAL CELLS

Nerve cells and neuroglial cells (except the microglia) differentiate from the epithelium of the neural tube according to the sequence shown in Figure 2–10. Although there are alternative routes of cell differentiation, the most important one in early stages is the differentiation of *medulloblasts* into *neuroblasts* and *spongioblasts.* Neuroblasts are capable of cell division and mature into neurons. The number of nerve cells is largely stabilized by the time of birth, but there are probably additions to the pools of interneurons during the first year or so of life. Spongioblasts divide and mature into *astroblasts,* and these differentiate into fibrous and protoplasmic astrocytes. Spongioblasts also differentiate into *oligodendroblasts,* followed by the mature oligodendrocytes.

The names of embryonic stages of cell

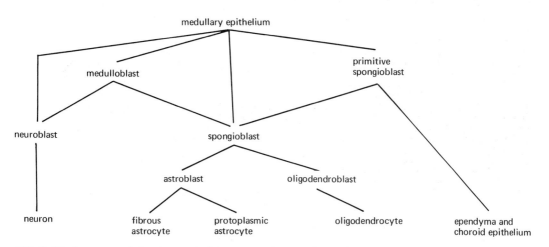

FIG. 2–10. Sequence of development of neurons and neuroglial cells.

maturation are of interest in neuropathology. The cells of tumors with malignant properties have certain characteristics of embryonic cells. The malignancy of a tumor is related to the maturity, or lack of maturity, of the tumor cells in relation to the cell lineage, i.e., the more primitive the appearance of the cells, the more malignant the tumor. The names of brain tumors (e.g., medulloblastoma) are therefore derived in part from the cell lineage in the embryonic brain.

SUGGESTIONS FOR ADDITIONAL READING

Barr ML: The significance of the sex chromatin. Int Rev Cytol 19:35–95, 1966

Bodian D: Synaptic types on spinal motoneurons: An electron microscopic study. Johns Hopkins Med J 119:16–45, 1966

Bourne GH (ed.): The Structure and Function of Nervous Tissue, Vol 1. New York, Academic Press, 1968

Bunge RP: Glial cells and the central myelin sheath. Physiol Rev 48:197–251, 1968

Droz B, Leblond CP: Axonal migration of proteins in the central nervous system and peripheral nerves as shown by radioautography. J Comp Neurol 121:325–346, 1963

Francoeur J, Olszewski J: Axonal reaction and axoplasmic flow as studied by radioautography. Neurology (Minneap) 18:178–184, 1968

Gray EG, Guillery RW: Synaptic morphology in the normal and degenerating nervous system. Int Rev Cytol 19:111–182, 1966

Haggar RA, Barr ML: Quantitative data on the size of synaptic end-bulbs in the cat's spinal cord. With a note on the preparation of cell models. J Comp Neurol 93:17–35, 1950

Herman CJ, Lapham LW: Neuronal polyploidy and nuclear volumes in the cat central nervous system. Brain Res 15:35–48, 1969

Hydén H (ed.): The Neuron. Amsterdam, Elsevier, 1967

Kruger L, Maxwell DS: Electron microscopy of oligodendrocytes in normal rat cerebrum. Am J Anat 118:411–435, 1966

Luse SA: Electron microscopic observations on the central nervous system. J Biophys Biochem Cytol 2:531–542, 1956

Mori S, Leblond CP: Identification of microglia in light and electron microscopy. J Comp Neurol 135:57–79, 1969

Mori S, Leblond CP: Electron microscopic features and proliferation of astrocytes in the corpus callosum of the rat. J Comp Neurol 137:197–225, 1969

Mori S, Leblond CP: Electron microscopic identification of three classes of oligodendrocytes and a preliminary study of their proliferative activity in the corpus callosum of young rats. J Comp Neurol 139:1–29, 1970

Mugnaini E: The relation between cytogenesis and the formation of different types of synaptic contact. Brain Res 17:169–179, 1970

Palay SL, Palade GE: The fine structure of neurons. J Biophys Biochem Cytol 1:69–88, 1955

Peters A, Palay SL, Webster HdeF: The Fine Structure of the Nervous System: The Cells and Their Processes. New York, Harper & Row, 1970

Siekevitz P: The organization of biologic membranes. N Eng J Med 283:1035–1041, 1970

Uchizono K: Characteristics of excitatory and inhibitory synapses in the central nervous system of the cat. Nature (London) 207:642–643, 1965

Windle WF (ed.): Biology of Neuroglia. Springfield, Ill., Thomas, 1958

Worthington WC Jr, Cathcart RS: Ependymal cilia: Distribution and activity in the adult human brain. Science 139:221–222, 1963

Wuerker RB, Palay SL: Neurofilaments and microtubules in anterior horn cells of the rat. Tissue Cell 1:387–402, 1969

3
Peripheral Nervous System

Certain aspects of the peripheral nervous system are especially pertinent to a study of the brain and spinal cord. These include the general sensory receptors, the motor endings, the histology of peripheral nerves, and the structure of ganglia. The following introductory comments refer to all spinal nerves and to those cranial nerves not concerned with the special senses. The structures discussed in this chapter are shown in Figure 3–1; this figure represents a spinal nerve in the thoracic and upper lumbar region in which neurons for visceral innervation are included.

The general sensory endings are scattered profusely throughout the body. These are biologic transducers, in which physical stimuli create an action potential in nerve endings. On reaching the central nervous system, the resulting nerve impulse gives rise to reflex responses, awareness of the stimulus, or both. Cutaneous endings are called *exteroceptors* and are sensitive to stimuli for pain, temperature, touch, and pressure. *Proprioceptors* in muscles, tendons, and joints provide data for reflex adjustments of muscle action and for awareness of position and movement.

Nerve impulses from exteroceptors and proprioceptors are conducted centrally by primary sensory neurons, whose cell bodies are located in dorsal root ganglia (or a cranial nerve ganglion). On entering the spinal cord, the dorsal root fibers divide into ascending and descending branches; these are distributed as necessary for reflex responses and for transmission of sensory data to the brain.

There is a third class of sensory endings, known as *interoceptors,* in the viscera. Central conduction is through primary sensory neurons like those noted above, except that the peripheral process follows a different route. The fiber reaches the sympathetic trunk through a white communicating ramus and continues to a viscus in a nerve arising from the sympathetic trunk. The spinal connections of these neurons are those required for visceral reflex responses and for transmission of data of visceral origin to the brain. There are therefore two broad categories of sensory endings and

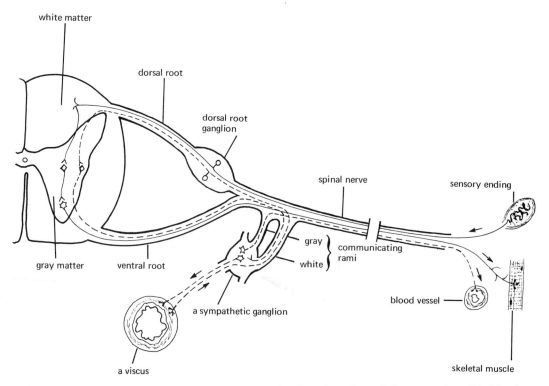

FIG. 3–1. Components of a spinal nerve between the first thoracic and the second or third lumbar segments.

afferent neurons, namely, *somatic afferents* for the body (soma) generally and *visceral afferents.*

There are also two categories of efferent or motor neurons. The cell bodies of *somatic efferent* neurons are situated in the ventral gray horns of the spinal cord and motor nuclei of cranial nerves. The axons of ventral horn cells traverse the ventral roots and spinal nerves, and terminate in motor end-plates on skeletal muscle fibers. The *visceral efferent* or autonomic system has a special feature in that two neurons take part in transmission from the central nervous system to the viscera. An example is the sympathetic division of the autonomic system. Here, the cell bodies of preganglionic neurons are located in the thoracic and upper lumbar segments of the spinal cord. The axons traverse the corre-

sponding ventral roots and white communicating rami, ending either in ganglia of the sympathetic chain or in prevertebral ganglia such as those found in the celiac and superior mesenteric plexuses of the abdomen. Axons of postganglionic cells in these locations proceed to smooth muscle or secretory cells of viscera and to the heart. Axons from some of the cells in sympathetic chain ganglia enter spinal nerves through gray communicating rami for distribution to blood vessels, sweat glands, and arrector pili muscles of hairs.

SENSORY ENDINGS

The sensory endings are supplied by nerve fibers differing in size and other characteristics. This is a matter of some importance, because there is a correlation between fiber diameter and the rate of conduction of the nerve impulse, and because different sensory endings tend to be supplied by fibers of different sizes.

A commonly used classification of peripheral nerve fibers is given in Table 3-1, which includes the sensory modalities and efferent neurons associated with the three main categories. The diameters of group A and group B fibers include the myelin sheaths. Group A is further subdivided into alpha, beta, gamma, and delta fibers in decreasing order of size. There is some overlapping of the size ranges of the A, B, and C groups because physiologic properties, especially the form of the spike potential and after-potential, are taken into consideration. In brief, the smallest fibers (group C) are unmyelinated and have the slowest conduction rate, while the myelinated fibers of group B and group A exhibit rates of conduction which increase progressively with increasing size of the fibers.

A second classification of nerve fibers applies specifically to somatic sensory fibers of the dorsal roots. Table 3-2 lists the receptors from which impulses traverse each of the four categories in the numerical system, together with the equivalents in the alternative classification.

It is customary to recognize two classes of sensory endings on a structural basis. *Nonencapsulated* endings are simple, undifferentiated terminal arborizations of the nerve fibers; they have a long phylogenetic history and respond to various forms of stimuli that are identified by the general senses. *Encapsulated* endings are more specialized, and of more recent phylogenetic origin.

NONENCAPSULATED ENDINGS

Sensory nerve terminals of the unencapsulated type are widely distributed throughout the body. They are present in epithelia, serous membranes, connective tissue, muscles, tendons, joints, periosteum, and viscera; as well as in special locations such

TABLE 3-1. CLASSIFICATION OF FIBERS IN PERIPHERAL NERVES

	Group	Diameter (μ)	Speed of impluse conduction (meters/sec)	Function
Myelinated	A ($\alpha, \beta, \gamma, \delta$)	1–20	5–120	Afferent fibers for proprioception, vibration, touch, pressure, pain, and temperature; somatic efferent fibers
Myelinated	B	1–3	3–15	Visceral afferent fibers; preganglionic visceral efferent fibers
Nonmyelinated	C	0.5–1.5	0.6–2.0	Afferent fibers for pain and temperature; postganglionic visceral efferent fibers

TABLE 3–2. CLASSIFICATION OF SOMATIC
DORSAL ROOT FIBERS

Number	Receptors	Letter equivalent
I.a.	Annulospiral ending of neuromuscular spindle	Aα
b.	Neurotendinous spindle	
II.	Flower spray ending of neuromuscular spindle; touch and pressure receptors	Aβ and γ
III.	Pain and temperature receptors	Aδ
IV.	Pain and temperature receptors	C

as the cornea, tympanic membrane, and dental pulp.

Simple nerve endings in the skin may be taken as the first example (Fig. 3–2A). Smaller fibers of group A and group C fibers form a plexus in the dermis and continue into the epidermis as unmyelinated fibers. They then divide into fine branches lying between the cells of the deep epidermal layers. These are endings for pain, among other senses, responding to stimuli that are damaging or potentially damaging to the skin. Endings such as these function in relation to pain in many tissues, including mucous membranes, joint capsules, dental pulp, and other sites known through experience to react painfully to trauma or disease. Reliable observations on the nature of sensory endings for temperature are scanty. Endings similar to those responding to painful stimuli are probably sensitive to changes of temperature, although more complex endings may also function in temperature sensibility. It is pertinent in this connection that sensations of pain and temperature both have protective functions; they give warning of real or potential injury and are hence known as *nociceptive*

senses (*noceo,* to injure). As such, they are phylogenetically old sensory modalities, and information concerning both pain and temperature reaches the brain through a common pathway in the spinal cord. Simple endings also respond to touch, as shown by the cornea, in which the sensory endings are all of this type.

Modifications of this simple type of nerve ending are sensitive to touch. In the first example, group A fibers of medium caliber pass from the dermal plexus into the epidermis and terminate as leaf-like, meniscal expansions, known as *Merkel's disks,* in contact with epidermal cells (Fig. 3–2B). There may be up to 50 Merkel's disks for a single nerve fiber, and they are confined to the deeper layers of the epidermis. The cells with which disks make contact are stained more darkly than neighboring epidermal cells because of an accumulation of glycoprotein granules in the cytoplasm. Merkel's disks are most numerous in the skin of the palm, sole, and nipple, but are also present at other sites, including the borders of the tongue.

The *hair follicle plexuses* (Fig. 3–2C), also known as peritrichial endings, are the second example of modified unencapsulated endings for the sense of touch. Hairs are present on most of the body surface and their role in man is that of touch receptors, aside from a cosmetic value in the head area. Depending on the size of the hair, from 2 to 20 fibers in the medium group A range approach a hair follicle deep to the sebaceous gland from various directions. The unmyelinated terminals wind around the follicle in its connective tissue sheath, giving off collateral branches to form a basket-like network. The hair is exquisitely sensitive to touch, acting as a lever in which slight changes in position produce an action potential in the nerve plexus.

Rather complicated terminal ramifica-

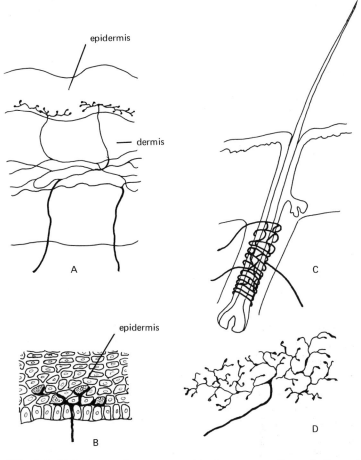

FIG. 3–2. Main types of nonencapsulated sensory endings. **A.** Dermal plexus and simple endings in the epidermis. **B.** Merkel's disks in the epidermis. **C.** Hair follicle plexus. **D.** Undifferentiated ending in deep somatic tissues or in viscera.

tions of sensory fibers occur in the ligaments of joints, and in periosteum, tendons, and fascia (Fig. 3–2D). These endings of group A fibers, especially those associated with joints, give precise information concerning the position and movements of parts of the body (proprioception). Non-encapsulated nerve terminals in the periosteum respond to vibration. Similar terminals of group B fibers are numerous in the viscera. These are sensory endings for vis-

ceral reflexes and for the sensation of fullness of the stomach, bladder, or rectum, together with general feelings of well-being or malaise.

In summary, the undifferentiated, nonencapsulated, sensory endings have a long evolutionary history and serve several modalities of sensation. Receptors for pain are entirely of this category. The simple endings also make important contributions to the senses of touch, proprioception, and vibration; probably to the sense of temperature; and to the visceral afferent system.

ENCAPSULATED ENDINGS

Meissner's Corpuscles

These sensors of touch are mainly in the skin, where they occur in the dermal papillae projecting into the epidermis (Fig. 3–3A). Meissner's corpuscles are most numerous and best developed on the palmar surface of the hand (especially the fingers) and on the plantar surface of the foot. They are present in smaller numbers in the volar surface of the forearm, around the mouth, in the tip of the tongue and margin of the eyelid, the nipple, and the external genitalia. The corpuscle is usually ovoid in shape and of the order of 50 by 100 μ in size; a thin capsule encloses epithelioid cells which tend to be arranged transversely. From one to four group A fibers, usually of large diameter, enter the deep pole of the corpuscle, give up their myelin sheaths, and pursue an irregular course among the epithelioid cells.

Meissner's corpuscles are exquisitely sensitive tactile endings that appeared rather late in evolution. They enable a person to detect that two points on the skin are touched, even though separated by millimeters (two-point discrimination). Among other properties, this delicate form of touch discrimination permits recognition of slight differences in the texture of surfaces.

Pacinian Corpuscles

Pacinian corpuscles, also called corpuscles of Vater–Pacini, are widely distributed. They are present (among other sites) in subcutaneous connective tissue, ligaments and joint capsules, the nipples, external genitalia, serous membranes and mesen-

teries, and some viscera. The corpuscles are typically ellipsoidal in shape and from 1 to 4 mm long. They are therefore visible to the naked eye; for this and other reasons the physiologic properties of pacinian corpuscles have been studied in considerable detail.

With light microscopy a pacinian corpuscle is seen to consist of a cylindrical core surrounded by numerous lamellae (Fig. 3–3B). A large group A nerve fiber enters the corpuscle at one pole, at which point the myelin sheath terminates, and continues along the central axis. Electron microscopy reveals further morphologic details. The central core consists of about 60 closely packed lamellae formed by much flattened cells, and the nerve fiber occupying the core is notable for containing an unusual concentration of mitochondria. In the immature corpuscle the core is surrounded by an intermediate growth zone containing numerous nuclei, but this is no longer a feature when full development has been reached. The peripheral zone which makes up the bulk of the corpuscle consists of 30 or more concentric lamellae, each consisting of flattened cells with greatly attenuated cytoplasm. The lamellae are bounded sparsely by collagen fibers and separated by spaces containing fluid. A few of the outer lamellae are close together and underlie a condensation of connective tissue which constitutes the external capsule of the corpuscle.

Pacinian corpuscles are considered to be mechanoreceptors and sensitive to light pressures. As such, they are able to serve several functions, depending on their location and the central connections of afferent neurons. Those in subcutaneous tissues respond to pressure on the skin. Pacinian corpuscles in and near joint capsules are proprioceptors; through excitation of these endings and nonencapsulated endings in the same tissues, there is accurate aware-

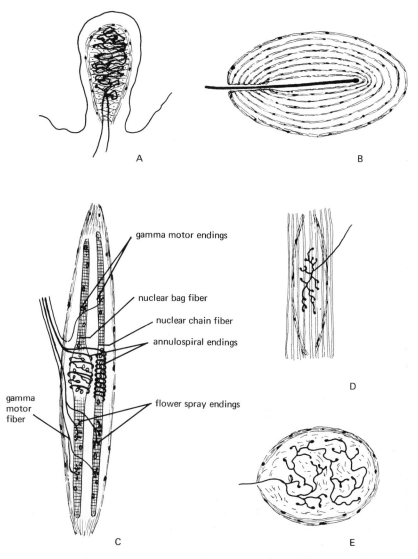

FIG. 3–3. Main types of encapsulated sensory endings. **A.** Meissner's corpuscle in a dermal papilla. **B.** Pacinian corpuscle. **C.** Neuromuscular spindle. **D.** Neuro-tendinous spindle. **E.** Sensory end-bulb.

ness of the position and movement of body parts (kinesthetic sense). Pacinian corpuscles serve as receptors for vibration. These corpuscles in viscera and mesenteries may contribute to sensations of fullness of hollow organs, as well as to the more generalized feelings of well-being or malaise.

Neuromuscular Spindles

The neuromuscular spindles (Fig. 3–3C) are the most complex of the receptors, both structurally and functionally. They provide sensory data for spinal reflex adjustments of muscle tonus, for the contribution of the cerebellum to motor functions, and for sensorimotor integration at the cerebral cortical level. Muscle spindles vary from simple to complex in structure; the following description applies in the main to fully developed spindles.

These slender spindles are a fraction of a millimeter wide and up to about 6 mm long. They are inserted in considerable numbers parallel with the fibers of voluntary muscles, being most numerous toward the tendinous insertion of a muscle. Each spindle consists of a fusiform-shaped capsule of connective tissue and from 2 to 10 intrafusal muscle fibers. The latter differ in several respects from the main or extrafusal fibers of the muscle; intrafusal fibers are considerably smaller than the extrafusal, the middle zone lacks cross-striations, and this region contains numerous nuclei which are not in the usual subsarcolemmal position characteristic of mature striated muscle. In some intrafusal fibers the midregion is expanded, while in others it is not; they are known as *nuclear bag fibers* and *nuclear chain fibers,* respectively.

Each neuromuscular spindle is supplied by two afferent nerve fibers. One of these is a large member of the A group; the myelin covering ends as the fiber pierces the capsule, and the dendrite winds spirally around the midportion of the intrafusal muscle fibers as the *annulospiral ending.* The second, slightly smaller, afferent fiber branches terminally and ends as varicosities on the intrafusal muscle fibers some distance from the midregion. The latter terminals are called *flower spray endings.* The annulospiral and flower spray terminals are also known as primary and secondary sensory endings of the spindle. The neuromuscular spindles are unique sensory endings in several respects, most significantly in having an efferent or motor innervation. The extrafusal fibers comprising the main mass of a muscle are innervated by large motor cells (alpha motor neurons),

whose axons are of alpha size in the A group. Smaller motor cells (gamma motor neurons), with axons of gamma size in the A group, supply the intrafusal muscle fibers of the spindle. There are end-plates on both ends of these fibers, probably because the midregion without cross-striations is not contractile.

Neuromuscular spindles contribute to muscle function in several ways, the simplest role being that of a receptor for the stretch or extensor reflex. Slight stretching of a muscle includes the intrafusal muscle fibers; the sensory endings are stimulated and a nerve impulse passes to alpha motor neurons supplying the main mass of the muscle. The latter thereupon contracts, in response to stretch, through a two-neuron reflex arc. Stimulation of the spindles ceases when the muscle contracts, because the spindle fibers are in parallel with the other muscle fibers. The stretch reflex is in almost constant use in the adjustment of muscle tonus. It also forms the basis of tests for tendon reflexes, such as the knee jerk test or extension at the knee on tapping the patellar tendon, which are standard items in a clinical examination.

The spindles also have an important role in muscle action resulting from neurologic processes in the brain. Certain nuclei in the brain stem have a motor function and come under the influence of such higher centers as the cerebral cortex, corpus striatum, and cerebellum. The entire complex is known as the extrapyramidal motor system to distinguish it from the more direct pyramidal motor system. Many of the fibers connecting brain stem nuclei with the spinal cord synapse with gamma motor neurons supplying the intrafusal muscle fibers. Contraction of the intrafusal muscle fibers in response to their stimulation by gamma motor neurons causes augmented firing of the sensory nerve terminals, partly through increasing the sensitivity of the spindle to stretch. This results in contraction of the regular muscle fibers through reflex stimulation of alpha motor neurons. The *gamma reflex loop* consists of the gamma motor neuron, neuromuscular spindle, afferent or sensory neuron, and the alpha motor neuron supplying extrafusal muscle fibers.

Neurotendinous Spindles

Neurotendinous spindles, also known as Golgi tendon organs or simply tendon spindles, are most numerous near the muscle attachment of the tendon. These receptors are relatively simple in structure, consisting of a thin capsule of connective tissue enclosing a few collagenous fibers of the tendon on which a nerve fiber ends (Fig. 3–3D). The latter is a large group A fiber (there may be more than one), which enters the spindle and breaks up into branches ending as varicosities on the intrafusal tendon fibers. These endings are stimulated by tension on the tendon, greater tension being required than for excitation of neuromuscular spindles by stretch. The afferent impulses reach intercalated neurons in the spinal cord. These have an inhibitory effect on alpha motor neurons, causing relaxation of the muscle to which the particular tendon is attached. The opposing functions of the neuromuscular spindles (excitatory) and the neurotendinous spindles (inhibitory) are in balance in the total integration of spinal reflex activity. By acting as constant monitors of tension, the inhibitory role of neurotendinous spindles also provides protection against damage to muscle or tendon because of excessive tension.

Four types of endings which serve as proprioceptors have now been discussed. These are the nonencapsulated endings and pacinian corpuscles in the regions of joints (both of which function elsewhere in other modalities of sensation), neuromuscular spindles, and Golgi tendon organs. All the above receptors provide data for motor responses of a reflex or automatic nature through pathways of varying degrees of complexity—from the simplest in the spinal cord to the more complicated connections inherent in circuits in the cerebellar and cerebral cortices. In addition, all of the receptors contribute to proprioception at the conscious level, i.e., to awareness of position and movement of body parts. However, the unencapsulated endings and pacinian corpuscles associated with joints are perhaps of special significance in this respect.

Sensory End-Bulbs

There is a group of sensory endings, known collectively as end-bulbs, which are difficult to appraise because their morphology and function are so poorly understood. The end-bulbs consist of a thin capsule enclosing poorly organized cellular and fibrous material (Fig. 3–3E). A group A fiber of small to medium caliber pierces the capsule, and the unmyelinated terminal forms an irregular pattern with numerous branches. The end-bulbs vary in size (many are of the order of 50–100 μ in diameter) and they are spherical, elongated, or irregular in shape. They also differ in the configuration of the intrinsic nerve fiber. End-bulbs have a wide distribution; being found in the dermis and subcutaneous tissue, mucous membranes and mucocutaneous junctions, glans of the clitoris and penis, the conjunctiva, serous membranes, and joint capsules. It has been supposed that specific end-bulbs could be identified histologically. These received names derived from their location or the investigator who described them—names such as mucocutaneous endings, genital corpuscles, and end-bulbs of Krause and Ruffini. It is doubtful that specific types of end-bulbs can be identified because there are so frequently intermediate types. It was thought at one time that end-bulbs of Krause were receptors for coolness and end-bulbs of Ruffini for warmth; but the evidence that these are special temperature sensors is no longer regarded as conclusive. These general sensory receptors are obviously in need of further study. They appear to participate in touch, pressure, temperature, and proprioceptive sensibilities; but definite correlations between modalities of sensation and specific end-bulbs have yet to be established.

MOTOR ENDINGS

The *motor end-plates* or *myoneural junctions* on extrafusal and intrafusal fibers of voluntary muscles are synapse-like structures with two components: the ending of a motor nerve fiber and the subjacent part of the muscle fibers. In regard specifically to the extrafusal fibers, the axon of an alpha motor neuron divides terminally to supply variable numbers of muscle fibers. A *motor unit* consists of a motor neuron and the muscle fibers innervated by that neuron. The number of muscle fibers in a motor unit varies from one to several hundred, depending on the size and function of the muscle. A large motor unit, in which a single neuron supplies many muscle fibers, is adequate for the functions of such muscles as those of the trunk and proximal portions of the extremities. However, in small muscles such as the extraocular and intrinsic hand muscles, which must function with precision, the motor units include only a few muscle fibers. Such an anatomic arrangement provides for intricate control of muscle action.

Each branch of the nerve fiber gives up its myelin sheath on approaching a muscle fiber and ends in the form of bulbous expansions which constitute the neural component of the end-plate (Fig. 3–4). The end-plate is typically 40–60 μ in diameter and is usually located midway along the length of the muscle fiber. Each peripheral nerve fiber is surrounded by two sheaths external to the myelin sheath. The neuro-

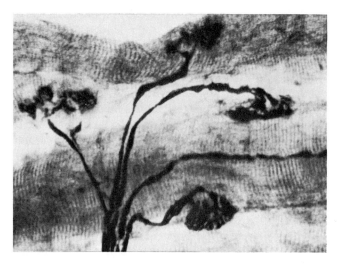

FIG. 3–4. Motor end-plates. Gold chloride chain. (Courtesy of R. Mitchell and Dr. A. S. Wilson) ×500

lemmal sheath consists of the nucleated cytoplasmic portions of Schwann cells, whose cell membranes wrap around the axon or axis cylinder to form the myelin sheath. The neurolemmal sheath continues around the terminal branches of the motor fiber after the Schwann cells cease to form a myelin sheath, but does not intervene between the nerve ending and the muscle fiber. The nerve fiber is surrounded outside the neurolemma by a delicate endoneurial sheath of connective tissue. The endoneurium is continuous at the motor end-plate with the thin endomysium or connective tissue sheath of the muscle fiber, forming a "tent" over the myoneural junction.

The ultrastructure of the axonal expansions within the end-plate is like that of a synaptic end-bulb, in that they contain synaptic vesicles and mitochondria. The surface of the muscle fiber is slightly elevated at the myoneural junction. The accumulation of sarcoplasm at this site constitutes the sole-plate, in which there are nuclei of the muscle fiber and mitochondria. Each neural expansion occupies a groove or trough on the surface of the sole-plate; there is an interval of 200–500 Å, constituting a synaptic cleft between the surface of the nerve terminal and that of the muscle fiber. The plasma membrane or sarcolemma of the muscle fiber has a wavy outline where it apposes the nerve terminal, the irregularities being known as junctional folds. The synaptic cleft contains glycoprotein material which is continuous with the boundary layer that invests the sarcolemma elsewhere.

Acetylcholine released from the synaptic vesicles by a nerve impulse traveling along the axon reduces the membrane potential of the sarcolemma, as in postsynaptic neuronal membranes. The resulting action potential is self-propagated over the sarcolemma and carried into the muscle fiber to the contractile myofibrils by means of an ultramicroscopic membrane system in the form of tubules (transverse tubular system). There is interference with the cholinergic excitation of muscle fibers in myasthenia gravis, a disorder characterized by impaired response of voluntary muscles, affecting at first small muscles such as those that move the eyes and raise the lids. Studies point to an autoimmune mechanism in which antibodies formed in the thymus affect proteins in the motor end-plates, suppressing cholinergic transmission in some manner which is not yet understood.

Postganglionic autonomic endings on smooth muscle and secretory cells are also similar to synapses. The fine axons make contact with the effector cell, and there is often a swelling along the course of the axon or at its end, which fits into a depression on the surface of the muscle or gland cell. The nerve fiber contains an accumulation of mitochondria at these sites, together with synaptic vesicles from which either noradrenaline or acetylcholine is released, according to whether the neuron is sympathetic or parasympathetic.

GANGLIA

The *spinal ganglia* are swellings on the dorsal roots of spinal nerves. They are situated in the intervertebral foramina, just proximal to the union of dorsal and ventral roots to form the spinal nerves. These ganglia contain the cell bodies of primary sensory neurons, mainly in a large peripheral zone. The center of the ganglion is occupied by nerve fibers, which are the proximal portions of peripheral and central processes of the nerve cells. Dorsal root ganglia and ganglia of cranial nerves involved with general sensation have the same histologic structure.

These sensory neurons develop from the

embryonal neural crests, which consist of ectodermal cells and lie along the dorso-lateral borders of the neural tube. The cells are bipolar at first, but the two processes soon unite to form the single process of this unipolar type of neuron. The processes arising from the smaller cell bodies are short and straight, while those given off by larger cells often wind at first around the parent cell body. In either case, the fiber divides into peripheral and central branches or processes; the former terminates in a sensory ending, and the latter enters the spinal cord through a dorsal root. The nerve impulse passes directly from the peripheral to the central process, thereby bypassing the cell body. Both processes have the structural characteristics of axons, although the peripheral one is a dendrite in the sense of conduction toward the cell body. Alternatively, the terminal part of the peripheral branch in the sensory ending may be considered as the dendrite. The major portion of the peripheral process and the central process then constitute a long axon, to which the cell body forms a necessary appendage with genetic and metabolic functions.

The spherical cell bodies vary from 20 to 100 μ in diameter; their processes are similarly of graded size, ranging from small unmyelinated fibers of the C group to the largest myelinated fibers in the A group. The large neurons are for proprioception and discriminative touch; those of intermediate size are concerned with simple touch, pressure, pain, and temperature; and the smallest neurons transmit impulses for pain and temperature. Each cell body is closely invested by a capsule consisting of two types of cells. An inner layer of satellite cells is continuous with the neurolemmal sheath that surrounds the processes. External to this, there are cells supported by connective tissue fibers, forming a layer of the capsule that is continuous with the endoneurial sheath of the processes. One of the most common disorders involving spinal or cranial nerve ganglia is herpes zoster (shingles), in which a virus infection of the ganglion causes pain and other sensory disturbances in the cutaneous area of distribution of the affected nerve.

Autonomic ganglia include ganglia of the sympathetic trunks along the sides of the vertebral bodies, collateral or prevertebral ganglia in plexuses of the thorax and abdomen (e.g., the cardiac, celiac, and mesenteric plexuses), and terminal ganglia in or near the viscera. The multipolar nerve cells of autonomic ganglia are 20–45 μ in diameter. The nucleus is often eccentric, and binucleate cells are encountered occasionally. The cell body is surrounded by satellite cells similar to those that form the inner capsular layer around the nerve cells of spinal ganglia. The dendrites, of which there are several, branch external to the capsule and are in synaptic contact with terminals of preganglionic fibers. The thin unmyelinated axon (group C fiber) takes the most convenient route to smooth muscle and gland cells in the viscera, to the heart, to blood vessels throughout the body, and to sweat glands and arrector pili muscles in the skin.

PERIPHERAL NERVES

The constituent fibers of all but the smallest peripheral nerves are arranged in bundles or fasciculi, and three connective tissue sheaths are recognized. The entire nerve is surrounded by an *epineurium;* the sheath enclosing a bundle of fibers is known as the *perineurium;* and individual nerve fibers have a delicate covering of connective tissue constituting the *endoneurium* or sheath of Henle.

NERVE FIBERS

A *nerve fiber* consists of the axon or axis cylinder, the myelin sheath in the case of fibers belonging to groups A and B, and the neurolemmal sheath (of Schwann). The *axis cylinder* has no features that are not shared with long axons in the central nervous system. Its cytoplasm (*axoplasm*) contains neurofilaments, microtubules, patches of smooth-surfaced endoplasmic reticulum, and mitochondria. The plasma membrane is called the *axolemma*.

Neurolemma and Myelin Sheath

The neurolemma and the myelin sheath have several points of interest, centering around the fact that both are components of Schwann cells. The myelin sheath has no significant intrinsic structure at the light microscope level (Fig. 3–5A). That it contains lipids has been obvious, since the myelin is dissolved by lipid solvents and stained black by osmic acid, which is known to react with lipids. Proteins were also known to be present in myelin; they remain as fibrillar material after the lipids have been dissolved.

The myelin sheath is interrupted at intervals by *nodes of Ranvier;* the length of an internode varies from 100 μ to about 1 mm, depending on the length and thickness of the fiber. Funnel-shaped clefts, called the *incisures of Schmidt-Lanterman,* are clearly visible in longitudinal sections of a nerve stained with osmic acid. (Incisures have not been seen in myelin sheaths in the central nervous system.) With light microscopy, the neurolemmal sheath is seen as a series of *Schwann cells,* one for each internode. Most of the cytoplasm is in the region of the ellipsoidal nucleus, but traces of cytoplasm and the plasma membrane closely surround the myelin sheath from one node of Ranvier to the next.

Observations on the growth of nerve fibers in culture and on regeneration of nerve fibers have established that Schwann cells are responsible for laying down the myelin sheath around the axis cylinder. X-ray diffraction studies have shown that the myelin consists of alternating protein and lipid layers, and the lipids have been identified chemically as cholesterol, phospholipids, and cerebrosides. More recently, the technique of electron microscopy has established that the myelin is not only formed by the Schwann cell, but consists of its plasma membrane wrapped around the axis cylinder. The term neurolemmal sheath or sheath of Schwann is used to distinguish the nucleated cytoplasmic layer from the layer of myelin. In fact, the Schwann cell is included in both sheaths, the cytoplasmic portion forming the neurolemma and an extensive proliferation of the plasma membrane constituting the myelin. The Schwann cells are continuous with satellite cells surrounding nerve cell bodies in cerebrospinal and autonomic ganglia. The cellular layer that is in such intimate relationship with all nerve fibers and ganglion cells of the peripheral nervous system originates mainly in the embryonal neural crest, but also includes a smaller number of cells which migrate from the neural tube along with growing motor fibers. Oligodendrocytes are the comparable cells in the central nervous system, the transition between oligodendrocytes and Schwann cells occurring at the junction of the nerve roots and spinal cord (or brain stem). Other oligodendrocytes lie close to neuronal cell bodies without forming a continuous layer like the satellite cells of peripheral ganglia.

Myelin sheaths are laid down during the latter part of fetal development and during the first year postnatally, in the manner shown diagrammatically in Figure 3–5B, C, and D. The ultrastructure of the myelin sheath is seen in Figure 3–6. In order to

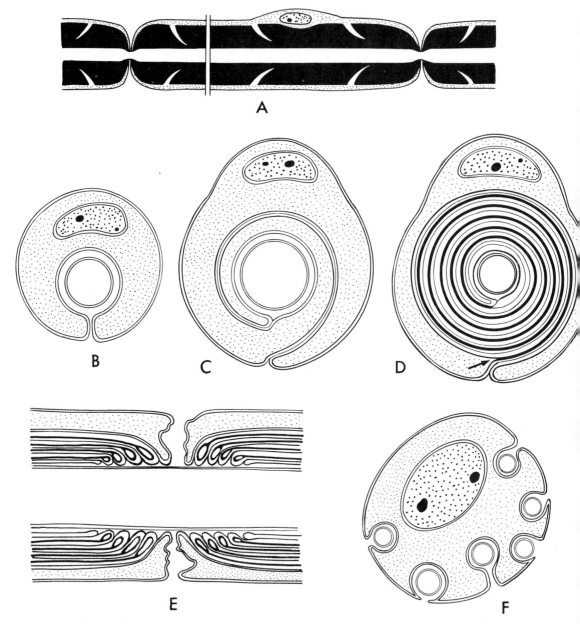

FIG. 3–5. A. The myelin sheath and neurolemmal sheath, as seen with light microscopy. **B, C, D.** Successive stages in the development of the myelin sheath from the plasma membrane of a Schwann cell. **E.** Ultrastructure of a node of Ranvier. **F.** Relation of a Schwann cell to several unmyelinated fibers.

explain the alternating layers of electron dense and less dense material, it is necessary to show the plasma membrane as a double line, representing outer and inner protein layers separated by an interval composed of lipids. Whether this trilaminar structure applies to the membrane of the Schwann cell generally, or only the extension of the membrane that constitutes the myelin sheath, is an open question.

The axis cylinder is first surrounded by the Schwann cell; the external plasma membrane is continuous with the membrane immediately around the axon through a *mesaxon*. Subsequent events could be explained by rotation of the Schwann cell around the axon, but the precise mechanism is not yet clear. The direction of the spiral is clockwise in some internodes and anticlockwise in others. In any event, the cytoplasm between the layers of cell membrane gradually disappears, except for surface cytoplasm which is most abundant in the region of the nucleus. The myelin sheath comes to consist of from a few to 50 turns of membrane, depending on the diameter and length of the axis cylinder. The major dense line, 25 Å in thickness, consists of two inner protein layers of the plasma membrane, which fuse along a line indicated by the arrow in Figure 3–5D. The less dense layer, about 100 Å wide, consists of a double thickness of the lipid layer of the cell membrane. The fused outer protein layers of the membrane become exceedingly thin, forming an inconspicuous intraperiod line in the middle of the lighter lipid layer (Fig. 3–6).

The node of Ranvier is the interval between the plasma membrane systems of two Schwann cells (Fig. 3–5E). The neurolemmal sheath portion of the adjoining Schwann cells has an irregular edge at the node. However, there is a space between the Schwann cells, through which the axolemma at the node is bathed by tissue fluid. The action potential skips electronically from node to node and the transmission of a nerve impulse along a myelinated fiber is therefore called saltatory conduction (*saltare*, to jump). The length of internodes has therefore a bearing on the conduction rate of the nerve impulse and the internodes are longer, up to a maximum of

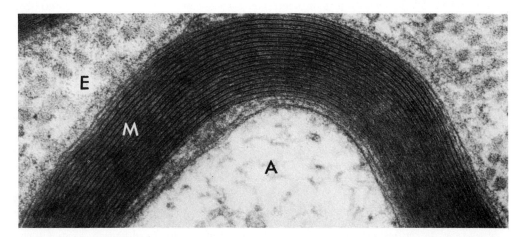

FIG. 3–6. Ultrastructure of the myelin sheath (*M*) consisting of alternating dense and less dense layers; the latter includes a thin intraperiod line. *A*, axoplasm; *E*, collagen fibers of the endoneurium. (Courtesy of Dr. R. C. Buck) ×107,500

about 1 mm, the thicker and longer the nerve fiber. The Schmidt–Lanterman incisures, which are of unknown functional significance, are formed by a loosening of the plasma membrane layers of the sheath with retention of cytoplasm between the membranes.

With respect to unmyelinated fibers, a Schwann cell envelops several (up to 15) thin axons, as shown in Figure 3–5F. Since the axon is surrounded by a single layer of the Schwann cell's plasma membrane, it is unmyelinated and there are no nodes of Ranvier. The nerve impulse is therefore a self-propagating action potential along the axolemma, without the accelerating factor of node-to-node or saltatory conduction. This accounts for the slow rate of conduction which is characteristic of unmyelinated fibers.

DISORDERS

The peripheral nervous system is subject to various disorders. Peripheral neuropathy (neuritis) is the most common of these and consists of degenerative changes in peripheral nerves, causing sensory loss and motor weakness. Distal portions of nerves are affected first, with symptoms in the hands and feet. There are multiple causes of peripheral neuropathy, including nutritional deficiencies, toxins of various kinds, and metabolic disorders such as diabetes. Regardless of the apparent etiological agent, it is likely that avitaminosis, especially for vitamin B, is the significant factor in many instances.

Damage to a peripheral nerve by a penetrating wound may result in an incapacitating disorder known as causalgia. There is severe pain in the affected limb, together with tropic changes in the skin. A nerve may be pressed upon where it passes through a restricted aperture; for example, the ulnar nerve is subject to pressure at the elbow and the median nerve in the carpal tunnel at the wrist. The resulting "entrapment syndrome" includes motor and sensory disturbances in the area of distribution of the nerve. The major plexuses, especially the brachial plexus, may be involved in a traumatic lesion, or there may be compression of major bundles of a plexus (as in crutch palsy). The nerve roots are involved in a variety of disorders (radiculopathy), causing motor and sensory disturbances. The latter may include pain in cutaneous areas and in muscles supplied by the affected nerve roots.

SUGGESTIONS FOR ADDITIONAL READING

Bodian D: The generalized vertebrate neuron. Science 137:323–326, 1962

Boyd IA: The structure and innervation of the nuclear bag muscle fibre system and the nuclear chain muscle fibre system in mammalian muscle spindles. Philos Trans Roy Soc (London) 245: 81–136, 1962

Bridgman CF: Comparisons in structure of tendon organs in the rat, cat and man. J Comp Neurol 138:369–372, 1970

Causey G: The Cell of Schwann. Edinburgh, Livingstone, 1960

Davis H: Some principles of sensory receptor action. Physiol Rev 41:391–416, 1961

Eames RA, Gamble HJ: Schwann cell relationships in normal human cutaneous nerves. J Anat 106: 417–435, 1970

Geren BB: Structural Studies of the Formation of the Myelin Sheath in Peripheral Nerve Fibers. In Rudnick D (ed.): Cellular Mechanisms in Differentiation and Growth, Chap. 10, pp. 213–220. Princeton, N.J., Princeton University Press, 1956

Keller JH, Moffett BC Jr: Nerve endings in the

temporomandibular joint of the Rhesus macaque. Anat Rec 160:587–594, 1968

Kennedy WR: Innervation of normal human muscle spindles. Neurology (Minneap) 20:463–475, 1970

Nishi K, Oura C, Pallie W: Fine structure of Pacinian corpuscles in the mesentery of the cat. J Cell Biol 43:539–552, 1969

Pease DC, Quilliam TA: Electron microscopy of the Pacinian corpuscle. J Biophys Biochem Cytol 3:331–350, 1957

Robertson JD: The ultrastructure of adult vertebrate peripheral myelinated nerve fibers in relation to myelinogenesis. J Biophys Biochem Cytol 1:271–278, 1955

Shantha TR, Bourne GH: The Perineural Epithelium: A New Concept. In Bourne GF (ed.): The Structure and Function of Nervous Tissue, Vol 1, pp. 379–495. New York, Academic Press, 1968

Sinclair DC: Cutaneous Sensation. London, Oxford University Press, 1967

Straile WE: Encapsulated nerve end-organs in the rabbit, mouse, sheep and man. J Comp Neurol 136:317–335, 1969

Thaemert JC: Ultrastructural interrelationships of nerve processes and smooth muscle cells in three dimensions. J Cell Biol 28:37–49, 1966

Winkelmann RK: Nerve Endings in Normal and Pathological Skin. Springfield, Ill., Charles C Thomas, 1960

4

Response of Nerve Cells to Injury; Nerve Fiber Regeneration; Neuroanatomic Methods

There are usually changes in the parent cell body following damage to an axon, and there are always degenerative changes in the nerve fiber distal to the injury. The effect on the cell body is called *axon reaction,* while the peripheral changes are known as *wallerian degeneration.* Axon reaction consists of the same sequence of events whether the traumatized fiber is in the central nervous system or in a peripheral nerve. However, there are significant differences in what happens in the distal portion of the severed fiber, more specifically with respect to regeneration, depending on whether the fiber is centrally or peripherally located. Nerve fibers in the central nervous system may be damaged by natural causes. Fibers may be included, for example, in a region of infarction caused by vascular occlusion or in a locus affected by one of the demyelinating diseases. Bundles of nerve fibers may also be interrupted by trauma, such as occurs in accidental injuries and neurosurgical procedures.

Lesions placed in specific locations are used widely in studies on experimental animals. Various forms of trauma (crushing, cutting, etc.) interrupt fibers of cerebrospinal nerves.

The sequelae of axon interruption, and regeneration of nerve fibers when this occurs, have important clinical implications. In addition, advantage is taken of wallerian degeneration to trace specific fiber pathways in the central nervous system.

AXON REACTION

The changes in the proximal portion of the affected neuron vary according to the type of neuron and the species, among other variables. Cells in some locations undergo progressive degeneration and ultimately disappear. Conversely, the proximal portion of the neuron may not be altered significantly by axon section. For example, the cell bodies of cerebrospinal ganglia react to section of their peripheral, but not their central, processes. Species differences include absence of axon reaction in motor cells of the spinal cord of the rat and rabbit, following peripheral nerve section; whereas typical reaction occurs in the same cells in most animals, including man. The cytologic details of axon reaction are best seen in large neurons of motor type, which contain coarse clumps of Nissl material. The following summary includes the more typical aspects of this fundamental response to injury in such cells.

The nerve fiber between the cell body and the lesion is not altered appreciably, except for traumatic degeneration immediately adjacent to the lesion. The structural changes in the cell body appear to reflect two overlapping types of responses. When stained by a basic dye (the Nissl method), the cells first show signs of reaction 24–48 hours after interruption of the axons. The coarse clumps of Nissl material are changed to a finely granular dispersion; this change, which is known as *chromatolysis,*

occurs first between the axon hillock and the nucleus, gradually spreading throughout the perikaryon. The nucleus assumes an eccentric position, moving away from the axon hillock, and the cell body swells, giving it a rounded contour (Fig. 4–1). This aspect of the reaction reaches a maximum 10–20 days after axon injury, and it is more severe the closer the injury to the cell body. The total amount of cytoplasmic RNA, as determined by cytochemical measurements, is not altered appreciably. Electron microscopy shows that there is disruption of the orderly array of the granular endoplasmic reticulum, with some loss of ribosomes from the outer surfaces of the cisternae and an increase in the number of free ribosomes in the cytoplasmic matrix. This early phase of reaction appears to be partly in the nature of cellular edema, which is a well known response of cells in general when affected by a harmful agent.

There are signs of recovery from the early effects of trauma to the axon, even while the above changes are in progress.

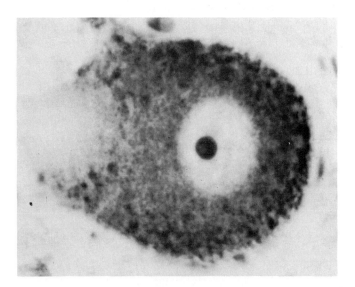

FIG. 4–1. Motor neuron undergoing axon reaction, 6 days after axon section. Cresyl violet stain. ×800

The nucleolus enlarges and dense basophilic caps are often seen on the cytoplasmic side of the nuclear membrane.
These are interpreted as evidence of accelerated RNA and protein synthesis, which
would favor regeneration of the axon when
circumstances make regeneration possible.
The recovery period is long, often several
months. The cell may pass through a phase
during which the RNA and protein contents are in excess of normal; normal levels
are then gradually restored, together with
the usual Nissl pattern for the type of cell.
The cell body is eventually smaller than
normal if the axon does not regenerate.
Histochemical studies show that there are
quantitative changes in cytoplasmic enzymes, including oxidative and hydro-
lytic enzymes, throughout the period of
morphologic alteration of the cell.

Reacting cells can be identified with little
difficulty, thus providing a method of determining the location of parent cell bodies
of interrupted fibers. The method has been
valuable in establishing the source of numerous fasciculi in the brain and spinal
cord, together with the cells of origin of
fibers in cerebrospinal nerves. In view of
the limitation of the method to large neurons, most of the information that can be
obtained from its use is now available.

WALLERIAN DEGENERATION IN A PERIPHERAL NERVE

The nucleus is essential for the synthesis of
cytoplasmic proteins, which are carried
distally in the axon by cytoplasmic flow,
replacing proteins that have been degraded
as part of the metabolic activity of the cell.
The axon therefore does not long survive
when separated from the cell body. Simultaneously throughout its length, that part
of the axon distal to the lesion becomes
slightly swollen and irregular within the
first day and breaks up into fragments by
the third to fifth day. Muscular contraction
on electrical stimulation of a degenerating
motor nerve ceases abruptly 2–3 days after
the nerve is interrupted. The degeneration
includes the neural component of sensory
and motor endings. The sheaths and other
nonnervous components of the endings remain intact for a considerable time and are
reinnervated under favorable circumstances.

The myelin sheath, which becomes converted into short ellipsoidal segments during the first few days after interruption of
the fiber, gradually undergoes complete
disintegration and the particles of degenerating myelin disappear over a period of
several weeks. While the axis cylinder and
myelin sheath are degenerating, or the axon
only in the case of unmyelinated fibers, the
Schwann cells become much altered. Each
cell loses the extensive membrane system
that constitutes the myelin sheath, leaving
only the part of the cell forming the neurolemmal sheath. The cells multiply by mitosis and fill the slightly contracted endoneurial sheath. The sheath and the altered
cells of Schwann occupying its lumen compose the *band fiber* or *band of von Büngner*. It has been assumed that the frag-
ments of axon and myelin are ingested by
tissue macrophages and macrophages of
hematogenous origin. However, there is
evidence that the Schwann cells take on
phagocytic properties and assist in removal
of myelin by autodigestion of the membrane systems that envelop the axis
cylinders.

REGENERATION OF PERIPHERAL NERVE FIBERS

If a nerve has been severed, regeneration of
fibers requires close apposition of the cut
ends by placing sutures through the outer

connective tissue sheaths. Assuming that this condition has been met, the following sequence of events takes place.

REGENERATION OF AXONS

During the first few days, proliferating Schwann cells fill the interval between the apposed nerve ends. Regenerating fibers begin to invade the region by about the fourth day, each fiber dividing into numerous branches with bulbous tips which grow along the clefts between Schwann cells. The rate of growth is slow at first; 2–3 weeks may elapse before the fibers have traversed the region of the lesion. The fine branches may then find their way into endoneurial tubes of the distal segment, these tubes now being the band fibers of von Büngner. Several filaments enter each tube, and the invasion of a particular endoneurial tube leading to a specific type of end-organ appears to be determined by chance alone. Many filaments fail to enter an endoneurial tube and grow into adjacent tissue. This is the fate of all regenerating axons if the severed ends are too widely separated or if connective tissue or extraneous material intervenes. Such fibers tend to form complicated whorls (spirals of Perroncito), producing a swelling or neuroma which may be a source of spontaneous pain. At the other extreme is the almost perfect regeneration of the nerve through the growth of each fiber along its original endoneurial tube. Such a regeneration may occur if the nerve is crushed just enough to interrupt axis cylinders without disruption of the connective tissue sheaths.

Having crossed the region of the lesion, the axonal filaments grow distally among the Schwann cells in the endoneurial tube. The regenerating fibers eventually reach motor and sensory endings; the proportion of endings that are reinnervated depends on conditions at the site of the original injury. The rate of growth is of the order of 2–4 mm daily. The number of days that will elapse between nerve suture and the beginning of functional return may be estimated on the basis of a regeneration rate of 1.5 mm daily. This value allows for the time required for the fibers to traverse the lesion and for reinnervation of the peripheral endings.

RECONSTITUTION OF NERVE FIBERS

Changes occur meanwhile along the course of the fibers. A myelin sheath is laid down by Schwann cells if the growing axon extends from a myelinated fiber in the proximal segment. Myelination begins near the lesion and proceeds in a proximodistal direction, the mechanism being like that described in the preceding chapter for myelination of fibers in the first instance. Of the several axons growing in an endoneurial tube, only one matures fully; the others gradually regress and disappear. The branching of axons as they begin to regenerate, the entry of branches from a single axon into a number of endoneurial tubes, and the presence of branches from several neurons in an individual endoneurial tube, all improve a neuron's chance of becoming reconnected with a suitable sensory or motor ending. The appropriate fiber for the ending persists, while others in the endoneurial tube regress. A regenerated fiber tends to have a diameter, internodal length, and conduction velocity that are about 80 percent of the corresponding values for the original fiber. The motor unit for a regenerated fiber is larger, compared with the preexisting motor unit; the axon supplies more muscle fibers than formerly. This contributes to less precise function of a reinnervated muscle. When all things are considered, it is understandable that there are limitations to functional recovery after peripheral nerve injuries.

The cut ends of a nerve can be placed in fairly accurate apposition by fine sutures inserted at intervals through the epineurium and including some subjacent perineurium. It may be desirable to postpone suturing for 2–3 weeks after the nerve is interrupted, but the delay should not extend much beyond 1 month. Later, there is atrophy of muscle fibers and end-organs and excessive shrinkage of endoneurial tubes. Delay beyond 6 months is likely to jeopardize seriously the chances of obtaining useful restoration of motor and sensory functions.

DEGENERATION AND REGENERATION IN THE CENTRAL NERVOUS SYSTEM

Following destruction of cell bodies or interruption of nerve fibers, degeneration of axis cylinders and myelin sheaths follows as in peripheral nerves. The presence of degenerative material serves as a stimulus to microglial cells, which then reveal their potentiality as macrophages and remove the debris by phagocytosis. Although severed axons regenerate in the central nervous system of fish and larval amphibia, regeneration is minimal at best in mammals. Instead, the affected region or fasciculus is converted into a special form of scar tissue by astroglial proliferation.

The histological, functional, and clinical events subsequent to wallerian degeneration in the brain and spinal cord are determined by the ineffectiveness of nerve fiber regeneration. Much of the research on this important problem has involved transection of the cord in experimental animals. The findings are in agreement that there is sprouting of axons and that regenerating fibers may traverse the cut and grow beyond it for a short distance. Whether there is any restoration of function is still contro-

versial; such recovery as has been described is slight in experimental animals, and there is no convincing evidence of clinically significant regeneration after transection of the human spinal cord. Several explanations have been offered. Endoneurial tubes are lacking for guidance of regenerating fibers; Schwann cells may have properties favorable to regeneration that are not shared with oligodendrocytes; and the glial reaction constitutes a barrier to regeneration. Moreover, the complexity of the central nervous system makes it unlikely that, even if the nerve fibers were to grow, they would establish appropriate synaptic connections with other neurons.

Nevertheless, the disability resulting from such injuries as compression of the spinal cord by a spinal fracture is so serious that any possibility of stimulating nerve fiber regeneration is of the first importance. Several chemicals have been investigated in the hope of reducing the glial reaction. They have been shown to improve the growth of axons through and beyond a cut made in the spinal cord of experimental animals, the effect being greater in young than in mature animals. Some regeneration also follows treatment with thyroid hormones, which probably act by increasing the rate of advancement of axon tips. The discovery of a "nerve growth factor" which can be extracted from mouse salivary glands and other sources has stimulated interest in future possibilities. The active substance, which consists of proteins, has the property of stimulating RNA and protein synthesis in sympathetic ganglion cells and cells of cerebrospinal ganglia *in vitro*. The cells increase in size and there is remarkable proliferation of their processes. An antiserum has been prepared by injecting the nerve growth factor into rabbits; cells of sympathetic and sensory ganglia are destroyed selectively when the antiserum is administered to young mice.

NEUROANATOMIC METHODS BASED ON WALLERIAN DEGENERATION

Advantage is taken of the structural and chemical changes in fibers undergoing wallerian degeneration to establish the position of fasciculi in the central nervous system and to trace the distribution of their constituent fibers. Two methods will be described: The first is applicable only to myelinated fibers, while the second method can be used to trace unmyelinated axons and the fine terminal branches of myelinated axons.

MARCHI TECHNIQUE

The *Marchi technique* (Fig. 4–2) for staining degenerating myelin sheaths has contributed a great deal to our understanding of the organization of the nervous system, and its usefulness is by no means exhausted. Fasciculi of myelinated fibers can be followed almost to the cells on which they synapse, i.e., to the point where the myelin sheaths cease. The principles of the technique are as follows.

As mentioned above, in the interval between 1 and 3 weeks of fiber degeneration the myelin is in the form of various sized

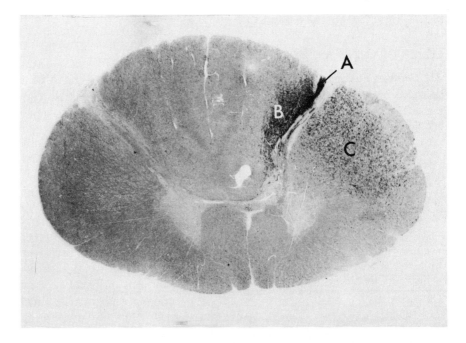

FIG. 4–2. Section of human spinal cord at the level of the third cervical segment. The patient succumbed 9 days after a traumatic lesion involved the dorsal roots of the second, third, and fourth cervical nerves on the right side, together with the dorsal portion of the lateral white column in the second cervical segment. There are the following areas of Marchi degeneration: *A,* entering fibers of the third cervical dorsal root; *B,* ascending branches of fibers that entered the spinal cord in the third and fourth cervical dorsal roots (branches of these fibers are seen entering the gray matter); *C,* descending corticospinal fibers in the lateral white column. Marchi preparation. ×10

droplets. The physical changes are accompanied by chemical degradation, the complex lipids being broken down into simpler compounds and ultimately fatty acids. Lipids are stained black by osmium tetroxide whether they are those of normal myelin or the chemically altered lipids of degenerating myelin. However, if the tissue is treated with osmium tetroxide and potassium chlorate simultaneously, only the hydrophobic cholesterol esters of unsaturated fatty acids in the degenerating myelin are stained. The degenerating fibers appear as black particles against a lighter background; their course can be followed with considerable precision by mapping the Marchi particles in sections taken at appropriate intervals.

SILVER STAINING METHODS

The use of solutions of silver nitrate forms the basis of most of the methods for staining degenerating unmyelinated fibers or the terminal branches of myelinated fibers. For example, the *Nauta technique* and its various modifications act by suppressing the argyrophilia of normal axons but not of those undergoing degeneration (Fig. 4–3). With these techniques, therefore, degenerating fibers have a beaded or fragmented appearance and are stained more darkly than normal fibers in the interval of 5–7 days following separation from the parent cell bodies. The degenerating fibers can be traced to the synaptic terminals with certain silver methods because the end-bulbs are first swollen and then fragmented, accompanied by an increase in affinity for silver nitrate. The above procedures offer rather precise and detailed information; they are therefore especially useful for the study of connections in the complex brain stem and diencephalon.

METHODS FOR NORMAL CYTOLOGY AND HISTOLOGY

The *Nissl method* employs basic aniline dyes, such as cresyl violet, toluidine blue, and thionine. Basophilic components of nerve cells are stained, i.e., parts of the cell containing nuclei acids (DNA and RNA). The Nissl method therefore stains the nucleus, nucleolus, and the granular endoplasmic reticulum or Nissl substance (Fig. 2–3). In addition to its use to show intrinsic cellular detail, the Nissl stain is used to establish the spatial pattern of nerve cells and to demonstrate functional groups of cells. Only the nuclei of neuroglial cells are stained by the Nissl method. These cells require special staining procedures, such as Cajal's gold chloride method for astrocytes and the silver carbonate staining method of Rio Hortega for microglia and, less usefully, for oligodendrocytes.

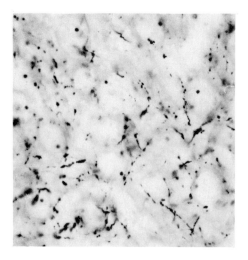

FIG. 4–3. Degenerating nerve fibers in the cerebral cortex, stained by a modification of the Nauta method. (Courtesy of Dr. Elizabeth Hall) ×320

In spite of its usefulness, the Nissl method has the drawback of leaving the nerve cell processes unstained. Of several techniques that have been devised to overcome this deficiency, the Golgi and Cajal methods are best known. In the *Golgi method,* small pieces of nervous tissue are fixed in potassium dichromate, then treated in a silver nitrate solution, following which sections are prepared. The nerve cells, including the finest branches of their dendrites, stand out as brownish-black silhouettes (Fig. 4–4). Only a proportion of the cells react to the Golgi process. This is a distinct advantage because the section would be too densely stained to be useful if all the nerve cells were blackened by the silver.

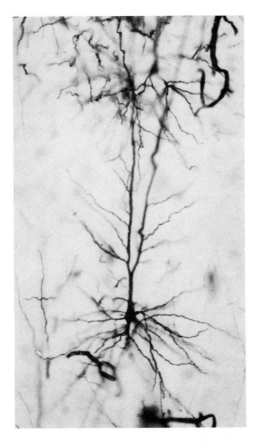

FIG. 4–4. Pyramidal cell in the cerebral cortex. Golgi technique. (Courtesy of Dr. E. G. Bertram) ×90

In the *Cajal method,* blocks of tissue are fixed in any one of a variety of solutions (e.g., alcohol, formalin, pyridine, or chloral hydrate), immersed for several days in a solution of silver nitrate, treated with a photographic reducing agent such as hydroquinone, and sectioned. The nerve cells are stained a golden-yellow color, the details varying according to the method of fixation. In general, the Cajal technique is useful for staining neurofibrils, the neuropil or complex mesh of fibers between cell bodies (Fig. 4–5), and synaptic end-bulbs (Fig. 4–6). Other silver methods accomplish similar purposes. Examples are the Bielschowsky method, in which an ammoniacal silver solution is used, and Bodian's method, which employs protargol, an organic silver compound.

The *Weigert method* is a stain for myelin sheaths and therefore for fiber bundles and white matter generally. The method is particularly useful in studying the intrinsic structure of the brain stem (Figs. 7–2 through 7–15). There are several modifications, but in the classic technique rather large blocks of nervous tissue are treated in a solution of potassium dichromate and embedded in celloidin; sections about 30 μ in thickness are stained with hematoxylin. The white matter takes on a bluish-black color. Luxol-fast-blue dyes for myelin are a useful alternative to the Weigert method. These dyes stain the protein-bound phospholipids of myelin; they are used for paraffin sections and these can be counterstained by the Nissl method for nerve cells.

Perfection of the *electron microscope* for biologic use made possible important advances in neurocytology and contributed to an integration of structure, function, and chemistry. A few examples will serve as illustrations. Electron microscopy has confirmed the Neuron Theory by demonstrating the synaptic cleft and has shown the

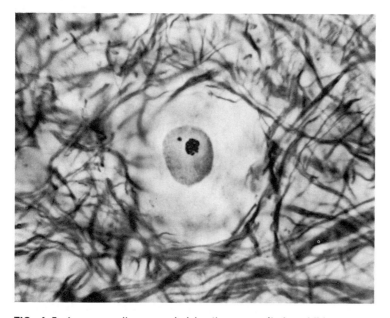

FIG. 4–5. A nerve cell surrounded by the neuropil. In addition to the nucleolus, the small accessory body of Cajal is seen in the nucleus. Cajal silver nitrate method (chloral hydrate fixation). ×1200

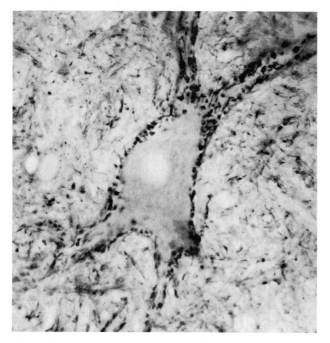

FIG. 4–6. A nerve cell surrounded by the neuropil; numerous synaptic end-bulbs are stained. Cajal silver nitrate method (formalin fixation). ×1000

synaptic vesicles which are thought to contain a chemical mediator for synaptic transmission. The myelin sheath is now known to consist of the Schwann cell membrane, wrapped in layers around the axis cylinder. Electron micrographs provide information concerning the volume of the extracellular space in the central nervous system. In view of the complexity of nervous tissue, a great deal of research at the ultrastructural level remains to be done.

ADDITIONAL METHODS OF VALUE IN NEUROANATOMY

The following lines of research have made valuable contributions to our understanding of the structure of the nervous system.

Embryologic studies have made a distinct contribution, in part because different fiber tracts of the brain and spinal cord are myelinated at different times. Certain pathways can therefore be traced in myelin-stained sections of the fetal nervous system at appropriate stages of development (the method of Flechsig). Once a cell group or fiber system has been acquired in the course of phylogeny, the structure persists, even though relegated to a minor role on being superseded by newer parts of the brain. For this reason, comparative neuroanatomy has been helpful in clarifying the significance of certain components of the human brain.

Procedures that originate in biochemis-
try, physiology, and pharmacology are complementary to those of morphology. Histochemical techniques help to identify the chemical constituents of the neuron and histochemical staining for cholinesterase and catecholamines is proving valuable in research on neurotransmitter substances. Autoradiography after administration of radioactive isotopes supplies information concerning metabolic processes in the cells of nervous tissue. A neuroanatomic method recently introduced consists of making a tritiated amino acid available to perikarya of neurons and tracing the intraaxonal transport of the radioactive amino acid to axon terminals by autoradiography. Nicotine has been used to block synapses and thus to establish their location, especially in autonomic ganglia. Anatomic studies of neuronal pathways are supplemented by stimulation of neurons and observing the destination of the nerve impulse by recording the "evoked potential" elsewhere. Accurate measurement of elapsed time between stimulation and recording gives information that may aid in determining the number of neurons, or synaptic delays, that are included in the pathway. The latter procedure is called "physiologic neuronography." It is the hope of neurologists that there will be an increasing convergence of structural, functional, biochemical, and pharmacologic approaches resulting in a unified basic neurologic science with close ties to clinical aspects of neurology.

SUGGESTIONS FOR ADDITIONAL READING

Angeletti PU, Gandini-Attardi D, Toschi G, Salvi, ML, Levi-Montalcini R: Metabolic aspects of the effect of nerve growth factor on sympathetic and sensory ganglia: Protein and ribonucleic acid synthesis. Biochem Biophys Acta 95:111–120, 1965

Bignami A, Ralston HJ, III: The cellular reaction to Wallerian degeneration in the central nervous system of the cat. Brain Res 13:444–461, 1969

Clemente CD: Regeneration in the vertebrate central nervous system. Int Rev Neurobiol 6:257–301, 1964

Cragg BG: What is the signal for chromatolysis? Brain Res 23:1–21, 1970

Edwards SB: The ascending and descending projections of the red nucleus in the cat: An experimental study using an autoradiographic tracing method. Brain Res 48:45–63, 1972

Guth L: Regeneration in the mammalian peripheral nervous system. Physiol Rev 36:441–478, 1956

Guth L, Windle WF: The enigma of central nervous regeneration. Exp Neurol Suppl 5:1–43, 1970

Heimer L: Silver impregnation of terminal degeneration in some forebrain fiber systems: A comparative evaluation of current methods. Brain Res 5:86–108, 1967

Johnstone G, Bowsher D: A new method for the selective impregnation of degenerating axon terminals. Brain Res 12:47–53, 1969

Levi-Montalcini R, Angeletti PU: Growth control of the sympathetic system by a specific protein factor. Q Rev Biol 36:99–108, 1961

Matthews MR, Cowan WM, Powell TPS: Transneuronal cell degeneration in the lateral geniculate nucleus of the macaque monkey. J Anat 94:145–169, 1960

Nandy K: Histochemical study on chromatolytic neurons. Arch Neurol (Chicago) 18:425–434, 1968

Nauta WJH, Gygax PA: Silver impregnation of degenerating axons in the central nervous system: A modified technic. Stain Technol 29:91–93, 1954

Olsson Y, Sjöstrand J: Origin of macrophages in Wallerian degeneration of peripheral nerves demonstrated autoradiographically. Exp Neurol 23:102–112, 1969

Parent A: Distribution of monoamine-containing nerve terminals in the brain of the Painted Turtle, *Chrysemys picta.* J Comp Neurol 148: 153–165, 1973

Ramón y Cajal S: Degeneration and Regeneration of the Nervous System. London, Oxford University Press, 1928

Silver A: Cholinesterases of the central nervous system, with special reference to the cerebellum. Int Rev Neurobiol 10:57–109, 1967

Smith AP, Varon S, Shooter EM: Multiple forms of the nerve growth factor protein and its subunits. Biochemistry (Wash) 7:3259–3268, 1968

Windle WF (ed.): Regeneration in the Central Nervous System. Springfield, Ill., Thomas, 1955

Windle WF (ed.): New Research Techniques of Neuroanatomy. Springfield, Ill., Thomas, 1957

Wolman L: Axon regeneration after spinal cord injury. Paraplegia 4:175–188, 1966

Regional Anatomy of the Central Nervous System

5

Spinal Cord

The spinal cord and dorsal root ganglia are directly responsible for innervation of the body, exclusive of most of the head. Afferent or sensory fibers enter the cord through the dorsal roots of spinal nerves, while efferent or motor fibers leave by way of the ventral roots (the Bell–Magendie Law). In addition to initiating spinal reflex responses, data originating in sensory endings are relayed to the brain stem and cerebellum, where they are utilized in various circuits, including those that influence motor performance. Sensory information is also transmitted to the thalamus and then the cerebral cortex where it becomes part of conscious experience, with the possibility of immediate or delayed behavioral responses. Motor neurons in the spinal cord are excited or inhibited by impulses originating at various levels of the brain from the medulla to the cerebral cortex. The spinal cord has therefore a complex internal structure.

As the fiber tracts of the spinal cord are identified, there will be reference to components of the brain that will be discussed in subsequent chapters. When the central nervous system is examined according to regions, it is necessary to probe ahead of the region under immediate consideration. An appreciation of the major systems is thus acquired step by step. The general sensory and motor systems are reviewed in later chapters of the book (Chapters 19 and 23).

GROSS FEATURES OF THE SPINAL CORD AND NERVE ROOTS

The spinal cord is a cylindrical structure, slightly flattened dorsoventrally, occupying the spinal canal of the vertebral column. Protection to the cord is provided not only by the vertebrae and their ligaments, but also by the meninges and a cushion of cerebrospinal fluid. The innermost menin-

57

geal layer of pia mater adheres to the surface of the cord. The outermost layer of thick dura mater forms a tube beginning at the level of the second sacral vertebra and extending up to the foramen magnum at the base of the skull, where it is continuous with the dura around the brain. The delicate arachnoid lies against the inner surface of the dura, forming the outer boundary of the fluid-filled subarachnoid space. The

spinal cord is suspended in the dural sheath by a *denticulate ligament* on either side. This ligament takes the form of a ribbon or shelf, which is attached along the lateral surface of the cord midway between the dorsal and ventral roots (Fig. 5–1). The lateral edge of the denticulate ligament is serrated. Twenty-one points or processes are attached to the dural sheath at intervals between the foramen magnum

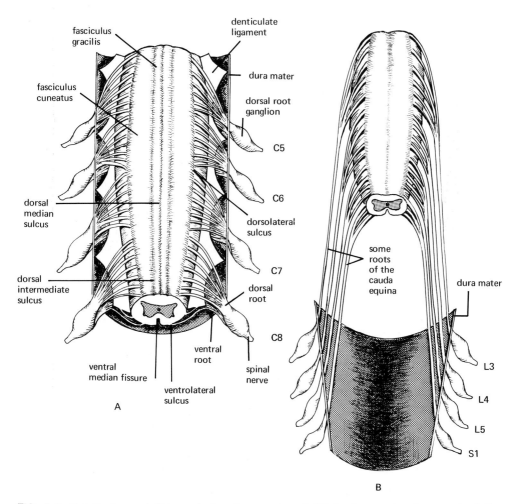

FIG. 5–1. Dorsal views of **(A)** cervical enlargement and **(B)** lumbosacral enlargement of the spinal cord and the corresponding nerve roots. In **(B)**, the dorsal and ventral roots appear to join one another close to the spinal cord. In fact, they unite just distal to the dorsal root ganglia to form the definitive spinal nerves.

and the level at which the dura mater is pierced by the roots of the first lumbar spinal nerve. An epidural space, filled with fatty tissue containing a venous plexus, occupies the interval between the dural sheath and the wall of the spinal canal.

The segmented nature of the spinal cord is demonstrated by the presence of 31 pairs of spinal nerves, but there is little indication of segmentation in its internal structure. Each dorsal root breaks up into a series of rootlets, which are attached to the cord along the corresponding segment (Fig. 5–1). The ventral root arises similarly as a series of rootlets. The spinal nerves are distributed as follows: cervical, 8; thoracic, 12; lumbar, 5; sacral, 5; coccygeal, 1. The first cervical nerves lack dorsal roots in 50 percent of individuals and the coccygeal nerve may be absent.

Segments of the neural tube (neuromeres) correspond in position with segments of the developing vertebral column (scleromeres) until the third month of fetal development. The vertebral column elongates more rapidly than the spinal cord during the remainder of fetal life. The cord, which is fixed at its rostral end, gradually advances; by the time of birth the caudal end is opposite the disk between the second and third lumbar vertebrae. A slight difference in growth rate continues during childhood, bringing the caudal end of the cord in the adult opposite the disk between the first and second lumbar vertebrae (Fig. 5–2). This is an average level, because the length of the spinal cord varies less from one individual to another than the length of the vertebral column. The caudal end of the cord may be as high as the twelfth thoracic vertebral body or as low as the third lumbar vertebra. In any event, the spinal cord occupies about the upper two-thirds of the spinal canal; the cord is ap-

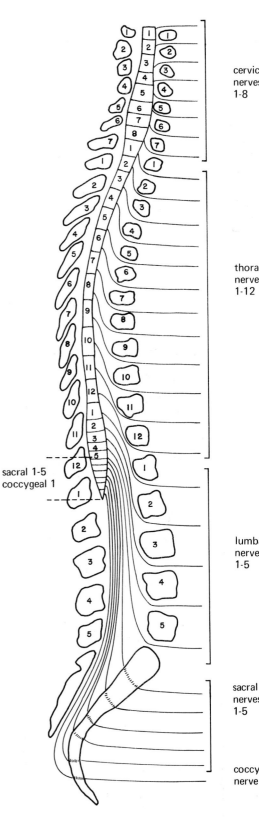

cervical nerves 1-8

thoracic nerves 1-12

sacral 1-5 coccygeal 1

lumbar nerves 1-5

sacral nerves 1-5

coccygeal nerve

FIG. 5–2. Relation of segments of the spinal cord and the spinal nerves to the vertebral column.

proximately 45 cm long in the adult male and 42 cm in the adult female.

The rostral shift of the cord during development determines the direction of spinal nerve roots in the subarachnoid space. As shown in Figure 5–2, spinal nerves from C1 through C7 leave the spinal canal through the intervertebral foramina above the corresponding vertebrae. (The first and second cervical nerves lie on the vertebral arches of the atlas and axis, respectively.) The eighth cervical nerve passes through the foramen between the seventh cervical and the first thoracic vertebrae, since there are eight cervical cord segments and seven cervical vertebrae. From that point caudally, the spinal nerves leave the canal through foramina immediately below the corresponding vetebrae. To be more precise, the nerves exit from the spinal canal by passing immediately inferior to the pedicles of the vertebrae and therefore slightly above the levels of the intervertebral disks.

The dorsal and ventral roots traverse the subarachnoid space and pierce the arachnoid and dura mater, at which point these meninges become continuous with the epineurium. After a short course in the epidural space, the roots reach the intervertebral foramina, where the dorsal root ganglia are located. The dorsal and ventral roots join immediately distal to a ganglion, forming the spinal nerve. The length and obliquity of the roots increase progressively in a rostrocaudal direction, because of the increasing distance between cord segments and corresponding vertebral segments (Figs. 5–1 and 5–2). The lumbosacral roots are of necessity the longest and constitute the *cauda equina* in the lower part of the subarachnoid space. The cord tapers into a slender filament called the *filum terminale,* which lies in the midst of the cauda equina and has a distinctive bluish-white color. The filum terminale picks up a dural investment opposite the second segment of

the sacrum and finally attaches to the dorsum of the coccyx. The filum terminale consists of pia mater and neuroglial elements; it has no functional significance.

Insertion of a needle into the subarachnoid space may be required to introduce air for diagnostic X-ray studies (pneumoencephalography), to obtain a sample of cerebrospinal fluid, or for other reasons. A lumbar spinal tap is the method of choice. There is little danger that the spinal puncture needle will damage the cord if it is inserted between the arches of the third and fourth lumbar vertebrae. It is helpful when examining a patient with a possible lesion involving the cord or nerve roots to determine the location of segments of the spinal cord in relation to vertebral spines or bodies. These relations are shown for reference in Figure 5–2.

The spinal cord is enlarged in two regions for innervation of the limbs. The cervical enlargement extends from C4 through T1 segments, most of the corresponding spinal nerves forming the brachial plexus for the nerve supply of the upper extremity. Segments L2 through S3 are included in the lumbosacral enlargement, and the corresponding nerves constitute most of the lumbosacral plexus for innervation of the lower extremity. Individual segments are longest in the thoracic region and shortest in the lower lumbar and sacral regions. The caudal end of the cord tapers rather abruptly, forming the *conus medullaris* from which the filum terminale arises.

The surface of the cord is marked off into dorsal, lateral, and ventral areas by longitudinal furrows. The deep *ventral median fissure* contains connective tissue of the pia mater and branches of the anterior spinal artery. The *dorsal median sulcus* is a shallow midline furrow. The *ventrolateral sulcus* is indistinct, but its position is indicated by the zone of attachment of the ventral roots. The *dorsolateral sulcus* marks the line of attachment of the dorsal roots. The dorsal area on either side is divided above the midthoracic level into a medial part containing the *fasciculus gracilis* and a lateral part containing the *fasciculus cuneatus.* The intervening groove is called the *dorsal intermediate sulcus* (Fig. 5–1).

GRAY MATTER AND WHITE MATTER

As seen in transverse section, the *gray matter* has a roughly H-shaped or butterfly outline (Figs. 5–3 through 5–5). The small central canal is lined by ependymal epithelium and the lumen may be obliterated in places. Thin *dorsal* and *ventral gray commissures* surround the central canal. The gray matter of either side consists of *dorsal* and *ventral horns* and an *intermediate zone.* A small *lateral horn,* containing sympathetic efferent neurons, is added in the thoracic and upper lumbar segments.

There are three main categories of neurons in the spinal gray matter. The smallest cells may be classified broadly as *internuncial neurons;* while they are most prevalent in the dorsal horn and intermediate zone, there are also many such cells in the ventral horn. Internuncial neurons receive afferents mainly from dorsal root fibers and fibers in descending fasciculi of the white matter. Their axons terminate for the most part on motor cells and tract cells. *Motor cells* of the ventral horn supply the skeletal musculature and consist of alpha and gamma motor neurons. The cells of the lateral horn and the sacral autonomic nucleus are preganglionic neurons of the sympathetic and parasympathetic divisions of the autonomic system, respectively. The cell bodies of *tract cells,* whose axons constitute the ascending fasciculi of the lateral and ventral white columns, are located mainly in the dorsal horn and the intermediate zone of gray matter.

The *white matter* consists of three columns or funiculi (Figs. 5–3 through 5–5). The *dorsal column* is bounded by the median septum and the dorsal gray horn. As noted above, this column consists of a *fasciculus gracilis* and a *fasciculus cuneatus* above the midthoracic level, the former corresponding with the entire dorsal column caudal to the midthoracic region. The two fasciculi are separated by a thin *dorsal intermediate septum.* The remainder of the white matter consists of *lateral* and *ventral columns,* between which there is no anatomic demarcation; they are sometimes combined under the heading of the ventrolateral white column. Nerve fibers decussate in the *ventral white commissure.* The *dorsolateral fasciculus* or *zone of Lissauer* lies in the interval between the apex of the dorsal horn and the surface of the cord. The white matter consists of partially overlapping fiber bundles (tracts or fasciculi), as will be described presently.

While the general pattern of gray matter and white matter is the same throughout the spinal cord, regional differences are apparent in the photographs of transverse sections (Figs. 5–3 through 5–8). For example, the amount of white matter increases in a caudal to rostral direction because fibers are added to ascending tracts, while fibers leave descending tracts to terminate in the gray matter. The main variation in the gray matter is caused by enlargements of the ventral horns in the cervical and lumbosacral regions for the motor supply of the limbs. The small lateral horn of gray matter is characteristic of the thoracic and upper lumbar segments.

CELL COLUMNS (NUCLEI) OF THE GRAY MATTER

Four cells columns are clearly delineated; these are the substantia gelatinosa and nucleus dorsalis in the dorsal horn, the

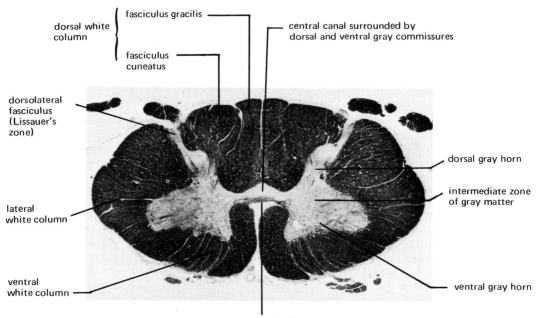

dorsal white column

fasciculus gracilis

central canal surrounded by dorsal and ventral gray commissures

fasciculus cuneatus

dorsolateral fasciculus (Lissauer's zone)

dorsal gray horn

intermediate zone of gray matter

lateral white column

ventral white column

ventral gray horn

ventral white commissure

FIG. 5–3. Seventh cervical segment. Weigert stain. ×7

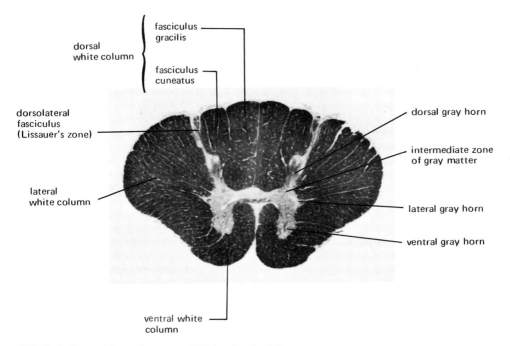

dorsal white column

fasciculus gracilis

fasciculus cuneatus

dorsolateral fasciculus (Lissauer's zone)

dorsal gray horn

intermediate zone of gray matter

lateral white column

lateral gray horn

ventral gray horn

ventral white column

FIG. 5–4. Second thoracic segment. Weigert stain. ×7

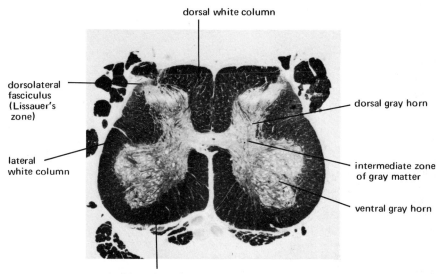

dorsal white column

dorsolateral
fasciculus
(Lissauer's
zone)

lateral
white column

dorsal gray horn

intermediate zone
of gray matter

ventral gray horn

ventral white column

FIG. 5–5. First sacral segment. Weigert stain. ×7

somatic motor cells of the ventral horn, and the visceral efferent cell column of the lateral horn. The remainder of the gray matter consists of a complex mixture of tract cells and internuncial neurons.

DORSAL HORN

The receptive or sensory part of the gray matter is in the dorsal horn and intermediate zone, in which most of the dorsal root fibers terminate. The following nuclei are recognized on the basis of cytoarchitecture and neuronal connections (Figs. 5–6 through 5–8).

Substantia Gelatinosa

The substantia gelatinosa of Rolando occupies the apex of the dorsal horn throughout the spinal cord; it is bounded externally by the dorsal white column and Lissauer's zone. The cells of the substantia gelatinosa are chiefly small neurons of the Golgi type

II variety whose axons terminate within the nucleus, often after traveling a distance of one to two segments in Lissauer's zone. Dendrites of neurons in the subjacent gray matter branch freely within the nucleus. Dorsal root fibers for pain and temperature in the zone of Lissauer terminate in the substantia gelatinosa, where they synapse with invading dendrites or with the intrinsic cells, which in turn synapse with these dendrites. In this manner conduction for pain and temperature is transferred to intercalated neurons on spinal reflex pathways and to tract cells for transmission to the brain. The cell bodies of second order neurons lay principally in the main part of the dorsal horn and the intermediate zone of gray matter.

However, the substantia gelatinosa is not to be conceived as simply a nucleus through which there is unaltered relay of pain and temperature data to higher centers. The nucleus also receives afferents from the dorsal white column, and by

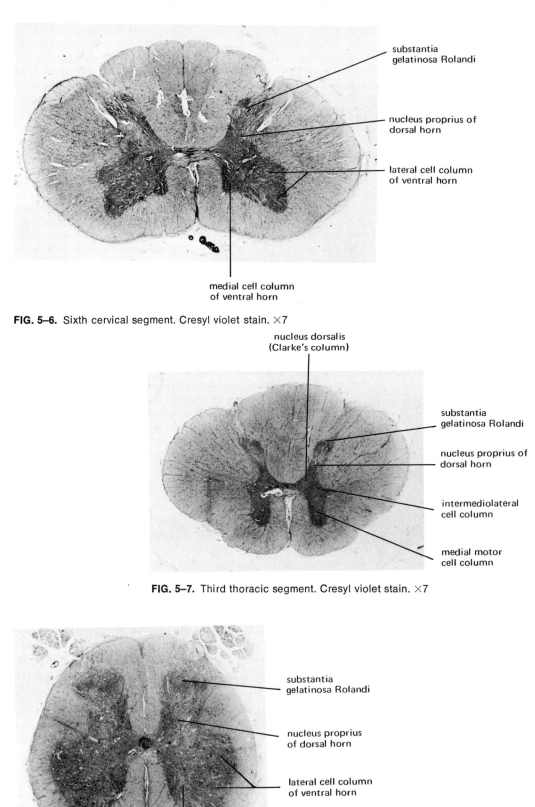

substantia
gelatinosa Rolandi

nucleus proprius of
dorsal horn

lateral cell column
of ventral horn

medial cell column
of ventral horn

FIG. 5–6. Sixth cervical segment. Cresyl violet stain. ×7

nucleus dorsalis
(Clarke's column)

substantia
gelatinosa Rolandi

nucleus proprius of
dorsal horn

intermediolateral
cell column

medial motor
cell column

FIG. 5–7. Third thoracic segment. Cresyl violet stain. ×7

substantia
gelatinosa Rolandi

nucleus proprius
of dorsal horn

lateral cell column
of ventral horn

FIG. 5–8. Third sacral segment. Cresyl violet stain. ×7

medial cell column
of ventral horn

means of this input transmission with respect to pain and temperature is thought to be modified by other modalities of general sensation. Further, fibers coming from the cerebral cortex enter the substantia gelatinosa from the lateral white column and this input may modify synaptic transmission by inhibition or excitation of intrinsic neuronal elements. The nucleus appears to have a complex function, therefore, which includes the modification or "editing" of pain and temperature data by concurrent stimulation of various types of general sensory receptors and by events occurring at any given moment in the cerebral cortex. This is a difficult area of research which is currently under investigation.

Nucleus Dorsalis

The nucleus dorsalis (Clarke's column) is a slender, yet well defined, column of cells in the ventromedial part of the dorsal horn. The nucleus extends from C8 through L2 or L3 segments and is largest in the twelfth thoracic and first lumbar segments. The cells are unusual in having an eccentric nucleus and diffuse Nissl material, giving the erroneous appearance of cells undergoing axon reaction. Impulses impinging on cells of Clarke's column originate in proprioceptive endings, including neuromuscular spindles, Golgi tendon spindles, and pacinian corpuscles, with a lesser contribution from touch and pressure receptors. The afferents to the nucleus are mainly collaterals of ascending and descending branches of dorsal column axons that entered the cord in the dorsal roots of spinal nerves. Fibers carrying data from the lower extremity reach the nucleus through ascending branches; this may account for the larger size of the caudal part of Clarke's column. The nucleus dorsalis receives no input from the upper four cervical spinal nerves, but descending branches of dorsal root fibers entering segments C5 through

C7 carry data to the upper part of Clarke's column. Axons from the nucleus dorsalis enter the lateral white column of the same side, where they form the dorsal spinocerebellar tract. This is therefore an important nucleus through which proprioceptive data, and to a lesser extent information derived from touch and pressure receptors, are sent on to the cerebellum.

Nucleus Proprius

All of the dorsal horn of gray matter, exclusive of the substantia gelatinosa and nucleus dorsalis, constitutes the nucleus proprius, also called the chief nucleus of the dorsal horn. This nucleus includes many internuncial neurons, together with tract cells whose axons contribute to ascending fasciculi in the white matter. Fibers enter the nucleus proprius from the dorsal white column, these being branches of dorsal root fibers for sensory modalities other than pain and temperature. Connections are thereby established for spinal reflexes and for transmission of sensory data to the brain. Many fibers of the lateral corticospinal tract, a large motor tract of the cord originating in the cerebral cortex, terminate on small neurons of the nucleus proprius. The latter cells in turn make synaptic contact with motor neurons of the ventral horn. The intermediate zone of gray matter between the dorsal and ventral horns is similar to the nucleus proprius with respect to constituent nerve cells and their connections.

Visceral Afferent Nucleus

Cells in the base of the dorsal horn make up a poorly defined visceral afferent nucleus, which receives impulses from visceral afferent fibers in the dorsal roots. The nucleus is present in the thoracic and upper lumbar segments, and in the second to fourth sacral segments, since visceral afferents are restricted to segments that give rise to autonomic efferent fibers. The visceral afferent nucleus projects to visceral efferent cells of the cord and to centers in the brain.

VENTRAL HORN

The efferent or motor part of the gray matter is included in the ventral horn, in which the large motor neurons are conspicuous. These are "lower motor neurons," in contrast to "upper motor neurons" whose cell bodies are in various gray areas of the brain. Dorsal root fibers and fibers of motor pathways from the brain excite or inhibit lower motor neurons, intercalated cells usually intervening, through synaptic end-bulbs numbering in the thousands for each motor cell. The motor neuron in the ventral horn therefore constitutes a "final common pathway" (Sherrington), through which impulses received from diverse sources are balanced one against the other, thus determining the constantly fluctuating activity of the muscle fibers included in a motor unit. The large cells of the ventral horn are cell bodies of alpha motor neurons for the main mass of muscle fibers. Inconspicuous but functionally important cells giving rise to gamma efferents for intrafusal fibers of neuromuscular spindles are scattered among the larger alpha cells.

Somatic Motor Cell Columns

Several columns of motor cells have been identified in the ventral horn, as summarized below (Figs. 5–6 through 5–8). Motor neurons, however, do not make up the whole of the ventral horn. There are also some tract cells, together with numerous small cells similar to those of the dorsal horn and intermediate gray matter. Many of these small cells are interposed between fibers of descending motor tracts and the motor neurons.

A *medial cell column* is present throughout the cord for innervation of the muscles of the neck and truck, i.e., muscles attached to the axial skeleton together with intercostal and abdominal muscles. A *lateral cell column* innervates the muscle of the limbs and is therefore present in the cervical and lumbosacral enlargements. The lateral column is further divided according to parts of the extremities innervated. The *ventrolateral nucleus* in segments C4 through C8 supplies muscles of the shoulder and upper arm, and in segments L2 to S2 this nucleus supplies muscles of the hip and thigh. The *dorsolateral nucleus*, which is present in segments C4 through T1 and L2 through S3, supplies the musculature of the forearm and hand and the leg and foot. There is a short *retrodorsolateral nucleus* in segments C8 and T1 and also in segments S1 through S3, for certain intrinsic muscles of the hand and foot. A *central group* of motor cells has been described in segments L2 through S2, but the distribution of axons from these cells is not known.

Special Golgi type II neurons, called *Renshaw cells*, have been identified by physiologic methods; they are located in the medial part of the ventral horn. These small nerve cells receive collateral branches from alpha motor cell axons; each Renshaw cell has a short axon which terminates on the particular motor cell from which the axon collateral arose or on a nearby alpha motor neuron. This would be an example of a feedback circuit, having an inhibitory effect on alpha motor neurons.

Phrenic and Spinal Accessory Nuclei

There are two additional motor nuclei in the cervical cord, one for the phrenic nerve and the other for the spinal root of the accessory nerve. The diaphragm develops from cervical myotomes and, although it migrates caudally during embryonic development, the origin of the diaphragm is reflected in its nerve supply. The phrenic nucleus is responsible for an enlargement of the medial group of ventral horn cells in segments C3 through C5, most prominently in C4. This nucleus receives afferents from higher motor centers, including the cerebral cortex, and from respiratory centers in the brain stem, for voluntary and automatic movements of the diaphragm, respectively.

The spinal accessory nucleus consists of motor cells in the lateral region of the ventral horn in the upper six cervical segments. The axons emerge as a series of rootlets along the lateral aspect of the cord, just behind the denticulate ligament. The rootlets converge to form the spinal root of the accessory nerve, which ascends along the side of the cord in the subarachnoid space and enters the posterior cranial fossa through the foramen magnum. The spinal root joins the cranial (medullary) root along the side of the medulla; the accessory nerve then leaves the posterior fossa through the jugular foramen, and the spinal component supplies the sterno-cleidomastoid and trapezius muscles.

LATERAL HORN

An *intermediolateral cell column* forms the small lateral horn of gray matter extending from segment T1 through L2 or L3. Consisting of motor-type cells smaller than the alpha cells of the ventral horn, the column gives rise to preganglionic sympathetic fibers. Stimuli are received from visceral afferents of the dorsal roots and from autonomic centers in the brain by way of fibers in the lateral white column. Similar cells in the base of the ventral horn in segments S2 through S4 constitute the *sacral autonomic nucleus,* from which arise the preganglionic fibers of the sacral portion of the parasympathetic system.

Certain data concerning the cell columns are summarized in Table 5–1.

LAMINAE OF REXED

Studies of the architecture of neurons (cytoarchitectonics) provide the basis for Rexed's laminar map of the spinal gray matter. This system of parceling the gray matter is useful in experimental work, providing a rather precise identification of areas in which there is terminal fiber degeneration following section of dorsal roots or descending fasciculi of the white matter. Briefly described, the 10 laminae are as follows (Fig. 5–9). The thin *lamina I,* consisting of medium-sized and large neurons, is superficial to the substantia gelatinosa. *Lamina II* corresponds with the substantia gelatinosa Rolandi. The chief nucleus of the dorsal horn is divided into *laminae III, IV, V,* and *VI. Lamina VII* includes most of the intermediate zone, together with the intervals between motor nuclei in the lateral part of the ventral horn. Similarly, *lamina VIII* consists of areas in the medial part of the ventral horn, in which motor neurons are few or absent. *Lamina IX* is made up of the motor nuclei of the ventral horn. Finally, *lamina X* consists mainly of neuroglial cells surrounding the central canal.

COURSE OF DORSAL ROOT FIBERS WITHIN THE CORD

Fibers of various calibers for the different modalities of general sensation are intermingled in the dorsal root. Just before reaching the spinal cord, however, unmyelinated and thinly myelinated fibers form a *lateral division* that enters the dorsolateral fasciculus or zone of Lissauer, while more heavily myelinated fibers form a *medial division* that continues into the dorsal white column. Fibers of the lateral division are concerned with conduction for pain and temperature, while those of the medial

TABLE 5–1. SUMMARY OF THE CHARACTERISTICS OF THE CELL COLUMNS

Cell column	Extent in cord	Function
Substantia gelatinosa Rolandi	Entire cord	Relay nucleus for pain and temperature, with modification of transmission of sensory input
Nucleus dorsalis (Clarke's column)	C8 through L2 or L3	Origin of dorsal spinocerebellar tract
Nucleus proprius of dorsal horn	Entire cord	Contains internuncial neurons, together with tract cells for ascending fasciculi of lateral and ventral white columns
Visceral afferent nucleus	T1 through L2 or L3; S2 through S4	Relay nucelus for visceral afferent impulses
Medial motor cell column	Entire cord	Supplies muscles of neck and trunk
Lateral motor cell column	C4 through T1; L2 through S3	Supplies muscles of extremities
Phrenic nucleus	C3 through C5	Motor innervation of diaphragm
Spinal accessory nucleus	C1 through C6	Origin of spinal root of accessory nerve
Intermediolateral cell column	T1 through L2 or L3	Source of preganglionic sympathetic fibers
Sacral parasympathetic nucleus	S2 through S4	Source of preganglionic parasympathetic fibers for pelvic viscera

division transmit impulses for touch (simple and discriminative), pressure, proprioception, and vibration.

ZONE OF LISSAUER

On entering *Lissauer's zone* (Fig. 5–10), dorsal root fibers divide into short ascending and descending branches. Each branch gives off numerous collaterals, and the entire fiber terminates in the substantia gelatinosa within the segment of entry or in the next rostral or caudal segment. Transmission within the substantia gelatinosa, as described above, provides connections for spinal reflex responses and transmission of pain and temperature data to the thalamus. The cell bodies of the tract cells concerned are located in the nucleus proprius and intermediate gray matter, their dendrites extending into the substantia gelatinosa. The axons of these cells cross to the opposite side of the cord, where they form the lateral spinothalamic tract. This tract traverses the brain stem and terminates in the general sensory nucleus of the thalamus. It is important to note that impulses for pain and temperature, in their passage from peripheral endings to the thalamus, cross to the opposite side, principally in the segment of entry into the spinal cord.

DORSAL COLUMN

The *dorsal white column* is constituted as follows. Fibers of the medial division of a dorsal root bifurcate on entering the cord just medial to Lissauer's zone. The ascending and descending branches run longitudinally on the lateral side of similar fibers that entered the cord in the segment just below. However, some of the descending fibers, which may be several segments in length, accumulate in the *fasciculus septomarginalis* in the lower half of the cord, and in the *fasciculus interfascicularis* in the upper half of the cord (Fig. 5–10). The descending fibers, which give off many collateral branches, synapse with tract cells, internuncial neurons, and motor cells.

Many of the ascending fibers of the dorsal column also end in the spinal gray matter, both as terminal fibers and as collateral branches. Some of these fibers, which vary in length from a few to many segments, are concerned with conduction for simple touch and pressure. Synaptic contacts are effected with internuncial neurons for spinal reflexes and with tract cells. Axons of the latter cells cross to the opposite side of the cord, where they form the ventral spinothalamic tract. The central pathway for simple touch and pressure is therefore ipsilateral for a considerable distance, as well as contralateral through the crossed ventral spinothalamic tract. Tract cells receiving afferents for simple touch and pressure contribute to additional as-

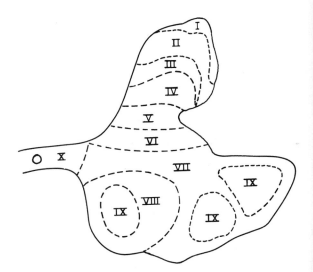

FIG. 5–9. Laminae of Rexed in the cervical enlargement.

cending fasciculi, as will be noted presently.

Other ascending branches of dorsal root fibers, specifically those transmitting impulses from the various proprioceptive endings, also give off branches to the gray matter as they traverse variable numbers of segments. These nerve fibers make synaptic contact with motor neurons, internuncial neurons, and tract cells, mainly for spinal reflexes and transmission of proprioceptive data to the cerebellum.

Finally, many dorsal root fibers in the dorsal white column continue upward into the medulla, where they terminate in two medullary nuclei—the nuclei gracilis and cuneatus. From the lower part of the cord, these fibers continue upward as the fasciculus gracilis, while fibers that enter the cord above the midthoracic level ascend in the fasciculus cuneatus. These long fibers reaching the medulla transmit impulses from proprioceptors, tactile endings, and endings that respond to vibration. Fibers from the nuclei gracilis and cuneatus cross the midline in the medulla and continue

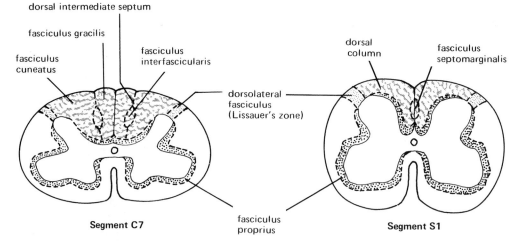

FIG. 5–10. Dorsal column, zone of Lissauer, and fasciculus proprius.

rostrally as the medial lemniscus, which terminates in the general sensory nucleus of the thalamus. The ascending pathway thus identified, which is completed by thalamocortical projections, is the main conduction pathway for detailed awareness of position and movement, discriminative touch, and vibration. The results of animal experiments and the study of effects of lesions restricted to the dorsal column in man suggest that these sensory modalities may also be transmitted to the thalamus and cortex, to some extent, through other ascending pathways.

There is a regular lamination of the dorsal white column according to segments in which the long ascending branches originate. At the level of the first cervical segment, for example, fibers that entered the cord in the lowest sacral segment are most medial; fibers from higher segments are progressively added in layers, and the newest upper cervical fibers are most lateral. Segments concerned with innervation of the limbs are well represented, while those for the trunk occupy a relatively small area adjacent to the dorsal intermediate septum. The size of the dorsal white

column increased with respect to other parts of the spinal cord in the course of vertebrate evolution, and the dorsal column is maximally represented in man.

FASCICULUS PROPRIUS

The *fasciculus proprius* (*fasciculus spinospinalis*) surrounds the gray matter, being rather thinner in the dorsal columns than elsewhere (Fig. 5–10). This zone of white matter consists of ascending and descending association fibers connecting different segments. The connections thus established are important in intersegmental spinal reflexes. The fasciculus proprius also forms a two-directional, polysynaptic pathway between the spinal cord and brain stem, providing a communication between the two that is additional to the uninterrupted tracts in the remainder of the white matter.

EXAMPLES OF SPINAL REFLEXES

Certain neuronal connections in the spinal cord form the basis of important spinal reflexes. The stretch reflex, gamma reflex loop, and flexor reflex will serve as examples.

The *stretch reflex* is based on a two-neuron or monosynaptic reflex arc (Fig. 5–11). Slight stretching of a muscle stimulates the sensory endings in neuromuscular spindles, and the resultant excitation reaches the cord by way of primary sensory neurons having large group A processes. Axons of these cells in the dorsal white column give off collateral branches that excite alpha motor neurons, causing the stretched muscle to contract. This is an important postural reflex. The afferent impulses originate as an asynchronous discharge from the neuromuscular spindles, which are delicate monitors of changes in the length of the muscle. The reflex alters tension in the muscle in such a way as to maintain a constant length. The stretch reflex forms the basis of the knee-jerk test and other tendon reflex tests that are used in a neurologic examination. A sharp tap on the patellar tendon causes synchronous discharges from the spindles in the quadriceps femoris muscle, with prompt reflex contraction of the muscle and extension of the leg at the knee.

The reflex arc just described forms part of the *gamma reflex loop,* through which muscle tension comes under the control of descending motor pathways (Fig. 5–12). Fibers of these pathways (e.g., reticulospinal, vestibulospinal, and others) excite gamma motor neurons, causing contraction of intrafusal muscle fibers and an increase in the rate of firing from sensory endings in the neuromuscular spindles. The impulses are conveyed to alpha motor neurons supplying the main muscle mass through the monosynaptic reflex arc described above for the stretch reflex.

The *flexor reflex,* which is protective as in withdrawal of the hand in response to a painful stimulus, is based on a series of at least three neurons and is therefore polysynaptic (Fig. 5–13). The cutaneous receptors are mainly unencapsulated endings in the epidermis, and the afferent fibers synapse in the substantia gelatinosa with dendrites of internuncial neurons. The latter neurons end on alpha motor cells in several segments because a withdrawal response requires the action of groups of muscles.

The tension on a muscle is monitored by Golgi tendon spindles as well as neuromuscular spindles. When the tension reaches a certain level, there is a distinct increase in the discharge from the tendon spindles. The resulting nerve impulses reach internuncial cells in the spinal gray matter, the latter cells inhibit alpha motor neurons, and relaxation of the muscle follows. This reflex therefore tends to prevent excessive tension on the muscle.

ASCENDING TRACTS OF THE LATERAL AND VENTRAL WHITE COLUMNS

The locations in a transverse section of most of the pathways conducting sensory information to the brain are shown in Figure 5–14. Since there is considerable intermingling of the fibers of adjacent tracts, both Figure 5–14 and Figure 5–15 indicate the sites in which fibers of a particular tract are most numerous. The cervical region of the cord is illustrated because not all tracts are present at lower levels.

The dorsal spinocerebellar tract originates in the distinctive nucleus dorsalis. Tract cells for the remaining ascending fasciculi are located primarily in the chief nucleus of the dorsal horn and the intermediate gray matter, with a few in the ventral gray horn.

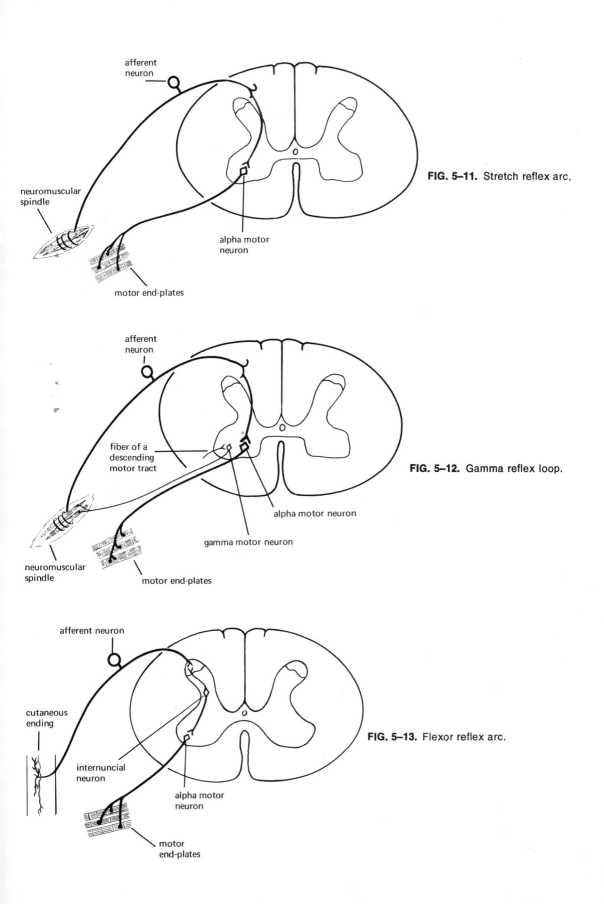

afferent
neuron

neuromuscular
spindle

alpha motor
neuron

motor end-plates

FIG. 5–11. Stretch reflex arc.

afferent
neuron

fiber of a
descending
motor tract

alpha motor neuron

gamma motor neuron

neuromuscular
spindle

motor end-plates

FIG. 5–12. Gamma reflex loop.

afferent neuron

cutaneous
ending

internuncial
neuron

alpha motor
neuron

motor
end-plates

FIG. 5–13. Flexor reflex arc.

SPINOTHALAMIC TRACTS

The *lateral spinothalamic tract* for pain and temperature is especially important clinically. The cells of origin receive afferents from the zone of Lissauer, small neurons of the substantia gelatinosa often intervening between the primary sensory neurons and the tract cells or second order sensory neurons. As noted above, the dorsal root fibers for pain and temperature in Lissauer's zone do not extend longitudinally for more than a segment beyond the segment of entry. Axons of the tract cells cross the midline in the ventral gray and white commissures, with a slight rostral inclination. The fibers then pass through the contralateral gray matter to reach the lateral spinothalamic tract. This fasciculus is present at all levels of the cord, fibers being added to the ventromedial aspect of the tract as they accumulate in a caudorostral direction. There is therefore a somatotopic arrangement of the constituent fibers. In the upper cervical region, for example, sacral segments are represented in the dorsolateral part of the tract, followed by fibers from lumbar and then thoracic segments, and fibers of cervical origin are in a ventromedial position. There is some indication that fibers for temperature are more dorsal than those for pain.

The lateral spinothalamic tract traverses the brain stem and ends in the general sensory nucleus of the thalamus. There is crude awareness of pain and temperature sensations, together with emotional responses, at the thalamic level. The somesthetic cortical area, to which the thalamic nucleus projects, adds discriminative qualities of localization and quantitative assessment. The lateral spinothalamic tract is the main central pathway for pain and temperature sensibilities. However, the study of patients following section of the tract (chordotomy) for relief of intractable pain suggests that there are additional routes for pain conduction to the thalamus; these may be provided by spinoreticular fibers, ascending visceral fibers, or the spinocervical tract (see below).

The *ventral spinothalamic tract* is a crossed pathway for simple touch and pressure, present at all levels of the cord. Some of the dorsal root fibers conveying data for these senses continue rostrally for considerable distances in the ipsilateral dorsal white column before synapsing with tract cells. The central pathway is therefore essentially bilateral; a unilateral cord lesion results in only slight and often undetectable impairment of simple touch and pressure sensations. The ventral spinothalamic tract terminates in the thalamic nucleus for general sensation, which in turn projects to the somesthetic cortex where the information thus conveyed enters into conscious experience.

Figures 5–14 and 5–15 show the lateral and ventral spinothalamic tracts separated by the spinotectal tract and the spino-oli-

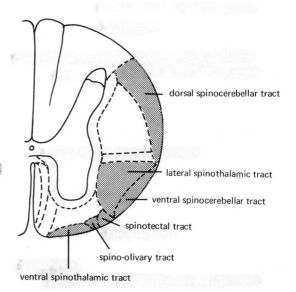

dorsal spinocerebellar tract

lateral spinothalamic tract

ventral spinocerebellar tract

spinotectal tract

spino-olivary tract

ventral spinothalamic tract

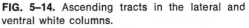

FIG. 5–14. Ascending tracts in the lateral and ventral white columns.

vary and olivospinal tracts. The latter tracts are small and for the most part limited to the cervical region. There is also considerable overlapping of fibers of adjoining tracts, as already mentioned. For these reasons, the lateral and ventral spinothalamic tracts form virtually a single system for conduction of exteroceptive data from the periphery to the brain.

The major pathways in the spinal cord, through which information collected from general sensory endings is transmitted to the thalamus and cerebral cortex, have now been noted. To recapitulate, the pathways are 1) the ipsilateral dorsal column for proprioception, discriminative touch, and vibratory sense; 2) the crossed lateral spinothalamic tract for pain and temperature; and 3) the dorsal column of the same side and the ventral spinothalamic tract of the opposite side for simple touch and pressure.

PATHWAYS TO THE CEREBELLUM

The *dorsal spinocerebellar tract* has its origin in the nucleus dorsalis (Clarke's column) of the same side and therefore begins in the upper lumbar segments. Afferents to the nucleus dorsalis come from the dorsal column of white matter, as described above, the impulses originating mainly in the various proprioceptive endings, with an additional contribution from touch and pressure receptors. The tract enters the inferior cerebellar peduncle from the medulla oblongata and the fibers terminate in the cerebellar cortex.

The *ventral spinocerebellar tract* first appears in the lower lumbar region of the cord. This is a crossed tract, a large proportion of the fibers originating in the lumbosacral enlargement, where the cells of origin are located in the ventral horn. The ventral spinocerebellar tract traverses most of the brain stem and enters the cerebellum through the superior cerebellar peduncle in

the region of the midbrain. The two spinocerebellar pathways differ in the location of their cells of origin, one is uncrossed and the other is crossed in the spinal cord, and they reach the cerebellum through different peduncles. However, they convey similar sensory data, which are predominantly proprioceptive, to the cerebellum. The part of the cerebellum receiving afferents from the spinal cord influences muscle tonus and maintains synergy among cooperating muscles, as appropriate in postural changes, locomotion, and other forms of movement.

The fibers of the small *spino-olivary tract,* whose caudal extent is uncertain, arise from the contralateral gray matter and mingle with olivospinal fibers. The inferior olivary complex of the medulla, in which the fibers terminate, consists of a prominent inferior olivary nucleus and small accessory olivary nuclei. The complex sends large numbers of fibers to the cerebellum through the opposite inferior cerebellar peduncle. The spino–olivary tract may therefore be related indirectly to cerebellar function.

OTHER ASCENDING FIBERS

A *spinocervical tract* has been demonstrated in the cat; it is said to be present, although small, in man. The constituent fibers originate from cells in the nucleus proprius of the dorsal gray horn at all levels of the cord. They are uncrossed fibers, situated in the most dorsal part of the lateral white column. The tract terminates in the lateral cervical nucleus which consists of a column of cells in the dorsal horn of the upper two cervical segments of the cord and extending for a short distance into the medulla. The axons of these cells cross the midline to the ventral white column and traverse the brain stem to reach the general sensory nucleus of the thalamus. The sensory modalities conveyed by this pathway appear to include touch, pressure, pain and temperature.

The *spinotectal tract* transmits general sensory data, originating principally in cutaneous receptors, to the roof (tectum) of the midbrain. This is a crossed tract, which has been identified most distinctly in the cervical region. The fibers end in a region of the tectum known as the superior colliculus, which also receives afferents from the visual and auditory systems. The superior colliculus serves as a midbrain center for reflex motor responses to various kinds of sensory stimuli.

Spinoreticular fibers are not well localized in the white matter and are therefore not shown in Figure 5–14. The reticular formation, which is discussed in Chapter 9, is a diffuse system of neurons in the brain stem, extending into the diencephalon. It has afferent and efferent connections with many parts of the central nervous system. Among other significant functions, the reticular formation constitutes an "activating system," which has an important influence on one's alertness and on levels of consciousness through projections to the diencephalon and cerebral cortex. The spinoreticular fibers convey data from general sensory receptors, both somatic and visceral, to the reticular formation. The pathway, which is for the most part uncrossed, consists of fibers scattered among the various tracts of the lateral and ventral white columns, together with spinospinalis relays.

An *ascending visceral system* of fibers is also poorly localized and is not entirely distinct from the spinoreticular system. The fibers, which are both crossed and uncrossed, originate in the visceral afferent nucleus and other parts of the dorsal horn. They run mainly in the deeper part of the lateral white column, and the system consists in part of chains of neurons (spinospinalis relays). This indefinite pathway transmits sensory data of visceral origin to

the reticular formation of the brain stem and to the diencephalon. Conduction for visceral pain appears to be a significant role of the ascending visceral fibers.

DESCENDING TRACTS OF THE LATERAL AND VENTRAL WHITE COLUMNS

The descending or motor tracts originate in the cerebral cortex and in various centers in the brain stem. The position of most of the tracts in the cervical region of the spinal cord is shown in Figure 5–15.

CORTICOSPINAL TRACTS

The *corticospinal tract* runs through a region of the ventral medulla known as the pyramid, hence the alternative name of *pyramidal tract.* The term *pyramidal system* includes, in addition to the corticospinal tract, the corticobulbar tract, which bears the same relationship to motor nuclei of cranial nerves as does the corticospinal tract to ventral horn motor cells.

Parent cell bodies of about 40 percent of corticospinal fibers are located in the primary motor cortex of the frontal lobe, and the remainder are in other cortical areas of the frontal and parietal lobes. At the lower end of the medulla, about 85 percent of the fibers cross into the opposite side of the cord through the pyramidal decussation. These crossed fibers constitute the *lateral corticospinal tract,* which extends throughout the cord. A few of the fibers synapse directly with alpha motor neurons, but the great majority (about 95 percent) terminate on internuncial neurons, which in turn synapse with alpha cells. The proportions of lateral corticospinal fibers terminating in the major regions of the cord are: cervical, 55 percent; thoracic, 20 percent; lumbosacral, 25 percent. The large proportion of fibers ending in the cervical cord probably reflects the role of the corticospinal tract with respect to nonstereotyped movements of the upper extremity, especially independent movements of the digits.

A few of the fibers not included in the decussation of the pyramids continue into the lateral corticospinal tract of the same side. However, most of the uncrossed fibers constitute the *ventral corticospinal tract,* whose fibers terminate in either ventral horn (mostly contralateral) of cervical and upper thoracic segments. Myelination of the corticospinal tracts begins in late fetal life and is not fully completed until the latter half of the second year of childhood.

TRACTS ORIGINATING IN THE BRAIN STEM

Motor tracts originating in brain stem nuclei convey impulses that impinge on gamma motor neurons as well as on alpha motor neurons, either directly or through

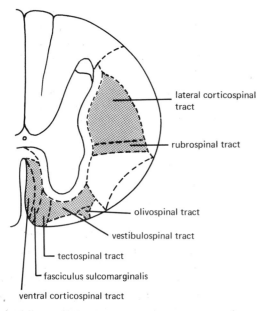

lateral corticospinal tract

rubrospinal tract

olivospinal tract

vestibulospinal tract

tectospinal tract

fasciculus sulcomarginalis

ventral corticospinal tract

FIG. 5–15. Descending tracts in the lateral and ventral white columns.

internuncial cells. Stimulation of alpha motor neurons through the gamma reflex loop is therefore an important aspect of the control of movements through extrapyramidal motor pathways. The relative contributions of the pyramidal and extrapyramidal systems to motor functions are discussed in Chapter 23.

Cell bodies for the *rubrospinal tract* are in the contralateral red nucleus of the midbrain; the fibers terminate in the cervical cord and the upper portion of the thoracic region. Among other functions, the red nucleus is included in a pathway through which the cerebellum and corpus striatum influence spinal motor neurons. The *tectospinal tract* is also a crossed fasciculus, originating in the contralateral superior colliculus of the midbrain tectum. This tract, which is limited to the cervical cord, is part of a reflex pathway for turning the head and perhaps moving the arms in response to visual, auditory, and cutaneous stimuli.

Three descending tracts originate in the medulla oblongata. The parent cell bodies of two of them are situated in the vestibular nuclear complex, which receives afferents from the vestibular portion of the inner ear and the cerebellum. The complex, one on either side, consists of four nuclei: the lateral, superior, medial, and inferior vestibular nuclei (Chapter 22). The cells of origin of the large *vestibulospinal tract* are in the lateral vestibular (Deiters') nucleus of the same side. The tract extends the length of the cord, most of the fibers ending in the ventral gray horn of the cervical and lumbosacral enlargements. The tonus of muscles is altered according to the position of the head and in response to head movements; the vestibulospinal tract is therefore important in the maintenance of equilibrium.

The *sulcomarginal fasciculus* (of Marie) includes fibers whose cell bodies are located mainly in the medial vestibular nuclei of both sides. The foregoing fibers make up the descending portion of a bundle in the brain stem known as the medial longitudinal fasciculus, of which the ascending component goes to cranial nerve nuclei that innervate the extraocular muscles. The descending fibers terminate in the ventral gray horn throughout the cervical cord, providing for changes in the tonus of neck muscles as required to support the head in various positions. The sulcomarginal fasciculus includes additional fibers with parent cell bodies in the reticular formation of the brain stem and in certain small nuclei of uncertain function in the midbrain.

A small *olivospinal tract* has been described as originating in the inferior olivary complex. The tract is said to be mainly crossed and limited to the cervical cord, where the constituent fibers intermingle with those of the spino-olivary tract. However, there is some doubt as to the existence of an olivospinal projection.

There remain two systems of descending fibers that are not sufficiently well localized to be shown in Figure 5–15. *Reticulospinal fibers* originate in the reticular formation of the brain stem and descend in the ventral and lateral white columns. Conduction is partly by means of long fibers and partly through polysynaptic relays in the fasciculus proprius. Among other functions, reticulospinal connections constitute an important system through which motor parts of the brain, notably the corpus striatum and cerebellum, are able to influence motor cells of the ventral horn. *Descending autonomic fibers* are not clearly marked off from reticulospinal fibers of the lateral white column. Most of the autonomic fibers originate in the reticular formation. They constitute a pathway through which the hypothalamus and visceral centers in the brain stem are brought into communication with the intermediolateral cell column

(sympathetic) and the parasympathetic nucleus in the sacral cord.

SOME ANATOMIC AND CLINICAL CORRELATIONS

Lesions of the spinal cord result from trauma, degenerative and demyelinating disorders, tumors, infections, and impairment of blood supply. Testing for impairment or loss of cutaneous sensation is an important part of the neurologic examination, being particularly useful in detecting the site of a lesion involving the spinal cord or nerve roots. The distribution of cutaneous areas (dermatomes) supplied by the spinal nerves is shown for reference in Figure 5–16. Cutaneous areas supplied by adjacent spinal nerves overlap. For example, the upper half of the area supplied by T6 is also supplied by T5, and the lower half by T7. There is therefore little sensory loss, if any, following interruption of a single spinal root.

Reflex contraction of muscles is also utilized in testing for the integrity of segments of the cord and the spinal nerves. The segments involved in the more commonly tested stretch or tendon reflexes are as follows: biceps reflex, C5 and C6; triceps reflex, C6 through C8; quadriceps reflex, L2 through L4; gastrocnemius reflex, S1 and S2.

Before specific pathologic conditions are mentioned, it should be pointed out that a distinction is made between the effects of a lesion involving lower motor neurons as opposed to upper motor neurons. Destruction or atrophy of lower motor neurons (in the present context those of the ventral horn) results in 1) flaccid paralysis of the affected muscles, 2) diminished or absent tendon reflexes, and 3) progressive atrophy of the muscles deprived of motor fibers. The term "upper motor neuron

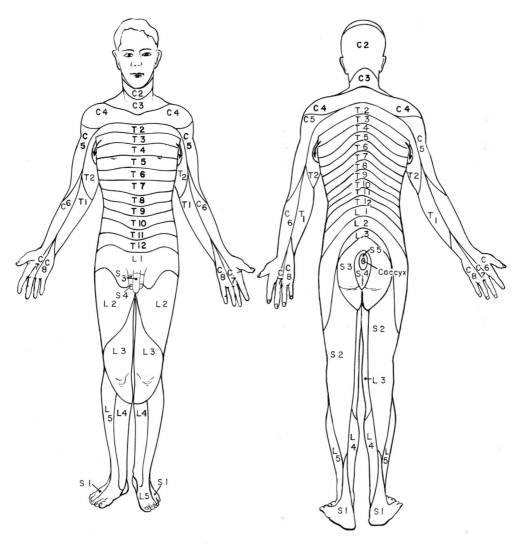

FIG. 5–16. Cutaneous distribution of spinal nerves (dermatomes).

lesion," although regularly used clinically, leaves much to be desired. The lesion may be in the cerebral cortex or another part of the cerebral hemisphere, in the brain stem, or in the spinal cord. Both pyramidal and extrapyramidal motor pathways are almost certain to be involved. In any event, the following signs are associated with an "upper motor neuron lesion" after the acute effects have worn off: 1) varying degrees of voluntary paralysis, which is most severe in the upper extremity; 2) the sign of Babinski (up-turning of the great toe and spreading of the toes on stroking the sole); and 3) spasticity with exaggerated tendon reflexes. The voluntary paralysis is now considered to be a result of both pyramidal and extrapyramidal dysfunction, the former being reflected especially in impairment of the more delicate, nonstereotyped movements such as independent use of the fingers. The Babinski sign is attributed to interruption of the pyramidal or cortico-spinal tract. (A sign of Babinski is normal in infants prior to myelination of the corti-cospinal tracts.) The muscle spasticity and hyperactive deep reflexes are thought to be caused by interruption of constituent fibers of extrapyramidal pathways. Such fibers project from the cerebral cortex to the corpus striatum and motor nuclei of the brain stem, while the latter nuclei influence ventral horn cells through such descending pathways as reticulospinal connections and the rubrospinal tract.

The following elementary notes on selected lesions will show the necessity of understanding the intrinsic anatomy of the spinal cord in order to interpret signs and symptoms.

The cord may be damaged by spinal fracture or dislocation, by penetrating wounds caused by projectile metal frag-ments, or by other traumatic events. Com-plete *transection* results in loss of all sensi-bility and voluntary movement below the lesion. The patient is quadriplegic (both arms and both legs paralyzed) if the upper cervical cord is transected, and paraplegic (both legs paralyzed) if the transection is between the cervical and lumbosacral en-largements. There is an initial period of spinal shock, lasting from a few days to several weeks, during which all somatic and visceral reflex activity is abolished. On return of reflex activity, there is spasticity of muscles and exaggerated tendon re-flexes. Bladder and bowel functions are no longer under voluntary control.

The events following partial section of the cord depend on the size and location of the lesion. *Hemisection*, although unusual, is an instructive lesion anatomically. The neurologic signs caudal to the hemisected region of the cord constitute the Brown–Séquard syndrome. Position sense and the feeling of vibration are lost *on the side of the lesion* because of interruption of the dorsal funiculus. There is anesthesia for pain and temperature *on the opposite side* because of interruption of the lateral spino-thalamic tract. Touch sensation is un-affected because of bilateral conduction through the dorsal column (uncrossed) and the ventral spinothalamic tract (crossed). The patient is hemiplegic if the lesion is in the upper cervical cord, while hemisection of the thoracic cord results in paralysis of the leg (monoplegia). The paralysis is *ipsilateral* to the lesion and is of the "upper motor neuron" type, as de-scribed above. A patient with hemisection of the cervical cord has a sympathetic dis-turbance, known as Horner's syndrome, on the side of the lesion. This syndrome is a sequel to interruption of descending auto-nomic fibers in the lateral white column, with withdrawal of stimuli to cells of the intermediolateral cell column. Horner's syndrome consists of 1) pupillary constric-tion due to paralysis of the dilator pupillae muscle; 2) slight lowering of the upper lid (ptosis) because of paralysis of the smooth muscle component (tarsal muscle) of the levator palpebrae superioris muscle; 3) slight enophthalmos resulting from paraly-sis of Müller's orbital muscle; and 4) in some cases, vasodilation and absence of sweating on the face and neck.

The following degenerative diseases also illustrate the anatomic basis of neurologic signs. In *subacute combined degeneration* there is bilateral demyelination and loss of nerve fibers in the dorsal column and the dorsal part of the lateral column. The prin-cipal etiologic factor is vitamin B_{12} defi-ciency, and the disorder is usually encoun-tered in association with pernicious anemia. The dorsal column lesion results in loss of the senses of position, discriminative touch, and vibration. The gait is ataxic (without coordination) because the patient is unaware of the position of the legs. However, the ataxia tends to be obscured by paraplegic signs caused by degeneration of the lateral corticospinal tracts and extrapyramidal pathways.

Friedreich's ataxia is a familial disease, usually beginning in childhood, in which the initial degenerative change affects Clarke's column and the dorsal spinocerebellar tract bilaterally. The dorsal white columns are involved to some extent, and the degenerative process spreads to the cerebellum and other parts of the brain. The characteristic sign of the disease is ataxia; disturbances of speech and other cerebellar signs are added, and there may be dementia late in the disease.

Amyotrophic lateral sclerosis is a bilateral degenerative disease of unknown origin. The degenerative process is restricted to the motor system, affecting the corticobulbar and corticospinal tracts along with motor nuclei of cranial nerves and ventral horn motor cells. The signs are therefore a combination of upper and lower motor neuron lesion effects.

Syringomyelia is a different disorder from those mentioned above, in that neuronal degeneration is not the primary pathology. The condition is characterized by central cavitation of the cord, usually beginning in the cervical region, with a glial reaction (gliosis) adjacent to the cavity. Decussating fibers for pain and temperature in the ventral gray and white commissures are interrupted early in the disease. The cavitation and gliosis spread into the gray matter and white matter, and also longitudinally, leading to variable signs and symptoms depending on the regions involved. The classic clinical picture is that of "yoke-like" anesthesia for pain and temperature over the shoulders and upper extremities, accompanied by lower motor neuron weakness and wasting of the muscles of the upper extremities. Spread of the cavitation and glial reaction into the lateral white columns may result in voluntary paresis of the "upper motor neuron" type, affecting especially the lower extremities. The etiology of syringomyelia is not known, although there are hypotheses based on neuropathologic studies. It has been suggested, for example, that the pulsatile circulation through the choroid plexuses produces pressure waves in the cerebrospinal fluid, that these are carried into the central canal from the fourth ventricle, and that in rare instances the eventual result is cyst formation and surrounding gliosis in the region of the central canal. Another suggestion is that when the cerebrospinal fluid pressure in the spinal canal is increased for any reason, the pressure is transmitted into the central canal of the cord through perivascular extensions of the spinal subarachnoid space.

SUGGESTIONS FOR ADDITIONAL READING

Austin G: The Spinal Cord: Basic Aspects and Surgical Considerations. Springfield, Ill., Thomas, 1961

Ball MJ, Dayan AD: Pathogenesis of syringomelia. Lancet 2:799–801, 1972

Barson AJ: The vertebral level of termination of the spinal cord during normal and abnormal development. J Anat 106:489–497, 1970

Calne DB, Pallis CA: Vibratory sense: A critical review. Brain 89:723–746, 1966

Eccles JC: Functional organization of the spinal cord. Anesthesiology 28:31–45, 1962

Gardner JW: Hydrodynamic mechanism of syringomyelia: Its relation to myelocele. J Neurol Neurosurg Psychiatry 28:247–259, 1965

Grant FC, Wood FA: Experiences with cordotomy. Clin Neurosurg 5:38–65, 1958

Ha H, Liu CN: Cell origin of the ventral spinocerebellar tract. J Comp Neurol 133:185–205, 1968

Heimer L., Wall PD: The dorsal root distribution to the substantia gelatinosa of the rat with a note on the distribution in the cat. Exp Brain Res 6: 89–99, 1968

Nathan PW, Smith MC: Fasciculi proprii of the spinal cord in man: Review of present knowledge. Brain 82:610–668, 1959

Oscarsson O: Functional organization of the spino- and cuneocerebellar tracts. Physiol Rev 45:495–522, 1965

Pearson AA: Role of gelatinous substance of spinal cord in conduction of pain. Arch Neurol Psychiatry 68:515–529, 1952.

Poirier LJ, Bertrand C: Experimental and anatomical investigation of the lateral spino-thalamic and spino-tectal tracts. J Comp Neurol 102:745–757, 1955

Renshaw B: Central effects of centripetal impulses in axons of spinal ventral roots. J Neurophysiol 9:191–204, 1946

Réthelyi M, Szentágothai J: The large synaptic complexes of the substantia gelatinosa. Exp Brain Res 7:258–274, 1969

Rexed BA: Cytoarchitectonic atlas of the spinal cord in the cat. J Comp Neurol 100:297–379, 1954

Scheibel ME, Scheibel AB: Spinal motoneurons, interneurons and Renshaw cells: A Golgi study. Arch Ital Biol 104:328–353, 1966

Smith MC: Observations on the topography of the lateral column of the human cervical spinal cord. Brain 80:263–272, 1957

Szentágothai J: Neuronal and synaptic arrangement in the substantia gelatinosa Rolandi. J Comp Neurol 122:219–239, 1964

Szentágothai J: Pathways and subcortical relay mechanisms of visceral afferents. Acta Neuroveg (Wien) 28:103–120, 1966

Teng P: Ligamentum denticulatum: An anatomical review and its role in various neurosurgical problems of the spinal cord. J Mount Sinai Hosp NY 32:567–577, 1965

Thomas RC, Wilson VJ: Precise localization of Renshaw cells with a new marking technique. Nature 206:211–213, 1965

Wall PD: The sensory and motor role of impulses travelling in the dorsal columns towards cerebral cortex. Brain 93:505–524, 1970

White JC: Conduction of pain in man: Observations on its afferent pathways within the spinal cord and visceral nerves. Arch Neurol Psychiatry 71:1–23, 1954

6

Brain Stem:
External Anatomy

The brain stem, as the term is used here, consists of the medulla, pons, and midbrain. Although each of the three regions has special features, they have certain fiber tracts in common and each region includes nuclei of cranial nerves. The fourth ventricle is partly in the medulla and partly in the pons. It is advantageous, therefore, to describe the medulla, pons, and midbrain together.

MEDULLA

The word medulla (marrow) referred in early usage to both the spinal cord and the caudal part of the brain stem, which were distinguished by calling them the medulla spinalis and the medulla oblongata. It is now customary to apply the term medulla specifically to the caudal part of the brain stem.

The *medulla* is about 3 cm long and widens gradually in a rostral direction. It rests on the basilar portion of the occipital bone (the clivus) and is concealed from above by the cerebellum. The junction of the spinal cord and medulla is at the upper rootlet of the first cervical nerve, which corresponds to the level of the foramen magnum. The spinal cord seems to pass imperceptibly into the medulla, in so far as surface markings are concerned, but there is in fact an abrupt and extensive rearrangement of the gray matter and white matter. The rostral limit of the medulla is clearly marked on the ventral surface by the border of the pons (Fig. 6–1). In dorsal view (Fig. 6–3), the medulla is seen to consist of a *closed portion* containing a continuation of the central canal of the cord, and an *open portion* in which part of the fourth ventricle is located. The ventricle results from a flexure of the neural tube with a dorsal concavity (the pontine flexure) and subsequent development of the large cerebellum with its thick peduncles. These events caused a divergence of the dorsal halves of the maturing neural tube, so that its lumen widened out to form the fourth ventricle bounded by the medulla, pons, and cerebellum. The junction of the medulla and pons dorsally may be taken as a line passing along the inferior edges of the middle cerebellar peduncles.

The longitudinal grooves previously described for the spinal cord continue on the medulla. The *ventral median fissure* is interrupted at the spinomedullary junction by small bundles of decussating fibers. These are corticospinal fibers crossing from the pyramid of the medulla to the opposite side of the cord where they constitute the lateral corticospinal tract. The *dorsal median sulcus* continues on the closed portion of the medulla, and the *ventrolateral* and *dorsolateral sulci* are in approximately the same position as they are in the spinal cord.

Three areas, all of which have important landmarks, are thus defined on either side. The ventral area is occupied by the *pyramid,* which consists of corticospinal fibers (Fig. 6–1). This is the origin of the term pyramidal tract as a synonym for corticospinal tract. The lateral area (Fig. 6–2) includes a prominent oval swelling, the *olive,* which marks the position of the inferior olivary nucleus. Rootlets of the accessory, vagus, and glossopharyngeal nerves are attached to the lateral area just dorsal to the olive. The *tuberculum cinereum* is that part of the lateral area intervening between the attachment of the above-mentioned nerves and the dorsolateral sulcus. The tuberculum cinereum marks the position of the spinal tract of the trigeminal nerve and the nucleus of the spinal tract, these being comparable to the zone of Lissauer and the substantia gelatinosa in the spinal cord. The dorsal spinocerebellar tract is superficial to the trigeminal spinal tract in the rostral part of the tuberculum cinereum, because the spinocerebellar fibers bend

dorsally at this point to enter the inferior cerebellar peduncle. The *fasciculi gracilis* and *cuneatus* continue from the spinal cord into the dorsal area of the medulla (Fig. 6–3). The *clava,* a slight elevation at the rostral end of the fasciculus gracilis, is produced by the nucleus gracilis, in which fibers of the fasciculus end. At a slightly more rostral level, the *cuneate tubercle* marks the position of the nucleus cuneatus or terminal nucleus of the fasciculus cuneatus. The apex of the V-shaped boundary of the inferior portion of the fourth ventricle is known as the *obex.*

Seven of the twelve cranial nerves are attached to the medulla or the junction of medulla and pons. Roots of the *hypoglossal nerve* emerge along the ventrolateral sulcus between the pyramid and the olive. The hypoglossal is a motor nerve, comparable in this respect to the ventral roots of spinal nerves. Roots of the *accessory nerve* (cranial division) and the *vagus* and *glossopharyngeal nerves* are attached to the medulla along a line between the olive and the tuberculum cinereum (the dorso-olivary sulcus). The accessory nerve is motor, while the vagus and glossopharyngeal nerves are mixed, with sensory and motor components. The four cranial nerves mentioned above have a relatively short course in the subarachnoid space. They leave the cranial cavity through foramina in the floor of the posterior fossa—the hypoglossal nerve through the hypoglossal foramen, and the accessory (spinal and cranial roots), vagus, and glossopharyngeal nerves through the jugular foramen.

The *vestibulocochlear* and *facial nerves* are attached to the brain stem at the caudal border of the pons well out laterally, the facial nerve being the more medial (Figs. 6–1 and 6–2). The facial nerve has two roots—motor and sensory. The sensory root lies between the larger motor root and the vestibulocochlear nerve; it is consequently

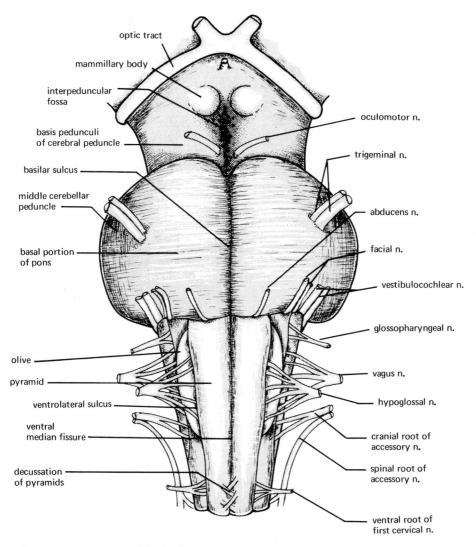

FIG. 6–1. Ventral aspect of the brain stem.

known as the *nervus intermedius* (of Wrisberg). The cochlear division of the vestibulocochlear nerve ends in the dorsal and ventral cochlear unclei, which are situated on the base of the inferior cerebellar peduncle (Fig. 6–3), while the vestibular division penetrates the brain stem deep to the root of the inferior peduncle. The vestibulocochlear and facial nerves enter the inter-

nal auditory meatus on the posterior surface of the petrous temporal bone.

Lastly, the *abducens nerve* emerges from the ventral surface, between the pyramid and the pons (Fig. 6–1). The nerve passes forward in the subarachnoid space beneath the pons, then traverses the cavernous venous sinus on the side of the sphenoid bone to reach the orbit.

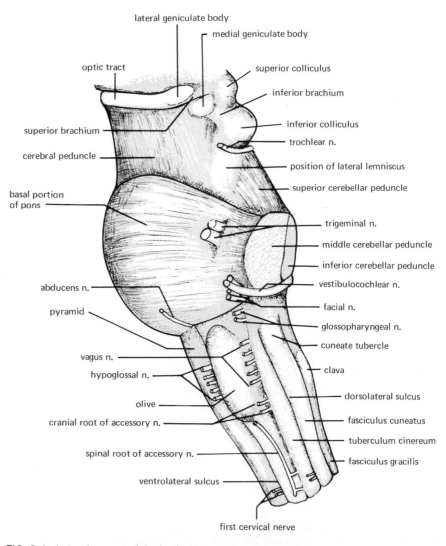

FIG. 6–2. Lateral aspect of the brain stem.

PONS

This part of the brain stem owes its name to the appearance presented on the ventral surface (Fig. 6–1), which is that of a bridge connecting the right and left cerebellar hemispheres. However, the appearance is deceptive as far as the constituent nerve fibers are concerned, as noted below.

The *pons* consists of two quite different parts, known as the basal and dorsal portions of the pons, as is seen clearly in sections (Figs. 7–8 and 7–9). The *basal portion* is distinctive of this part of the brain stem. Fibers from the cerebral cortex terminate ipsilaterally on nerve cells composing the pontine nuclei, and axons of the latter cells constitute the contralateral middle cerebellar peduncle. In effect, the basal pons is a large synaptic or relay sta-

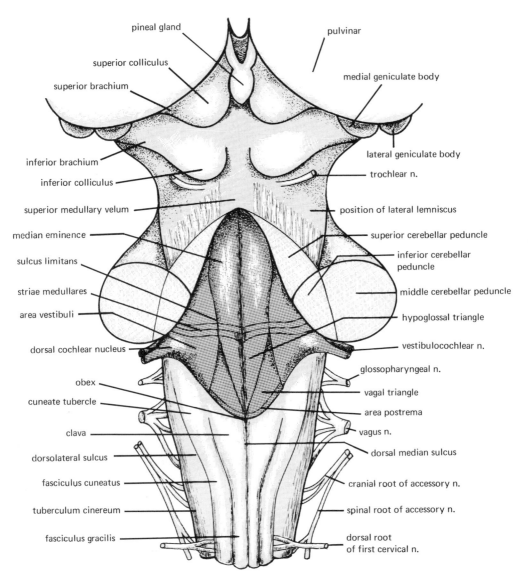

FIG. 6–3. Dorsal aspect of the brain stem.

tion, providing a connection between the cortex of a cerebral hemisphere and that of the opposite cerebellar hemisphere as part of a circuit contributing to maximal efficiency of voluntary movements. The cerebral cortex, basal pons, and cerebellum all increased in size during mammalian phylogeny and are best developed in the human brain. The corticospinal tracts traverse the basal portion of the pons before entering the pyramids.

The *dorsal portion* or *tegmentum* of the pons is similar to the medulla and midbrain, in that it contains ascending and descending tracts and nuclei of cranial nerves. The dorsal surface of the tegmentum contributes to the floor of the fourth ventricle.

The pons is about 2.5 cm long and lies on the clivus, formed by the occipital and sphenoid bones. A shallow groove, the basilar sulcus of the pons, runs along the ventral surface in the midline. The pons merges laterally into the middle cerebellar peduncles, the attachment of the *trigeminal nerve* marking the transition between the pons and the peduncle (Figs. 6–1 and 6–2). The motor root of the trigeminal nerve is rostromedial to the larger sensory root. The trigeminal nerve enters the middle cranial fossa at the medial end of the petrous temporal bone, where the trigeminal (semilunar) ganglion is located. The three divisions of the nerve diverge from the ganglion, embedded in the dura mater. The ophthalmic division passes through the superior orbital fissure to reach the orbit. The maxillary division traverses the foramen rotundum, and the mandibular division the foramen ovale, both foramina being in the floor of the middle cranial fossa.

The rostral part of the pons is also known as the *isthmus of the brain stem.* A slight, band-like elevation runs obliquely across the dorsolateral surface of the isthmus toward the inferior colliculus of the midbrain (Fig. 6–2). This elevation is produced by the underlying lateral lemniscus, which is the main auditory tract of the brain stem.

FOURTH VENTRICLE

The *floor of the fourth ventricle (rhomboid fossa)* is broad in its midportion, narrowing toward the obex and the aqueduct of the midbrain (Fig. 6–3). The floor is divided into symmetrical halves by a *median sulcus;* the *sulcus limitans* further divides each half into medial and lateral areas. The vestibular nuclear complex lies beneath most of the lateral area, which is therefore known as the *vestibular area* of the rhomboid fossa. Motor nuclei are located be-

neath the medial area, the caudal part of which is marked by two triangles. Of these, the *hypoglossal triangle* indicates the position of the rostral end of the hypoglossal nucleus, while the rostral end of the dorsal motor nucleus of the vagus nerve lies beneath the *vagal triangle* (ala cinerea). The appearance of this part of the rhomboid fossa suggested the tip of a pen to early anatomists, and the term calamus scriptorius (writing pen) was therefore applied.

The *area postrema* is a narrow strip between the vagal triangle and the margin of the ventricle. The tissue immediately beneath this area consists of neuroglial cells, a few nerve cells, and many blood vessels.

The *facial colliculus,* a slight swelling at the lower end of the median eminence, is formed by fibers from the motor nucleus of the facial nerve looping over the abducens nucleus. There is a small pigmented area, the *locus ceruleus* (blue place), at the forward end of the sulcus limitans, indicating the site of a cluster of nerve cells containing melanin pigment. Delicate strands of nerve fibers emerge from the median sulcus, run laterally over the floor of the ventricle as the *striae medullares,* and enter the inferior cerebellar peduncle. The floor of the fourth ventricle is covered by ependymal epithelium, such as lines the whole of the ventricular system and the central canal of the spinal cord.

The tent-shaped roof of the fourth ventricle protrudes into the cerebellum. The forepart of the roof is formed on either side by the superior cerebellar peduncles, which consist mainly of fibers proceeding from cerebellar nuclei into the midbrain. The V-shaped interval between the converging peduncles is bridged by the *superior medullary velum,* a thin sheet of tissue consisting of a layer of pia mater and one of ependyma, with some nerve fibers in between. The caudal or inferior part of the roof consists of a thin pia-ependymal membrane, the *inferior medullary velum,* which often adheres to the undersurface of the cerebellum. A deficiency of variable size in the latter membrane constitutes the *median aperture of the fourth ventricle,* alternatively known as the *foramen of Magendie,* which provides the principal communication between the ventricular system and the subarachnoid space (Fig. 6–4).

The lateral walls of the fourth ventricle include the inferior cerebellar peduncles, which curve from the medulla into the cerebellum on the medial aspects of the middle peduncles (Fig. 6–3). Lateral recesses of the ventricle extend around the sides of the medulla and open ventrally as the *lateral apertures of the fourth ventricle* or the *foramina of Luschka,* through which cerebrospinal fluid enters the subarachnoid space (Fig. 6–5). These foramina are situated at the junction of the medulla, pons, and cerebellum (the cerebellopontine angles) near the attachment to the brain stem of the glossopharyngeal, vestibulocochlear, and facial nerves. The choroid plexus of the fourth ventricle is suspended from the inferior medullary velum; the plexus extends into the lateral recesses, and tufts even protrude into the foramina of Luschka.

MIDBRAIN

The ventral surface of the *midbrain* extends from the pons to the mammillary bodies of the diencephalon (Fig. 6–1). The prominent elevation on either side is formed by the *basis pedunculi,* which consists of fibers of the pyramidal motor system and corticopontine fibers. Many small blood vessels penetrate the midbrain in the floor of the *interpeduncular fossa,* and this region is therefore known as the *posterior perforated substance.* The *oculomotor nerve* emerges from the side of the inter-

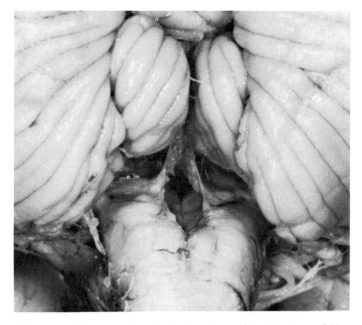

FIG. 6–4. Median aperture of the fourth ventricle (foramen of Magendie), opening from the fourth ventricle into the cerebellomedullary cistern of the subarachnoid space. ×2½

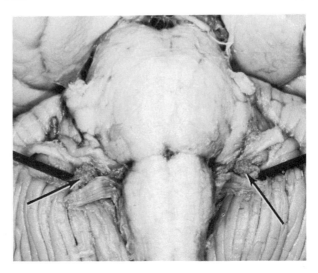

FIG. 6–5. Lateral apertures of the fourth ventricle (foramina of Luschka). Tufts of choroid plexus (*arrows*) occupy the foramina, into which *marker sticks* have been inserted. ×1⅕

peduncular fossa and continues forward through the cavernous venous sinus into the orbit.

The dorsal surface of the midbrain bears four rounded elevations, the paired *inferior* and *superior colliculi* (corpora quadrigemina) (Figs. 6–2 and 6–3). The colliculi make up the *roof* or *tectum* and indicate the extent of the midbrain on the dorsal surface (about 1.5 cm long). The major role of the inferior colliculus is that of a relay nucleus on the auditory pathway to the thalamus and thence to the cerebral cortex. Fibers connecting the inferior colliculus with the specific thalamic nucleus for hearing (medial geniculate nucleus) form an elevation known as the *inferior brachium* (Figs. 6–2 and 6–3). The superior colliculus is primarily a reflex center for movements of the eyes and head in response to visual and other stimuli. The *superior brachium* contains fibers proceeding from cortex of the occipital lobe and from the retina to the superior colliculus. Other fibers in the superior brachium

terminate in the pretectal nucleus just in front of the superior colliculus; the latter fibers are part of a pathway from the retina for the pupillary light reflex. The *trochlear nerve* emerges from the brain stem immediately behind the inferior colliculus, curves around the midbrain, and enters the orbit after traversing the cavernous venous sinus.

The lateral surface of the midbrain (Fig. 6–2) is formed mainly by the *cerebral peduncle*, which constitutes the major portion of this region of the brain stem on either side.

The posterior part of the thalamus grows beyond the plane of transition between the diencephalon and midbrain during maturation of the brain (Fig. 6–3). Consequently, transverse sections at the level of the superior colliculi include thalamic nuclei, in particular the medial and lateral geniculate nuclei and a prominent nucleus of the thalamus known as the pulvinar (Figs. 7–14 and 7–15).

7

Brain Stem: Nuclei and Tracts of the Medulla, Pons, and Midbrain

The principal nuclei and fiber tracts of the brain stem are identified and discussed in the present chapter. Long fiber tracts that traverse all, or most, of the brain stem are noted successively in the medulla, in the pons, and again in the midbrain. A regional presentation of such tracts is not wholly desirable, and some pathways are reviewed as functional systems in Chapters 19 and 23. The larger nuclei of cranial nerves are included among the cell groups identified, although a description of the functional components of the cranial nerves is reserved for Chapter 8.

Sections stained by the Weigert method are used as illustrations, the levels of the sections being shown in Figure 7–1. The course of individual tracts, except for the very large ones, is not easily followed in the normal brain. The position of these tracts has been established with reasonable certainty by means of experimental studies in laboratory animals and by clinicopathologic correlations in man. In the illustrations,

therefore, the sites of some tracts are indicated although they cannot be distinguished clearly from adjacent fasciculi.

The reticular formation is again mentioned briefly at this point because it is necessary to use the term in the present chapter. The reticular formation of the brain stem consists of neurons in areas not occupied by prominent nuclei or tracts. Many of the constituent cells defy organization into easily identifiable groups, and histologic analysis therefore presents a formidable problem. The reticular formation has several functions of the first importance. These include the following, among others: 1) an influence on levels of consciousness and degrees of alertness (reticular activating system); 2) a role in the extrapyramidal motor system through afferents from the cerebral cortex and several motor nuclei and through efferents to motor neurons of cerebrospinal nerves; and 3) a contribution to the autonomic nervous system through groups of neurons that

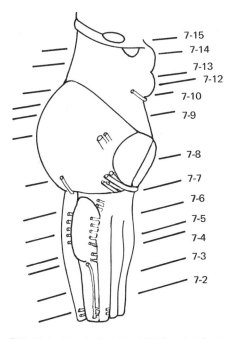

7-15
7-14
7-13
7-12
7-10
7-9
7-8
7-7
7-6
7-5
7-4
7-3
7-2

FIG. 7–1. Key to levels of Weigert-stained sections of the brain stem shown in Figures 7–2 through 7–10 and 7–12 through 7–15.

function as cardiovascular and respiratory centers. In view of its special histologic characteristics and functional importance, the reticular formation is discussed separately in Chapter 9.

MEDULLA

There is an extensive rearrangement of gray matter and white matter in the transitional zone between the spinal cord and medulla, this zone being coextensive with the pyramidal decussation. The ventral gray horns continue into the region of the decussation, where they include motor cells for the first cervical nerve and the spinal root of the accessory nerve, and where the gray matter is traversed obliquely by bundles of fibers passing from the pyramids to the lateral corticospinal tracts

(Figs. 7–2 and 7–3). Dorsal expansions of the gray matter at the level of the pyramidal decussation form the nuclei gracilis and cuneatus. The medulla has a complex internal structure above the decussation, a structure that is entirely different from that of the spinal cord (Figs. 7–4 through 7–7). The inferior olivary nucleus is the most prominent feature of the upper half of the medulla. Near the pons, the base of the inferior cerebellar peduncle appears as a distinctive area of white matter in the dorsolateral part of the medulla (Fig. 7–7).

ASCENDING PATHWAYS TO THE THALAMUS AND TECTUM

Dorsal Column—Medial Lemniscus System

It will be recalled that long dorsal column fibers reaching the medulla oblongata transmit impulses for discriminative touch, proprioception, and vibratory sense as an ipsilateral pathway. The *fasciculus gracilis* is concerned with these sensations for the leg and lower trunk, while impulses from the upper trunk, arm, and neck are transmitted in the *fasciculus cuneatus*.

The *nucleus gracilis*, in which fibers of the corresponding fasciculus terminate, is present throughout the closed portion of the medulla. The fibers of the fasciculus cuneatus end in the *nucleus cuneatus*, which first appears slightly above the beginning of the nucleus gracilis and continues beyond the latter nucleus. There is a somatotopic representation in these dorsal column nuclei, i.e., fibers entering the cord in a specific segment synapse with a specific group of cells in the nuclei. Such a point-to-point projection of fibers on sensory nuclei is characteristic of pathways to the thalamus and cerebral cortex, forming an anatomic basis for recognition of the source of stimuli. The less the convergence from primary to secondary to tertiary neurons in the pathway, the greater is the precision of localization and the quality of discrimination, maximal discrimination obviously being achieved by a 1:1:1 ratio. The system for fine touch, position and movement, and vibration is the most discriminative of the general sensory systems. There is therefore little convergence between successive neurons that constitute the pathway to the cerebral cortex.

The myelinated axons of cells in the dorsal column nuclei pursue a curved course to the median raphe as *internal arcuate fibers,* which are shown especially well in Figure 7–4. After crossing the midline in the *decussation of the medial lemniscus,* the fibers immediately turn rostrally in the *medial lemniscus.* This is one of the more substantial tracts of the brain stem, occupying the interval between the median raphe and the inferior olivary nucleus in the medulla (Figs. 7–4 through 7–7). Fibers conducting data from the foot are most ventral, i.e., adjacent to the pyramid. The body is then represented sequentially, and fibers for the neck are in the most dorsal part of the lemniscus. After traversing the pons and midbrain, the tract ends in the thalamic nucleus for general sensation, which is the ventral posterior nucleus of the thalamus.

Spinothalamic and Spinotectal Tracts

The *lateral spinothalamic tract* for pain and temperature and the *ventral spinothalamic tract* for simple (light) touch and pressure, from the opposite side of the body, continue into the lower medulla without appreciable change in position. This is also true of the *spinotectal tract,* which carries somesthetic data to the superior colliculus of the midbrain. The position of ventral spinothalamic fibers in the more rostral portion of the medulla has not been

demonstrated satisfactorily in man. Some have placed them in or near the dorsal part of the medial lemniscus. However, the weight of evidence indicates that the lateral and ventral spinothalamic tracts and the spinotectal tract traverse the lateral area of the medulla, dorsal to the inferior olivary nucleus. They are so close to one another that the combined tracts are called the *spinal lemniscus* in this location (Figs. 7–4 through 7–7) and throughout the remainder of the brain stem. The spinothalamic tracts terminate with the medial lemniscus in the ventral posterior thalamic nucleus.

SPINORETICULAR FIBERS

Spinoreticular fibers in the ventrolateral white matter of the cord continue into the brain stem and terminate on neurons of the reticular formation, mainly in the lateral area of the medulla. One group of reticular neurons in this area forms a nucleus of sufficient size to be seen in Weigert-stained sections. This is the *lateral reticular nucleus,* which is situated dorsal to the inferior olivary nucleus and near the surface of the medulla (Figs. 7–4 through 7–6). Spinoreticular fibers transmit somesthetic data, especially of cutaneous origin, and data from the viscera. Their distribution in the cord and medulla is diffuse, and some spinoreticular fibers intermingle with fibers of the spinal lemniscus. The number of such fibers leaving the spinal lemniscus in the medulla is sufficiently large to cause a significant decrease in the size of the lemniscus rostral to the medulla. In addition, lemniscal fibers give off collateral branches to the reticular formation. Cells of the reticular formation project to various parts of the diencephalon including thalamic centers known as intralaminar nuclei, which in turn influence neuronal activity throughout the cerebral cortex.

There are, therefore, alternative routes for exteroceptive somesthetic conduction from the spinal cord to the thalamus. The direct lemniscal route proceeds without interruption to the ventral posterior thalamic nucleus. This is the more recent pathway, which became increasingly important as the thalamus and cerebral cortex increased in size and functional significance during mammalian phylogeny. Alternatively, exteroceptive data reach intralaminar thalamic nuclei through a polysynaptic, extralemniscal route involving the reticular formation. Although the latter pathway is related to early stages of phylogeny, it has attained importance in man as part of the reticular activating system which has an important influence with respect to levels of consciousness and degrees of alertness.

SPINOCEREBELLAR TRACTS

The *dorsal* and *ventral spinocerebellar tracts* traverse the medulla in the periphery of the lateral area (Figs. 7–2 through 7–6). It will be recalled that the dorsal tract, which is uncrossed, originates in the nucleus dorsalis (Clarke's column) of the thoracic and upper lumbar segments of the spinal cord. The ventral tract, on the other hand, is crossed, and many of the cells of origin are in the lumbosacral enlargement of the cord. The dorsal spinocerebellar fibers enter the inferior cerebellar peduncle (Figs. 7–7 and 7–8), while the ventral spinocerebellar tract continues through the pons and enters the cerebellum by way of the superior cerebellar peduncle.

MEDULLARY NUCLEI CONNECTED WITH THE CEREBELLUM

Inferior Olivary Complex

Several nuclei in the medulla receive afferents from various sources and project to the cerebellum. These nuclei include the components of the inferior olivary complex. The largest component of the complex is the *inferior olivary nucleus,* which is shaped like a crumpled bag or purse with the hilus facing medially (Figs. 7–5 through 7–7). The *medial accessory olivary nucleus* lies between the medial lemniscus and the inferior olivary nucleus, while the *dorsal accessory olivary nucleus* is immediately dorsal to the inferior olivary nucleus (Fig. 7–6). The relatively small accessory nuclei are phylogenetically older than the inferior olivary or principal nucleus.

The *central tegmental tract,* which will be identified in the pons and midbrain, is the largest afferent pathway to the inferior olivary complex. The constituent fibers originate in the corpus striatum, the red nucleus of the midbrain (both are motor nuclei), and probably at other sites that have not yet been identified. The terminal portion of the central tegmental tract forms a dense layer on the dorsal surface of the inferior olivary nucleus, best seen in Figure 7–7. The central tegmental tract contains fibers other than those ending in the inferior olivary complex; more specifically, these include ascending fibers from cells in the reticular formation.

Other afferents to the inferior olivary complex come from the cerebral cortex and the spinal cord. *Cortico–olivary fibers* originate in the sensorimotor strip of cerebral cortex, which borders the boundary between the frontal and parietal lobes. These fibers, which terminate mainly in the principal nucleus, accompany the corticospinal tract through the midbrain and pons. The *spino–olivary tract* continues from the cord into the ventrolateral area of the medulla (Figs. 7–2 and 7–3), and most of the fibers end in the accessory olivary nuclei.

Olivocerebellar fibers constitute the main projection from the inferior olivary complex. Fibers from the principal nucleus

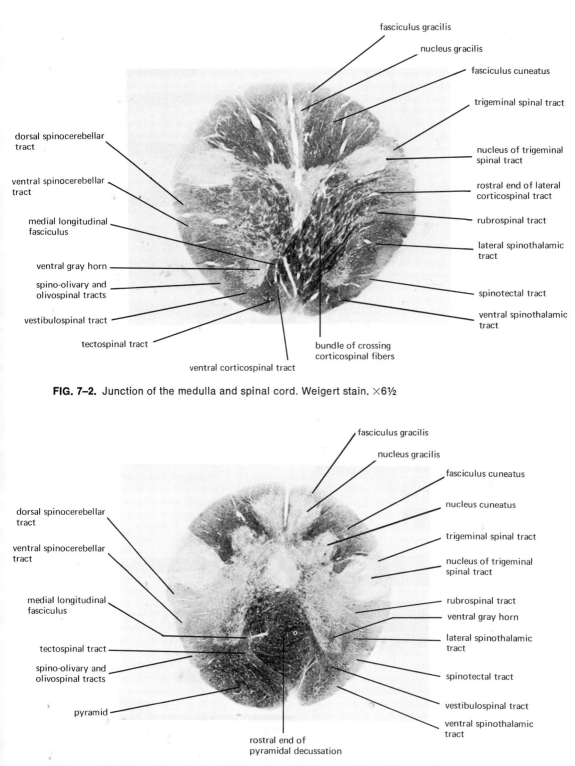

fasciculus gracilis

nucleus gracilis

fasciculus cuneatus

trigeminal spinal tract

nucleus of trigeminal spinal tract

rostral end of lateral corticospinal tract

rubrospinal tract

lateral spinothalamic tract

spinotectal tract

ventral spinothalamic tract

dorsal spinocerebellar tract

ventral spinocerebellar tract

medial longitudinal fasciculus

ventral gray horn

spino-olivary and olivospinal tracts

vestibulospinal tract

tectospinal tract

bundle of crossing corticospinal fibers

ventral corticospinal tract

FIG. 7–2. Junction of the medulla and spinal cord. Weigert stain. ×6½

fasciculus gracilis

nucleus gracilis

fasciculus cuneatus

nucleus cuneatus

trigeminal spinal tract

nucleus of trigeminal spinal tract

rubrospinal tract

ventral gray horn

lateral spinothalamic tract

spinotectal tract

vestibulospinal tract

ventral spinothalamic tract

dorsal spinocerebellar tract

ventral spinocerebellar tract

medial longitudinal fasciculus

tectospinal tract

spino-olivary and olivospinal tracts

pyramid

rostral end of pyramidal decussation

FIG. 7–3. Medulla at the rostral end of the pyramidal decussation. Weigert stain. ×5½

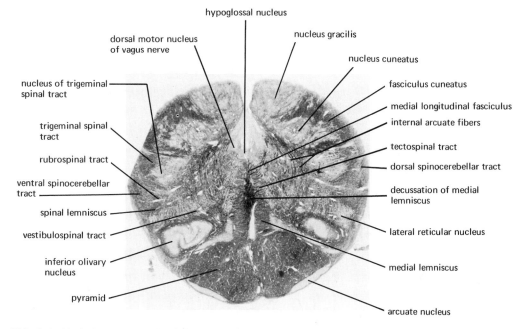

FIG. 7–4. Medulla at the caudal limit of the inferior olivary nucleus. Weigert stain. ×4⅘

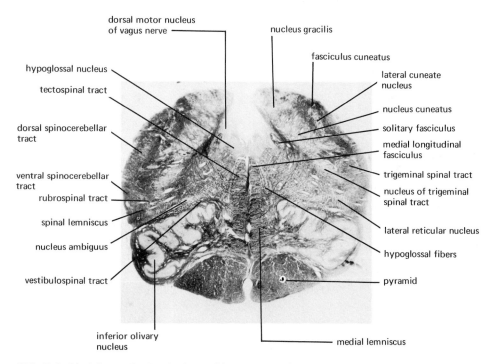

FIG. 7–5. Medulla at the level of transition between its closed and open portions. Weigert stain. ×4

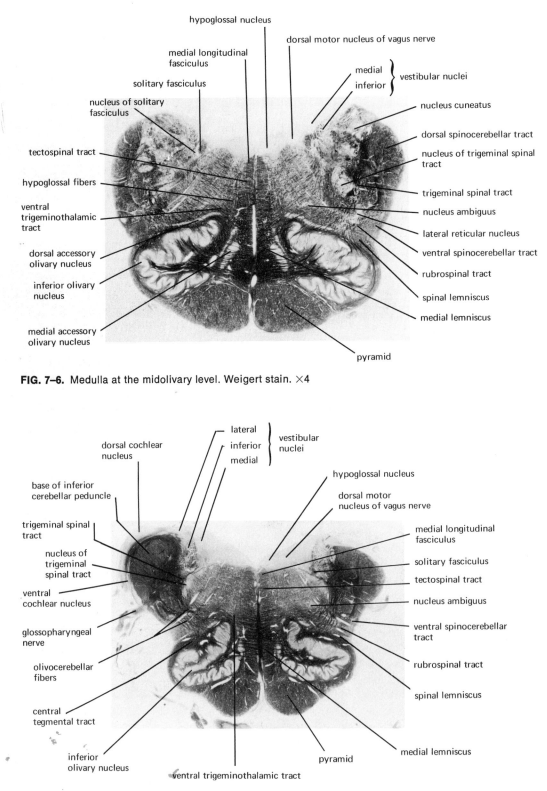

FIG. 7–6. Medulla at the midolivary level. Weigert stain. ×4

In Fig. 7–6, the following labels appear:

hypoglossal nucleus

dorsal motor nucleus of vagus nerve

medial longitudinal fasciculus

medial ⎫
inferior ⎭ vestibular nuclei

solitary fasciculus

nucleus cuneatus

nucleus of solitary fasciculus

dorsal spinocerebellar tract

tectospinal tract

nucleus of trigeminal spinal tract

hypoglossal fibers

trigeminal spinal tract

ventral trigeminothalamic tract

nucleus ambiguus

lateral reticular nucleus

dorsal accessory olivary nucleus

ventral spinocerebellar tract

inferior olivary nucleus

rubrospinal tract

spinal lemniscus

medial lemniscus

medial accessory olivary nucleus

pyramid

In Fig. 7–7, the following labels appear:

lateral ⎫
inferior ⎬ vestibular nuclei
medial ⎭

dorsal cochlear nucleus

hypoglossal nucleus

dorsal motor nucleus of vagus nerve

base of inferior cerebellar peduncle

medial longitudinal fasciculus

trigeminal spinal tract

solitary fasciculus

nucleus of trigeminal spinal tract

tectospinal tract

ventral cochlear nucleus

nucleus ambiguus

glossopharyngeal nerve

ventral spinocerebellar tract

olivocerebellar fibers

rubrospinal tract

central tegmental tract

spinal lemniscus

inferior olivary nucleus

medial lemniscus

ventral trigeminothalamic tract

pyramid

FIG. 7–7. Rostral end of the medulla. Weigert stain. ×3

occupy its interior and leave through the hilus. After decussating in the median raphe, the strands of myelinated olivocerebellar fibers curve in a dorsolateral direction and enter the inferior cerebellar peduncle, of which they are the largest single component (Fig. 7–7). The phylogenetically older accessory olivary nuclei project to correspondingly older regions of the cerebellum. These regions constitute the archicerebellum, which is concerned with the maintenance of equilibrium, and the paleocerebellum, which functions in relation to the generally stereotyped movements of postural changes and locomotion. The inferior olivary nucleus projects to the neocerebellum—the major part of the cerebellum of man. Its role is to ensure efficiency of voluntary movements, especially those requiring precision. The exact location, within the complex, of cell bodies for *olivospinal fibers* is not known; in fact, even the existence of an olivospinal tract has been questioned. Most of the fibers are said to cross to the opposite side of the medulla, intermingle with spino-olivary fibers (Figs. 7–2 and 7–3), and terminate in the ventral gray horn of the cervical cord.

In spite of the large size of the inferior olivary nucleus in man, its function and that of the accessory nuclei are poorly understood. Data received by the inferior olivary complex from various sources are no doubt integrated and modified before transmittal to the cerebellum. The termination of olivocerebellar fibers on Purkinje cells throughout the cerebellar cortex and in the central nuclei of the cerebellum, and the possible role of the olivocerebellar input on neuronal activity in the cerebellum are discussed in Chapter 10.

Information is also scanty with respect to the effects of lesions involving the inferior olivary complex. A curious clinical observation is that of rhythmic movement of the soft palate (palatal myoclonus) when a degenerative lesion of the brain stem includes the inferior olivary nucleus. Instances of degeneration of the olivary nuclei, nuclei of the basal pons, and the cerebellum are well documented, although the etiology is unknown. The patients show a combination of motor deficits, including ataxia, that are characteristic of cerebellar dysfunction.

Arcuate Nucleus

The arcuate nucleus lies on the surface of the pyramid (Fig. 7–4) and receives collateral branches of corticospinal fibers. Fibers from the nucleus enter the cerebellum by way of the inferior cerebellar peduncle, which they reach by two routes. Some of them travel over the lateral surface of the medulla; the remainder run dorsally in the median raphe and then laterally in the striae medullares on the floor of the fourth ventricle. The connections of the arcuate nucleus are like those of the cell groups in the basal portion of the pons—both receive afferents from the cerebral cortex and project to the cerebellum.

Lateral Cuneate Nucleus

The lateral cuneate nucleus is embedded in the fasciculus cuneatus external to the cuneate nucleus (Fig. 7–5). The afferents to the lateral cuneate nucleus are fibers of the fasciculus cuneatus that entered the cord in cervical dorsal roots; many such afferents are in fact collateral branches of fibers ending in the main cuneate nucleus. Efferents from the lateral cuneate nucleus, accompanied by a few fibers from the main nucleus, enter the cerebellum by way of the inferior peduncle. These cuneocerebellar fibers reinforce the dorsal spinocerebellar tract as a pathway from proprioceptive and other sensory endings in the neck and upper extremity. They provide the main route to the cerebellum for impulses entering the cord in the upper four cervical nerves, from which no fibers reach Clarke's column.

DESCENDING TRACTS

Corticospinal Tract

The corticospinal (pyramidal) tract is among the larger and more important tracts of the human brain and spinal cord. About 40 percent of the parent cell bodies are situated in the upper two-thirds of the primary motor area (a strip of cortex along the posterior boundary of the frontal lobe), while the remainder are in the premotor area of the frontal lobe and cortex of the parietal lobe. The corticospinal fibers traverse the medullary center of the cerebral hemisphere and the internal capsule to reach the brain stem. The fibers continue as a compact fasciculus in the basis pedunculi of the midbrain, but the tract is broken up into many small bundles on entering the basal portion of the pons. The bundles coalesce in the caudal pons and the corticospinal tract is again a compact fasciculus in the pyramid of the medulla (Figs. 7–7 through 7–4).

Each pyramid contains approximately 1 million fibers of varying size. About 50 percent of the fibers are fine and very thinly myelinated, measuring 1 μ in diameter, and the width of 90 percent of the fibers is 4 μ or less. However, approximately 35,000, or roughly 3 percent, of the pyramidal fibers are thickly myelinated and of the order of 10 μ in diameter. The latter rapidly conducting fibers are considered to come from the giant pyramidal cells of Betz in the primary motor area.

The proportion of fibers that cross over in the *decussation of the pyramids* varies among individuals, but on the average about 85 percent of the fibers enter the decussation. The upper limit of the pyramidal decussation appears in Figure 7–3; although many of the fibers have crossed the midline, the gray matter is not disrupted because of the caudal slope of the decussating bundles. A bundle of fibers passing through the gray matter, from a pyramid to the opposite lateral corticospinal tract, is included in Figure 7–2. A few pyramidal fibers enter the lateral corticospinal tract of the same side. With this exception, the 15 percent of nondecussating fibers continues into the ventral white column of the cord as the ventral corticospinal tract. The bundles of corticobulbar fibers destined for motor nuclei of cranial nerves in the medulla are small and inconstant in position; no attempt has been made to identify them in the illustrations.

Tracts Originating in the Midbrain

The *rubrospinal tract* arises from the red nucleus and crosses to the opposite side of the brain stem at the level of origin. The tract runs caudally in the lateral area, dorsal to the inferior olivary nucleus, throughout most of the medulla (Figs. 7–7 through 7–4). The fibers of the pyramidal decussation turn caudally immediately dorsal to the rubrospinal tract (Fig. 7–2), and the lateral corticospinal and rubrospinal tracts continue into the lateral white column of the cord in this relationship.

The *tectospinal tract* originates in the superior colliculus of the midbrain, and the fibers cross at that level to the opposite side of the brain stem. The tract lies next to the median raphe and dorsal to the medial lemniscus throughout most of the medulla (Figs. 7–7 through 7–4). The decussating corticospinal bundles pass dorsal to the tectospinal tract, which is therefore deflected ventrally (Figs. 7–3 and 7–2) to take up a position in the ventral white column of the cord.

NUCLEI OF CRANIAL NERVES AND ASSOCIATED TRACTS

Hypoglossal, Accessory, Vagus, and Glossopharyngeal Nerves

The *hypoglossal nucleus* for innervation of the tongue consists of a column of motor cells near the midline and coextensive with the inferior olivary nucleus. The hypoglossal nucleus is situated in the central gray matter in the closed part of the medulla (Fig. 7–4) and beneath the hypoglossal triangle of the rhomboid fossa (Figs. 7–5 through 7–7). The medullated axons from the nucleus are directed ventrally between the medial lemniscus and the inferior olivary nucleus (Figs. 7–5 and 7–6), then lateral to the pyramid, emerging as the hypoglossal nerve roots along the ventrolateral sulcus. The *nucleus ambiguus* is situated dorsal to the inferior olivary nucleus in the position shown in Figures 7–5 through 7–7. This important cell column supplies muscles of the soft palate, pharynx, larynx, and upper esophagus through the cranial division of the accessory nerve and the vagus and glossopharyngeal nerves. The *dorsal motor nucleus of the vagus nerve* is the largest of the parasympathetic nuclei in the brain stem, supplying smooth muscle and glandular elements of thoracic and abdominal viscera, as well as the heart. The nucleus lies lateral to the hypoglossal nucleus in the gray matter surrounding the central canal (Fig. 7–4), continuing forward beneath the vagal triangle of the rhomboid fossa (Figs. 7–5 through 7–7).

There is a bundle of visceral afferent fibers known as the *solitary fasciculus*, which lies along the lateral side of the dorsal motor nucleus of the vagus nerve (Figs. 7–5 through 7–7). This fasciculus consists of caudally directed fibers, whose cell bodies are in the inferior ganglia of the vagus and glossopharyngeal nerves and the geniculate ganglion of the facial nerve. The fibers terminate in the *nucleus of the solitary fasciculus*, a column of cells that lies adjacent to, and partly surrounds, the fasciculus. The vagal and glossopharyngeal afferents have an important role in visceral reflexes and transmit impulses for taste from the epiglottis and posterior third of the tongue. The fibers contributed by the facial nerve are for taste in the anterior two-thirds of the tongue and in the palate.

Vestibulocochlear Nerve

Nuclei in which the cochlear and vestibular divisions of the eighth cranial nerve terminate are situated in the most rostral part of the medulla. The *dorsal cochlear nucleus*, lying on the base of the inferior cerebellar peduncle, is shown in Figure 7–7, and a portion of the *ventral cochlear nucleus* appears lateral to the peduncle in the same figure. Fibers leaving the cochlear nuclei are noted later in the description of the pons. The *vestibular nuclear complex*, situated beneath the vestibular area of the rhomboid fossa, is divided into *superior, lateral, medial,* and *inferior vestibular nuclei* on the basis of cytoarchitecture and connections. The superior nucleus is in the pons, in the position shown in Figure 7–8, while the remaining nuclei are situated in the medulla (Figs. 7–6 and 7–7). The vestibular nerve penetrates the brain stem deep to the fibers of the inferior cerebellar peduncle. This occurs slightly rostral to the attachment of the cochlear nerve and the vestibular nerve is therefore not included in Figure 7–7. Some vestibular nerve fibers enter the cerebellum through the inferior peduncle while the majority terminate in the vestibular nuclear complex. Descending branches of vestibular nerve fibers that terminate in the inferior vestibular nucleus give this nucleus a stippled appearance in sections (Fig. 7–7).

In addition to the primary vestibulocerebellar fibers just mentioned, numerous secondary fibers proceed from the vestibular nuclei into the cerebellum through the inferior peduncle. Vestibular nuclei project to spinal motor neurons by means of two tracts. The larger of these is the *vestibulospinal tract,* for which the cells of origin are in the lateral vestibular (Deiters') nucleus. Vestibulospinal fibers run caudally, dorsal to the inferior olivary nucleus, in the position indicated in Figures 7–5 and 7–4. The tract is deflected ventrally at the level of the pyramidal decussation (Figs. 7–3 and 7–2) and continues into the ipsilateral ventral white column of the cord.

Fibers from all the vestibular nuclei form the *medial longitudinal fasciculus,* which extends rostrally and caudally adjacent to the midline. The ascending fibers are identified later in the pons and midbrain. The parent cell bodies of the descending fibers are mainly in the medial vestibular nucleus; they are both crossed and uncrossed, but predominantly the latter. The fasciculus is dorsal to the tectospinal tract until the level of the pyramidal decussation is reached (Figs. 7–7 through 7–4). The decussating pyramidal fibers intervene between the gray matter around the central canal and the medial longitudinal fasciculus, so that the latter assumes a more ventral position (Figs. 7–3 and 7–2) and continues into the spinal cord as a major component of the fasciculus sulcomarginalis in the ventral white column. The tectospinal tract is similarly deflected ventrally by the pyramidal decussation. The fibers of the medial longitudinal fasciculus and the tectospinal tract are joined by the ventral corticospinal tract below the decussation, and there is considerable intermingling of the three categories of fibers in the ventral white column of the cervical cord.

Trigeminal Nerve

The trigeminal nerve contributes an important tract and nucleus to the internal structure of the medulla. Many of the fibers of the trigeminal sensory root turn caudally on entering the pons. These fibers constitute the *trigeminal spinal tract,* so named because some of the fibers extend caudally as far as the third cervical segment of the spinal cord. The spinal tract transmits data for pain, temperature, simple touch, and pressure from the extensive area of distribution of the trigeminal nerve. The fibers terminate in the subjacent *nucleus of the trigeminal spinal tract.* The tract and nucleus lie deep to the root of the inferior cerebellar peduncle and the dorsal spinocerebellar tract in the rostral part of the medulla (Figs. 7–7 through 7–4). More caudally, they lie under the surface area of medulla known as the tuberculum cinereum (Figs. 7–3 and 7–2). Many of the spinal tract fibers are unmyelinated or thinly myelinated, and the nucleus consists principally of small neurons. The trigeminal spinal tract and its nucleus are, therefore, similar in some respects both structurally and functionally to the dorsolateral fasciculus and substantia gelatinosa of the spinal cord. The *ventral trigeminothalamic tract* (Fig. 7–6) is a crossed fasciculus, which projects from the nucleus of the spinal tract (and the chief sensory nucleus in the pons) to the ventral posterior nucleus of the thalamus. Conducting sensory data from the head, the ventral trigeminothalamic tract is comparable functionally to the spinothalamic pathways for the body generally.

PONS

The major landmarks in Weigert-stained sections through the pons are 1) the division of the pons into basal and dorsal regions, and 2) the prominent cerebellar peduncles (Figs. 7–8 and 7–9). The basal portion consists of longitudinal fiber bundles, transverse fibers, and collections of nerve cells in the intervals between longitudinal and transverse fasciculi. The longitudinal bundles are numerous and small at rostral levels (Figs. 7–9 and 7–10), while many of them coalesce as they approach the medulla (Fig. 7–8). The inferior and middle cerebellar peduncles appear in Figure 7–8, and the superior peduncles in Figure 7–9.

DORSAL PORTION (Tegmentum) OF THE PONS

The *pontine tegmentum* is similar structurally to the medulla and midbrain. There are therefore tracts that were described in the medulla to identify, together with components of several cranial nerves.

Ascending Tracts; Inferior and Superior Cerebellar Peduncles

The *medial lemniscus* "rotates" in passing from the medulla into the pons, where it takes up a position in the most ventral part of the tegmentum. The lemniscus has a roughly oval outline at the level shown in Figure 7–8; it moves laterally further forward and becomes strap-like in shape (Figs. 7–9 and 7–10). The medial lemniscus rotates in such a way that fibers from the nucleus cuneatus are medial to those from the nucleus gracilis. The somatotopic representation is therefore neck, arm, trunk, and leg, in a medial to lateral sequence. The *spinal lemniscus* is situated near the lateral edge of the medial lemniscus throughout the pons (Figs. 7–8 through 7–10). The *ventral spinocerebellar tract* traverses the most lateral part of the tegmentum (Fig. 7–8), then curves dorsally

and enters the cerebellum through the superior peduncle (Figs. 7–9 and 7–11).

The *inferior cerebellar penduncles* enter the cerebellum from the caudal part of the pons. In this location, the inferior peduncle lies on the medial aspect of the middle cerebellar peduncle, forming the lateral wall of the fourth ventricle. The main part of the inferior cerebellar peduncle consists of the *restiform body* (Fig. 7–8), in which olivocerebellar fibers are the most numerous, followed by fibers of the dorsal spinocerebellar tract. Smaller components are contributed by cuneocerebellar fibers from the lateral cuneate nucleus, fibers from the arcuate nucleus and the reticular formation of the medulla, and others from the chief sensory nucleus and nucleus of the spinal tract of the trigeminal nerve. The region of the inferior cerebellar peduncle immediately adjoining the fourth ventricle is known as the *juxtarestiform body* (Fig. 7–8) and includes fibers entering the cerebellum from the vestibular nerve and vestibular nuclei. The juxtarestiform body also contains cerebellar efferents from portions of the cerebellum that are concerned with maintaining equilibrium; these fibers terminate in vestibular nuclei and in the reticular formation of the medulla and pontine tegmentum.

The *superior cerebellar peduncles* (Fig. 7–9) consist mainly of cerebellar efferent fibers, which constitute the *brachia conjunctiva*. The brachia originate in the central nuclei of the cerebellum and enter the brain stem behind the inferior colliculi of the midbrain. The constituent fibers cross the midline at the level of the inferior colliculi in the *decussation of the brachia conjunctiva* (Figs. 7–10, 7–12, and 7–13), continuing forward to a thalamic nucleus, from which fibers project to motor areas of frontal lobe cortex. A minority of fibers of the brachia terminate in the red nuclei. In addition to the brachium conjunctivum, the

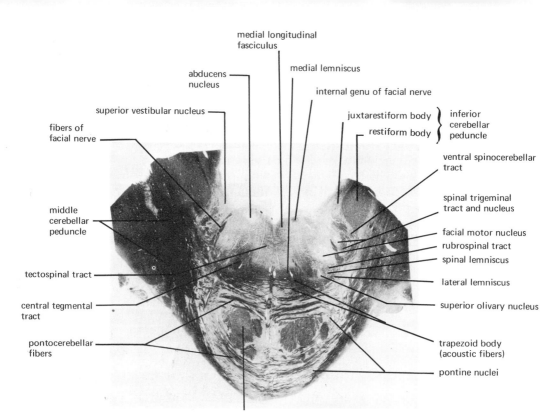

FIG. 7–8. Caudal region of the pons. Weigert stain. ×2⅖

FIG. 7–9. Pons at approximately midlevel. Weigert stain. ×2⅓

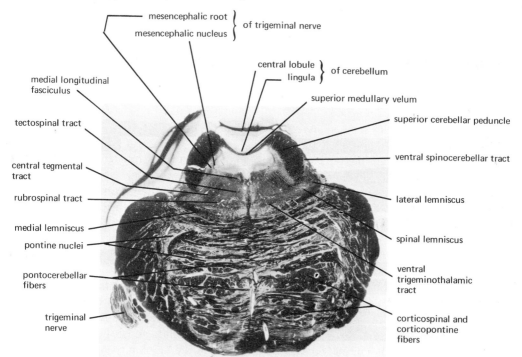

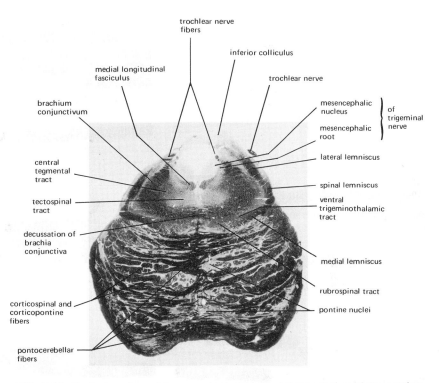

trochlear nerve
fibers

inferior colliculus

medial longitudinal
fasciculus

trochlear nerve

brachium
conjunctivum

mesencephalic
nucleus

of
trigeminal
nerve

mesencephalic
root

central
tegmental
tract

lateral lemniscus

spinal lemniscus

tectospinal
tract

ventral
trigeminothalamic
tract

decussation of
brachia
conjunctiva

medial lemniscus

corticospinal and
corticopontine
fibers

rubrospinal tract

pontine nuclei

pontocerebellar
fibers

FIG. 7–10. Rostral portion of the pons including the isthmus region of the pontine tegmentum. Weigert stain. ×2⅕

superior cerebellar peduncle contains fibers entering the cerebellum. These consist of the ventral spinocerebellar tract, a few fibers from the red nucleus, and fibers from a trigeminal nucleus known as the mesencephalic nucleus of the trigeminal nerve (see below).

Descending Tracts

Fibers from the red nucleus, corpus striatum, and probably other gray areas run in the *central tegmental tract* to the inferior olivary complex. This tract is situated medial to the fibers of the brachium conjunctivum at the level of the pontine isthmus (Fig. 7–10), in the central area of the tegmentum at midpons levels (Fig. 7–9), and just dorsal to the medial lemnis-

cus in the caudal region of the pons (Fig. 7–8). As noted previously the central tegmental tract also includes fibers ascending from the reticular formation of the brain stem to the diencephalon.

The *rubrospinal tract* is situated deeply in the tegmentum; the tract shifts from a position near the midline to the lateral area of the tegmentum while descending through the pons from its origin in the contralateral red nucleus (Figs. 7–10 through 7–8). The rubrospinal tract and the spinal lemniscus are close to one another at lower pontine levels. The *tectospinal tract* from the contralateral superior colliculus of the midbrain is situated near the midline in the pontine tegmentum (Figs. 7–10 through 7–8), a position that is maintained throughout the course of the tract in the medulla and spinal cord. Corticobulbar fibers proceeding to motor nuclei of cranial nerves in the pons and medulla are present in the tegmentum, but they are difficult to identify in Weigert-stained preparations.

Nuclei of Cranial Nerves and Associated Tracts

Vestibulocochlear Nerve. Fibers from the cochlear nuclei cross the pons to ascend in the lateral lemniscus of the opposite side. These slender bundles of auditory (acoustic) fibers are directed across the brain stem in the deepest part of the tegmentum, and it is difficult to distinguish them from nearby fascicles of pontocerebellar fibers. The transverse strands of acoustic fibers, some of which intersect the medial lemniscus, are known as the *trapezoid body* (Fig. 7–8). A proportion of fibers from the cochlear nuclei end in the *superior olivary nucleus* (Fig. 7–8) of either side, from which efferent fibers are added to the auditory pathway. Fibers originating in the cochlear and superior olivary nuclei turn rostrally in the lateral part of the tegmentum to form the *lateral lemniscus* (Fig. 7–8). This tract is situated at the lateral edge of the medial lemniscus in the first part of its course (Fig. 7–9), then moves dorsally and ends in the inferior colliculus (Fig. 7–10). The auditory pathway continues through the inferior brachium to the medial geniculate nucleus of the thalamus, and then to the auditory area of cortex in the temporal lobe.

Of the four vestibular nuclei, only the *superior vestibular nucleus* is as far rostral as the level shown in Figure 7–8. Fibers from all the vestibular nuclei, some crossed and some uncrossed, ascend in the *medial longitudinal fasciculus,* which runs near the midline and close to the floor of the fourth ventricle throughout the pons (Figs. 7–8 through 7–10). The fibers terminate in the abducens, trochlear, and oculomotor nuclei; the connections thereby established have the important function of coordinating movements of the eyes with movements of the head.

Facial and Abducens Nerves. The *motor nucleus of the facial nerve* for the muscles of expression consists of a prominent group of typical motor neurons in the ventrolateral part of the tegmentum (Fig. 7–8). Fibers from the nucleus pass first in a dorsomedial direction, then form a compact bundle, the *internal genu,* which loops over the abducens nucleus beneath the facial colliculus of the rhomboid fossa. The bundle of fibers forming the genu first runs forward along the medial side of the abducens nucleus, then curves over its rostral end, where it appears on the right-hand side of Figure 7–8. After leaving the genu, the fibers pass between the nucleus of origin and the trigeminal spinal nucleus, emerging as the motor root of the facial nerve at the junction of the pons and medulla.

The *abducens nucleus,* for innervation of the lateral rectus muscle of the eye, is located beneath the facial colliculus, as noted above (Fig. 7–8). The efferent fibers of the nucleus proceed in a ventral direction, with a caudal inclination, and leave the brain stem as the abducens nerve between the pons and the pyramid of the medulla.

Trigeminal Nerve. The *spinal trigeminal tract* and *nucleus* are situated in the lateral part of the tegmentum of the caudal portion of the pons (Fig. 7–8). The pontine tegmentum also contains two additional trigeminal nuclei, the chief sensory and motor nuclei (Fig. 7–11). The *chief sensory nucleus,* which receives trigeminal sensory root fibers for touch (especially discriminative touch), lies at the rostral end of the spinal trigeminal nucleus. Fibers from the

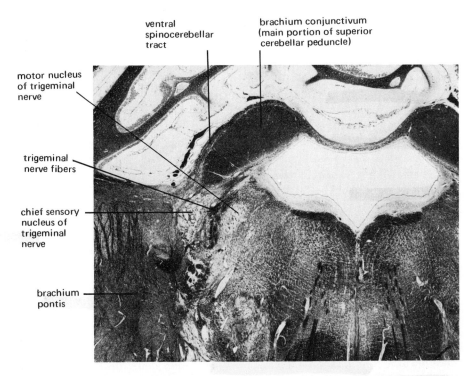

ventral
spinocerebellar
tract

brachium conjunctivum
(main portion of superior
cerebellar peduncle)

motor nucleus
of trigeminal
nerve

trigeminal
nerve fibers

chief sensory
nucleus of
trigeminal
nerve

brachium
pontis

FIG. 7–11. Portion of a section through the middle of the pons, at the level of the chief sensory and motor nuclei of the trigeminal nerve. (This particular level was missing from the series of Weigert-stained sections that illustrate this chapter. Figure 7–11 is therefore substituted from another brain specimen.) ×5½

chief sensory nucleus project to the thalamus, along with fibers from the spinal nucleus, in the *ventral trigeminothalamic tract* (Figs. 7–9 and 7–10). A *dorsal trigeminothalamic tract,* consisting of crossed and uncrossed fibers, has been described as originating in the chief sensory nuclei exclusively. Although not as well documented as its ventral counterpart, the dorsal tract appears to lie in a more dorsal position in the tegmentum, as its name suggests. The *motor nucleus,* which is situated medial to the chief sensory nucleus and separated from the latter by trigeminal nerve fibers, consists of typical lower motor neurons for the muscles of mastication.

The *mesencephalic nucleus of the trigeminal nerve* is a slender column of cells beneath the rostral part of the fourth ventricle (Figs. 7–9 and 7–10) and extending into the midbrain. These cells are unusual because they are cell bodies of primary sensory neurons and the only such cells that are not in cerebrospinal ganglia. Fibers from the nucleus form the *mesencephalic root of the trigeminal nerve* (Figs. 7–9 and 7–10), and most of the constituent fibers are distributed through the mandibular division of the nerve to proprioceptive endings in the muscles of mastication and around the temporomandibular joint.

BASAL PORTION OF THE PONS

The *basal pons* (Figs. 7–8 through 7–10) is especially large in man because of its relationship to those parts of the cortex of the cerebral and cerebellar hemispheres that

The sensory nucleus extends thruout the whole brainstem and into the upper cervical segments. The mesencephalic part extends thruout the midbrain, lying lateral to the cerebral aqueduct. Its cell bodies are of first order neurons that passed thru the trigeminal ganglion without synapsing. The divisions of V register on the spinal nucleus upside down, V₃ in upper medulla, V₂ in closed medulla V₁ in cervical cord.

increased in size and functional importance during mammalian phylogeny.

The longitudinal fasciculi consist of fibers that entered the pons from the basis pedunculi of the midbrain. Many of them are *corticospinal fibers* passing through the pons to the pyramids of the medulla. The fasciculi also contain a large number of *corticopontine fibers,* which originate in widespread areas of cerebral cortex and establish synaptic connections with cells of the *pontine nuclei* of the same side. Except in the caudal third of the pons, in which there are large regions of pontine gray matter (Fig. 7–8), the pontine nuclei consist of small groups of cells between the longitudinal and transverse fasciculi (Figs. 7–9 and 7–10). The pontine nuclei consist of small and medium-sized polygonal cells. Their axons cross the midline, forming the conspicuous transverse bundles of *pontocerebellar fibers*, and enter the cerebellum through the *middle cerebellar peduncle* (*brachium pontis*). These fibers are distributed to the cortex of the cerebellar hemispheres (*neocerebellum*). Corticopontine and pontocerebellar fibers are not myelinated until some time after birth. Data from the cerebral cortex, in which most of the neural events underlying volitional movements take place, are made available to the cerebellar cortex through the relay in the pontine nuclei. Activity in the neocerebellar cortex influences the motor areas in the frontal lobe of the cerebral hemisphere through a pathway that includes the dentate nucleus of the cerebellum and a thalamic nucleus. The well developed circuit linking the cerebral and cerebellar cortices provides for precision and efficiency of voluntary movements.

MIDBRAIN

The internal structure of the midbrain is illustrated in Figures 7–12 through 7–15.

The sections shown in Figures 7–12 and 7–13 are through the inferior colliculi. The plane of the sections is such that Figure 7–12 includes the basal pons and Figure 7–13 shows the extreme rostral lip of the basal pons (see Fig. 7–1). Figures 7–14 and 7–15 illustrate more rostral levels that include the superior colliculi; the latter figure also includes certain thalamic nuclei that are in the transverse plane of the rostral midbrain.

For purposes of description, the midbrain is divided into the following regions (Fig. 7–14 may be referred to for their identification). 1) The *tectum* or *roof,* which is special to this part of the brain stem, consists of the paired inferior and superior colliculi (corpora quadrigemina). 2) The *basis pedunculi* is a dense band of descending fibers. 3) The *substantia nigra,* a motor nucleus, appears as a prominent zone of gray matter, immediately dorsal to the basis pedunculi. 4) The remainder of the midbrain comprises the *tegmentum,* which contains fiber tracts, the prominent red nuclei, and a poorly organized region of gray matter surrounding the cerebral aqueduct (of Sylvius). The term *cerebral peduncle* refers to all of the midbrain, on either side, exclusive of the tectum.

TECTUM AND ASSOCIATED TRACTS

Inferior Colliculus

The inferior colliculus, which consists of a large nucleus made up of small and medium-sized cells, is incorporated in the auditory pathway to the cerebral cortex. Fibers of the lateral lemniscus envelop the nucleus and enter it from superficial and deep aspects (Fig. 7–12). The pathway continues through the *inferior brachium* to the *medial geniculate nucleus* of the thalamus (Figs. 7–13 through 7–15), and thence to the auditory cortical area of the temporal lobe. There are commissural fibers between the inferior colliculi, accounting in part for the bilateral cortical projection from either ear.

Some fibers from the inferior colliculus also pass forward into the superior colliculus. From the latter site, nerve impulses reach cranial nerve nuclei supplying the extraocular muscles and spinal motor neurons in the cervical region. A reflex pathway is thereby established for turning the eyes and head toward the source of a sound. Tectocerebellar fibers from the inferior colliculi enter the cerebellum by way of the superior medullary velum between the superior cerebellar peduncles and are distributed to the cerebellar cortex. The inferior colliculi evolved as increasingly significant structures in mammals concurrent with the development of the cortical area for hearing.

Superior Colliculus

The superior colliculi (Figs. 7–14 and 7–15) differ from the inferior colliculi in phylogenetic background and function. The optic lobes of the midbrain in lower animals are homologues of the superior colliculi, and the optic lobes constitute an important integrating center for visual, auditory, and somesthetic data. The visual pathway to the cerebral cortex bypassed the superior colliculi during mammalian phylogeny. Although the superior colliculi are relegated to the role of reflex centers, the importance of the optic lobes in lower animals leaves an imprint in the form of a complex histologic structure, consisting of seven alternating layers of white matter and gray matter.

The cortex of the occipital lobe is the most important source of afferent fibers to the superior colliculus in man. These corticotectal fibers come mainly from visual association cortex in the occipital lobe; the latter cortex surrounds the primary visual

area on which the retina projects after a synaptic relay in the lateral geniculate nucleus of the thalamus. Corticotectal fibers make up most of the *superior brachium*, which reaches the superior colliculus by passing between the pulvinar and the medial geniculate nucleus (Figs. 7–14 and 7–15). Through collicular efferents to be described, the above connection between the cortex and the superior colliculus is responsible for reflex movements of the eyes and head—as in following objects passing across the visual field (automatic scanning movements). Corticotectal connections also appear to be of significance in the ocular responses for accommodation to near objects; these responses consist of convergence of the eyes, thickening of the lens, and pupillary constriction. A few fibers of the optic tract, originating in the retina, bypass the lateral geniculate nucleus and reach the superior colliculus by way of the superior brachium. These fibers constitute the afferent limb of a reflex arc that allows turning of the eyes and head toward the source of a sudden visual stimulus, together with closing the eyelids and perhaps raising the arms for protection against an approaching object.

Other afferents to the superior colliculus are indicative of its role as a sensory integrative center in lower forms. As previously mentioned, fibers from the inferior colliculus convey impulses of cochlear origin. In addition, spinotectal fibers terminate in the superior colliculus, transmitting data from general sensory endings, of which cutaneous endings are the most important. Reflex connections are thereby established for directing the eyes and head toward the source of auditory and cutaneous stimuli.

Efferents from the superior colliculus are distributed to the spinal cord and nuclei of the brain stem. Fibers destined for the spinal cord curve around the periaqueductal gray matter, cross to the opposite side in the *dorsal tegmental decussation of*

lat. geniculate gang. ──────→ *occipital cortex*

retina *sudden visual stimuli* ─────→ *automatic scanning* ─ *turn eyes and head towards stimulus*

cutaneous stimuli → (*S.C*) ──→ *maybe raise arm*

spinotectal tract *sound stimulus* ─ *maybe close eyelids.*

I.C cochlear info

Meynert, and continue caudally near the midline as the *tectospinal tract* (Figs. 7–12 and 7–13). Efferents to the brain stem (tectobulbar fibers) are directed for the most part bilaterally. Some of them go to the oculomotor, trochlear, and abducens nuclei for eye movement responses (mainly scanning) and to the facial nucleus for protective closure of the eyelids when there is a sudden visual stimulus. Still other efferents terminate in the red nucleus, substantia nigra, and reticular formation. A projection to the cerebellum consists of tectopontine fibers to the dorsolateral region of the nuclei pontis (basal pons) and pontocerebellar fibers in the middle cerebellar peduncle. The connections of the superior colliculus with various motor nuclei are indicative of its earlier role as an important sensory integrative center.

The superior colliculi are interconnected by the *commissure of the superior colliculi* (Figs. 7–14 and 7–15). The *posterior commissure* is a robust bundle running transversely, just dorsal to the transition between the cerebral aqueduct and the third ventricle. A small piece of the commissure in the midline is included in the section illustrated in Figure 7–15. In spite of the large size of the posterior commissure, the source and termination of its constituent fibers are not well known. The superior colliculi of the two sides are interconnected by some of the fibers; others appear to originate in the habenular nuclei, which are in the diencephalon just in front of the tectum.

Pretectal Nucleus

The pretectal nucleus is a small group of cells situated immediately in front of the lateral edge of the superior colliculus; the nucleus receives fibers from the retina by way of the optic tract and superior brachium. Fibers leaving the pretectal nucleus pass around the periaqueductal gray matter to the Edinger–Westphal nucleus, a parasympathetic component of the oculomotor nuclear complex. The pretectal nucleus is part of a reflex pathway for the pupillary response to light, the pupil becoming smaller as the intensity of light increases.

TEGMENTUM

Fasciculi Proceeding to the Thalamus

The *medial lemniscus* continues to be a readily identifiable fasciculus as it traverses the midbrain in the lateral area of the tegmentum (Figs. 7–13 through 7–15). The *spinal lemniscus* is dorsolateral to the medial lemniscus, this spatial relationship being carried forward from the pontine tegmentum. Spinotectal fibers leave the spinal lemniscus to enter the superior colliculus; the lateral and ventral spinothalamic fibers continue into the diencephalon, where they end in the ventral posterior nucleus of the thalamus.

Red Nucleus and Associated Tracts

The red nucleus is a prominent motor component of the tegmentum. The nucleus is egg-shaped (round in transverse section), extending from the caudal limit of the superior colliculus into the subthalamic region of the diencephalon. The nucleus has a pinkish hue in a fresh specimen because it is more vascular than the surrounding tissue. Myelinated nerve fibers entering and leaving the nucleus give it a punctate appearance in Weigert-stained sections (Figs. 7–14 and 7–15).

The red nucleus is differentiated into two regions that differ in cytoarchitecture and connections. The caudal region is the older part phylogenetically; it consists of large cells in the midst of small neurons and is

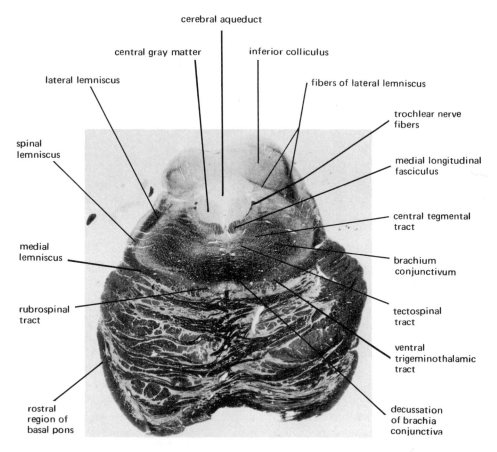

FIG. 7–12. Section through the basal pons and inferior colliculi of the midbrain. Weigert stain. ×3

known as the *pars magnocellularis*. The newer rostral portion is especially well developed in man; consisting of small cells only, it is called the *pars parvicellularis*.

While some of the connections of the red nucleus are well known, the evidence for others is equivocal and they are still under investigation. Afferents from the cerebellum and the cerebral cortex are best documented. Fibers originating in cerebellar nuclei constitute the brachium conjunctivum and enter the midbrain. Some of these fibers terminate in the red nucleus, especially the pars magnocellularis. The majority of the fibers of the superior bra-

chium pass through and around the red nucleus en route to a thalamic nucleus (the ventral lateral nucleus) which in turn projects to motor areas of the frontal lobe. These same areas give rise to numerous corticorubral fibers. Tectorubral fibers from the superior colliculus have been described. The pallidorubral connection, coming from the globus pallidus of the corpus striatum, appears to be largely indirect through a synaptic relay involving cells in the prerubral area of the subthalamus.

Of efferent connections of the red nucleus, fibers of the rubrospinal tract originate in the pars magnocellularis and cross

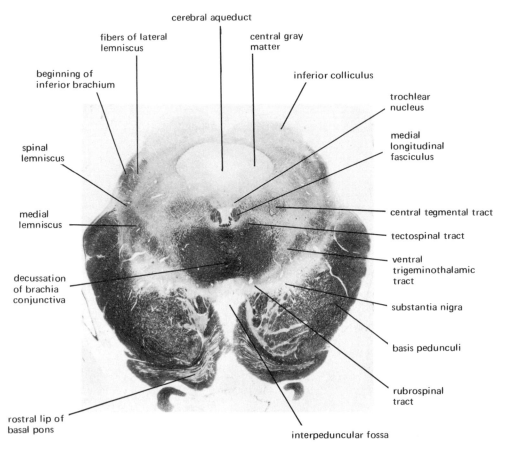

FIG. 7–13. Midbrain at the level of rostral portions of the inferior colliculi. Weigert stain. ×3

the midline at the level of the nucleus in the *ventral tegmental decussation of Forel.* Impulses of motor significance from the various sources projecting to the red nucleus are also relayed to lower motor neurons through rubroreticular and reticulospinal connections. Numerous rubro-olivary fibers arise from the pars parvocellularis and proceed to the inferior olivary complex through the central tegmental tract. The red nucleus sends a few fibers to cerebellar nuclei through the superior peduncle, and there is some evidence for reciprocal connections between the red nucleus and the substantia nigra. A projection from the red

nucleus to the ventral lateral nucleus of the thalamus has been described, but the existence of such fibers has not been substantiated by recent experimental work.

Nuclei of Cranial Nerves and Associated Fasciculi

Vestibulocochlear Nerve. Certain tracts originating in sensory nuclei of cranial nerves run forward into the midbrain and two such fasciculi are associated with the vestibulocochlear nerve. Of these, the *lateral lemniscus* for auditory conduction was identified when discussing the

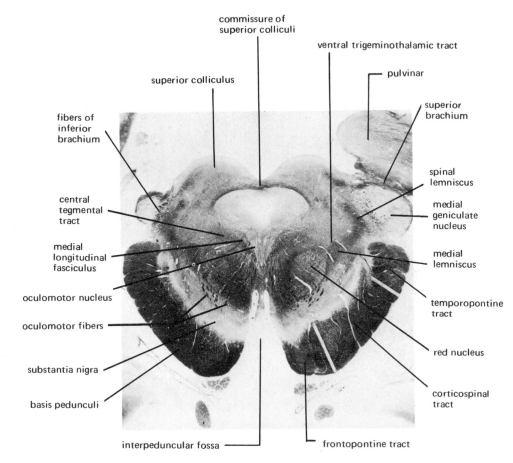

commissure of
superior colliculi

ventral trigeminothalamic tract

superior colliculus

pulvinar

fibers of
inferior
brachium

superior
brachium

spinal
lemniscus

central
tegmental
tract

medial
geniculate
nucleus

medial
longitudinal
fasciculus

medial
lemniscus

oculomotor nucleus

oculomotor fibers

temporopontine
tract

substantia nigra

red nucleus

basis pedunculi

corticospinal
tract

interpeduncular fossa

frontopontine tract

FIG. 7–14. Midbrain at the level of the superior colliculi. Weigert stain. ×3

inferior colliculus. The *medial longitudinal fasciculus is* situated adjacent to the midline (Figs. 7–12 through 7–15), in the same general position as at lower brain stem levels. Most of the constituent fibers of the latter fasciculus originate in vestibular nuclei, and those reaching the midbrain terminate in the trochlear and oculomotor nuclei. The fasciculus also contains association fibers connecting nuclei of the abducens, trochlear, and oculomotor nerves.

Trigeminal Nerve. The *ventral trigeminothalamic tract,* which arises from the nucleus of the spinal tract and the chief

sensory nucleus, continues through the midbrain near the medial lemniscus (Figs. 7–12 through 7–15). *Dorsal trigeminothalamic fibers* from the chief sensory nuclei of both sides run forward through the midbrain tegmentum some distance dorsal to the ventral tract. The *mesencephalic nucleus* of the trigeminal nerve continues from the pons into the lateral region of the periaqueductal gray matter throughout most of the midbrain.

Trochlear and Oculomotor Nerves. The *trochlear nucleus* is in the central gray matter at the level of the inferior colliculus,

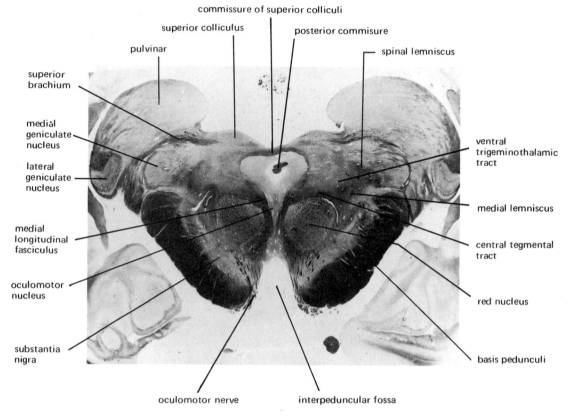

commissure of superior colliculi

superior colliculus

posterior commisure

pulvinar

spinal lemniscus

superior brachium

medial geniculate nucleus

lateral geniculate nucleus

ventral trigeminothalamic tract

medial longitudinal fasciculus

medial lemniscus

central tegmental tract

oculomotor nucleus

red nucleus

substantia nigra

basis pedunculi

oculomotor nerve

interpeduncular fossa

FIG. 7–15. Midbrain at the level of the rostral portions of the superior colliculi. Weigert stain. ×2

where it lies just dorsal to the medial longitudinal fasciculus (Fig. 7–13). Fibers from the nucleus curve dorsally around the central gray matter, with a caudal slope (Figs. 7–12 and 7–10). On reaching the dorsal surface of the brain stem, the fibers decussate in the superior medullary velum and emerge as the trochlear nerves just behind the inferior colliculi. The trochlear nerve supplies the superior oblique muscle of the eye.

The *oculomotor nucleus* is in the ventral area of the central gray matter and coextensive with the superior colliculus; the paired nuclei have a V-shaped outline in sections (Figs. 7–14 and 7–15). Bundles of fibers from the nucleus pursue a curved course through the tegmentum, many of

them traversing the red nucleus (Fig. 7–14), then emerge along the side of the interpeduncular fossa to form the oculomotor nerve (Fig. 7–15). The oculomotor nerve supplies the extraocular muscles, with the exception of the lateral rectus and superior oblique muscles, together with the striated fibers of the levator palpebrae superioris muscle. The oculomotor nucleus includes a parasympathetic component, the *Edinger–Westphal nucleus*, for the ciliary and constrictor pupillae muscles of the eye.

SUBSTANTIA NIGRA

The *substantia nigra* is a large motor nucleus, situated between the tegmentum and the basis pedunculi throughout the midbrain (Figs. 7–13 through 7–15) and extending into the subthalamic region of the diencephalon. The nucleus is rudimentary in lower vertebrates, makes its first definitive appearance in mammals, and is largest in the human brain. The neurons are multipolar and of medium size. The cells composing the *compact zone* adjacent to the tegmentum contain cytoplasmic inclusion granules of melanin pigment. These pigment-containing cells are most numerous in primates, especially in man. Melanin granules are scanty at birth, increase rapidly during childhood, and then more slowly throughout life. The pigment is said to be present in albinos. The region of the nucleus bordering the basis pedunculi is called the *reticular zone;* the cells here are lacking in pigment but contain significant amounts of iron compounds.

The connections of the substantia nigra have not been fully worked out, mainly because of technical difficulties. Corticonigral fibers from the frontal, parietal, and occipital lobes are rather numerous. Reciprocal connections between the substantia nigra and the corpus striatum, the red nucleus, and the reticular formation have been established with varying degrees of certainty. A projection from the substantia nigra to thalamic nuclei (ventral lateral and ventral anterior) has been described, but perhaps confirmation is needed.

In spite of the gaps in anatomic knowledge the importance of the substantia nigra as a motor center is manifest when one considers the disturbances of motor function in paralysis agitans or Parkinson's disease. In this crippling disorder, there is muscular rigidity, a fine tremor, a slow and shuffling gait, mask-like facies, and other abnormalities. The most consistent pathologic finding in Parkinson's disease is degeneration of the melanin-containing cells in the compact portion of the substantia nigra. Biochemical and histochemical studies offer a lead to therapy. Under normal circumstances the chemical dihydroxytyramine (dopamine) is present in the pigmented cells of the substantia nigra and in the corpus striatum, while there is virtual absence of dopamine at these sites in Parkinson's disease. These observations led to the suggestion that the substantia nigra may have, as part of an undoubtedly complex role, an inhibitory effect on nuclei to which it projects (especially the corpus striatum) through release of dopamine. Administration of dopamine is an obvious form of biochemical therapy to explore. However, dopamine does not cross the blood-brain barrier, so a metabolic precursor that does gain access to brain tissue is used instead. This precursor is dihydroxyphenylalanine (dopa). The administration of L-dopa, which crosses the blood–brain barrier more readily than D-dopa and has fewer side effects, shows considerable promise as a therapeutic agent for ameliorating some of the abnormalities of motor function in Parkinson's disease.

The significance of melanin in the substantia nigra is not known. However, melanin is related chemically to the metabolic sequence that includes dopamine. This sequence, carried out by means of the appropriate enzyme at each step, is: phenylalanine, tyrosine, dihydroxyphenylalanine (dopa), dihydroxytyramine (dopamine), norepinephrine, and epinephrine. Melanin pigment is produced by the action of the enzyme tyrosinase on dopa; this is the basis of the "dopa reaction" for the identification of melanocytes, or melanin-producing cells, in the skin or elsewhere. Melanocytes contain tyrosinase, and melanin is formed when dopa is made available as a substrate to tissue sections. Melanin pigment may be an inert byproduct of the essential biochemical reactions in the substantia nigra. The increase in amount of pigment with age is consistent with such a hypothesis.

BASIS PEDUNCULI

The *basis pedunculi* consists of fibers of the pyramidal and corticopontine systems (Figs. 7–13 through 7–15). Pyramidal fibers, most of them *corticospinal,* make up the middle three-fifths of the basis pedunculi. The somatotopic arrangement of corticospinal fibers, in a medial to lateral direction, is that of fibers for the neck, arm, trunk, and leg. *Corticobulbar fibers* for the oculomotor and trochlear nuclei proceed to these nuclei through the tegmentum of the midbrain; some of the corticobulbar fibers for other cranial nerves also leave the basis pedunculi and continue to their destination through the tegmentum of the midbrain and pons. Such corticobulbar fibers as remain continue caudally in the basis pedunculi, where they are situated between the corticospinal and frontopontine tracts. *Corticopontine fibers* are divided into two large fasciculi. The *frontopontine tract* occupies the medial one-fifth of the basis pedunculi. The lateral one-fifth consists of the *temporopontine tract*, which is inappropriately named because most of the constituent fibers originate in the cortex of the parietal lobe.

VISCERAL PATHWAYS IN THE BRAIN STEM

Central pathways related to visceral innervation are less well defined anatomically than many of the somatic sensory and motor pathways. For these reasons, and because many of the constituent fibers are unmyelinated, identification of visceral pathways has presented technical problems.

Primary visceral afferent neurons at spinal cord levels accompany the parasympathetic division of the autonomic system in the sacral region and the sympathetic division in the thoracic and upper lumbar regions. In addition to their involvement in spinal visceral reflexes, the sacral afferents convey information related to the feeling of fullness in the bladder and rectum, and perhaps pain in pelvic viscera. The thoracic and upper lumbar afferents are concerned with pain of visceral origin, in addition to visceral reflex responses. The *ascending visceral pathway,* which consists in part of spinospinalis relays in the cord, continues through the brain stem as polysynaptic relays involving cells of the reticular formation. By this means, data of visceral origin reach the ventral posterior thalamic nucleus, intralaminar nuclei of the thalamus, and the hypothalamus.

The more important visceral afferents physiologically reach the nucleus of the solitary tract in the medulla by way of the vagus and glossopharyngeal nerves. These nerves include general visceral afferents for visceral reflexes, in which the dorsal motor nucleus of the vagus is the principal efferent component. The nucleus of the solitary tract also receives afferents for taste through the vagus, glossopharyngeal, and facial nerves. Data for taste (a special visceral sense) are relayed to parasympathetic nuclei of the brain stem, notably the salivatory nuclei and the dorsal motor nucleus of the vagus nerve. In addition to the above reflex connections, fibers from the nucleus of the solitary tract join the internal arcuate fibers and ascend in the contralateral brain stem. These fibers travel rostrally near the medial lemniscus, probably in the region of the ventral trigeminothalamic tract, conduction along this route being supplemented by relays in the reticular formation. The principal destinations are the hypothalamus and the ventral posterior thalamic nucleus. From the latter site, information with respect to taste is relayed to a cortical taste area in the parietal lobe.

There are two descending fasciculi, whose cells of origin are located in the hypothalamus. *Mammillotegmental fibers* originate in the mammillary nucleus of the hypothalamus; they are distributed to the reticular formation of the midbrain, which has connections with autonomic nuclei throughout the neuraxis. Fibers from other hypothalamic nuclei run caudally in the *dorsal longitudinal fasciculus* (of Schütz), a bundle of unmyelinated fibers in the periaqueductal gray matter of the midbrain, and terminate in the autonomic nuclei and reticular formation of the brain stem. (Some of the ascending visceral fibers going to the hypothalamus are also in the dorsal longitudinal fasciculus.) Impulses of hypothalamic origin reach the intermediolateral cell column of the cord and the sacral parasympathetic nucleus by way of reticulospinal connections.

ANATOMIC AND CLINICAL CORRELATIONS

Of the various types of pathology affecting the brain stem, vascular lesions are among the more important. Hemorrhage into the brain stem usually has serious consequences because of the presence of nuclei that control the vital functions of respiration and circulation. The neurologic signs resulting from vascular occlusion depend on the location and size of the affected region. The following examples are presented to show the correlation between neurologic signs and the location of the lesion.

The *medial medullary syndrome* results from occlusion of a medullary branch of the vertebral artery; the size of the infarction depends on the distribution of the

particular artery involved. In the example shown in Figure 7–16, the affected area includes the pyramid and most of the medial lemniscus on one side. The lesion extends far enough laterally to include fibers of the hypoglossal nerve as they pass between the medial lemniscus and the inferior olivary nucleus. A patient with this particular lesion has contralateral hemiparesis; there is loss of sensations of position and movement, discriminative touch, and vibration on the opposite side of the body. Paralysis of the tongue muscles is ipsilateral, however, and the tongue deviates to the affected side on protrusion because the action of the healthy genioglossus muscle is unopposed. This is an example of crossed or alternating paralysis, in which the body is affected on the side opposite the lesion, while muscles supplied by a cranial nerve are affected on the same side as the lesion. The condition is therefore known as *alternating hypoglossal hemiplegia*.

Occlusion of a vessel supplying the lateral area of the medulla results in the *lateral medullary* or *Wallenberg's syndrome*. The occluded vessel may be the posterior inferior cerebellar artery, or medullary branches of this artery or the vertebral artery. The extent of the infarcted area is typically that shown in Figure 7–17. Inclusion of the spinal trigeminal tract and its nucleus is responsible for ipsilateral loss of pain and temperature sensibility in the area of distribution of the trigeminal nerve. Pain and temperature sensibility is absent on the opposite side of the body because of interruption of fibers of the lateral spinothalamic tract in the spinal lemniscus. The medial lemniscus being intact, touch sensation is diminished rather than abolished. Destruction of the nucleus ambiguus causes paralysis of muscles of the soft palate, pharynx, and larynx on the side of the lesion, with difficulty in swallowing and

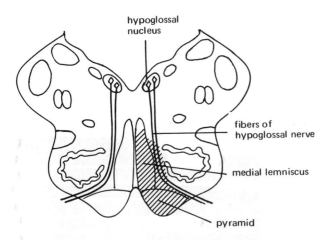

FIG. 7–16. Site of a lesion producing the medial medullary syndrome.

speaking. The pathway from the hypothalamus to the intermediolateral cell column of the cord through the reticular formation may be included in the area of degeneration. The signs of a lateral medullary lesion may therefore include Horner's syndrome which consists of a small pupil, slight drooping of the upper eyelid (pto-sis), slight enophthalmos, and sometimes warm, dry, skin of the face, all on the side of the lesion. The infarcted region may extend dorsally to include the base of the inferior cerebellar peduncle and vestibular nuclei causing dizziness, cerebellar ataxia, and nystagmus. Cerebellar signs are more pronounced, of course, if infarction of part

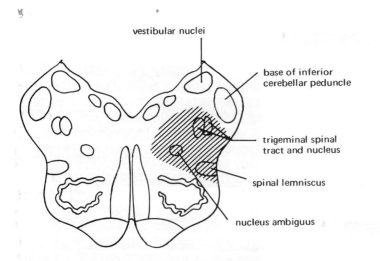

FIG. 7–17. Site of a lesion producing the lateral medullary syndrome.

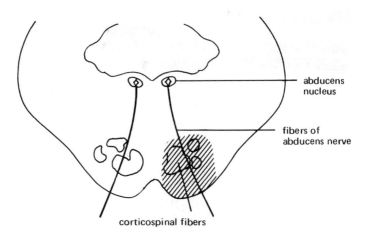

FIG. 7–18. Site of a basal pontine lesion involving the pyramidal tract and abducens nerve.

of the cerebellum is added to that of the medulla (posterior inferior cerebellar artery thrombosis).

Lesions in the basal region of the pons or midbrain may produce alternating paralysis, similar to that described in the first example. Figure 7–18 illustrates an area of infarction in one side of the caudal region of the pons, resulting from occlusion of a pontine branch of the basilar artery. Interruption of corticospinal fibers causes contralateral hemiparesis, while inclusion of abducens nerve fibers in the lesion causes paralysis of the lateral rectus muscle on the ipsilateral side and an internal strabismus or squint.

The position of a vascular lesion in the basal region of a cerebral peduncle, such as might follow occlusion of a branch of the posterior cerebral artery, is shown in Figure 7–19. A lesion at this site causes *Weber's syndrome,* in which there is con-

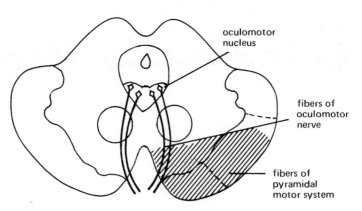

FIG. 7–19. Site of a lesion in the midbrain involving the pyramidal tract and oculomotor nerve.

tralateral hemiparesis, due to interruption of pyramidal tract fibers, and ipsilateral paralysis of ocular muscles because of inclusion of oculomotor nerve fibers in the infarcted area. There is paralysis of all the extraocular muscles except the lateral rectus and superior oblique muscles. The most obvious signs are external strabismus and loss of ability to raise the upper eyelid, together with dilation of the pupil because of interruption of parasympathetic fibers supplying the constrictor pupillae muscle.

SUGGESTIONS FOR ADDITIONAL READING

Barbeau A: L–dopa therapy in Parkinson's disease: A critical review of nine years' experience. Can Med Assoc J 101:791–800, 1969

Calne DB, Sandler M: L–dopa and Parkinsonism. Nature (London) 226:21–24, 1970

Cooke JD, Larson B, Oscarsson O, Sjölund B: Origin and termination of cuneocerebellar tract. Exp Brain Res 13:339–358, 1971

Costa E, Côté LJ, Yahr MD (eds.): Biochemistry and Pharmacology of the Basal Ganglia. New York, Raven Press, 1965

Courville J: Connections of the red nucleus with the cerebellum and certain caudal brain stem structures: A review with functional considerations. Rev Can Biol 27:127–144, 1968

Crosby EC, Humphrey T, Lauer EW: Correlative Anatomy of the Nervous System. New York, Macmillan, 1962

Currier RD, Giles CL, DeJong RN: Some comments on Wallenberg's lateral medullary syndrome. Neurology (Minneap) 11:778–791, 1961

Edwards SB: The ascending and descending projections of the red nucleus in the cat: An experimental study using an autoradiographic tracing method. Brain Res 48:45–63, 1972

Falck B: Observations on the possibilities of the cellular localization of monoamines by a fluorescence method. Acta Physiol Scand 56 (Suppl 197): 1–25, 1962

Kuypers HGJM, Lawrence DG: Cortical projections to the red nucleus and the brain stem in the rhesus monkey. Brain Res 4:151–188, 1967

Lassek AM: The Pyramidal Tract. Springfield, Ill., Thomas, 1954

Marsden CD: Pigmentation in the nuclei substantiae nigrae of mammals. J Anat 95:256–261, 1961

Massion J: The mammalian red nucleus. Physiol Rev 47:383–436, 1967

Miller RA, Burack E: Atlas of the Central Nervous System in Man. Baltimore, Williams & Wilkins, 1968

Olszewski J, Baxter D: Cytoarchitecture of the Human Brain Stem. Basel, Karger, 1954

Poirier LJ: Experimental and historical study of midbrain dyskinesias. J Neurophysiol 23:534–551, 1960

Poirier LJ, Bouvier G: The red nucleus and its efferent nervous pathways in the monkey. J Comp Neurol 128:223–243, 1966

Pollack M, Hornabrook RW: The prevalence, natural history and dementia of Parkinson's disease. Brain 89:429–448, 1966

Riley HA: An Atlas of the Basal Ganglia, Brain Stem and Spinal Cord. New York, Hafner, 1960

Rinvik E: The cortico-nigral projection in the cat: An experimental study with silver impregnation methods. J Comp Neurol 126:241–254, 1966

Stern G: The effects of lesions in the substantia nigra. Brain 89:449–478, 1966

Truex RC, Carpenter MB: Human Neuroanatomy, 6th ed. Baltimore, Williams & Wilkins, 1969

Voorhoeve PE: Some neurophysiological aspects of Parkinson's disease. Psychiatr Neurol Neurochir 73:329–338, 1970

8
Cranial Nerves

The cranial nerves, listed in the order in which numbers are assigned to them, are as follows:

1. Olfactory
2. Optic
3. Oculomotor
4. Trochlear
5. Trigeminal
6. Abducens
7. Facial
8. Vestibulocochlear
9. Glossopharyngeal
10. Vagus
11. Accessory
12. Hypoglossal

In addition to motor and general sensory functions, five systems for the special senses are served by various cranial nerves. In these, the receptors are localized and highly specialized, in contrast to general sensory endings, which are scattered throughout the tissues of the body and are relatively simple in structure. Of the special senses, the olfactory system is an integral part of the forebrain and is discussed in Chapter 17. Discussion of the optic and vestibulocochlear nerves is set aside for the section on systemic neuroanatomy, in which the visual, auditory, and vestibular systems are described (Chapters 20, 21, and 22). There remains the special sense of taste (gustatory system), certain aspects of which are included in the present chapter because the primary sensory neurons for taste are included with sensory neurons having other functions in the facial, glossopharyngeal, and vagus nerves.

OCULOMOTOR, TROCHLEAR, AND ABDUCENS NERVES

The third, fourth, and sixth cranial nerves supply the extraocular muscles with motor fibers; their nuclei therefore consist of multipolar motor neurons and receive afferents from the same sources. The oculomotor nucleus includes a parasympathetic component (the Edinger–Westphal nucleus) for the constrictor pupillae and ciliary muscles of the eye.

119

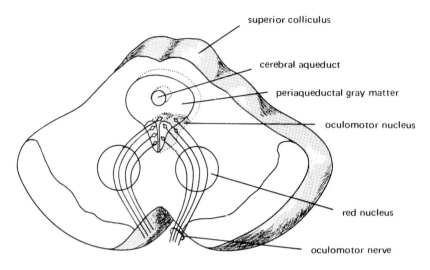

FIG. 8–1. Components of the oculomotor nerve in the midbrain.

OCULOMOTOR NERVE

The *oculomotor nucleus* is situated in the periaqueductal gray matter of the midbrain, ventral to the aqueduct and coextensive with the superior colliculus (Fig. 8–1). The paired nuclei have a triangular outline in transverse section and are bounded by the medial longitudinal fasciculi. (The reader may wish to refer to illustrations in the preceding chapter for the topography of cranial nerve components in Weigert-stained sections.) The cells for individual extraocular muscles (including the levator palpebrae superioris muscle) are localized in longitudinal groups; these subnuclei are represented bilaterally, except for one, which is situated dorsocaudally in the midline. According to Warwick's schema for the oculomotor nucleus of the monkey (Fig. 8–2), there are three laterally disposed cell groups, which supply the in-

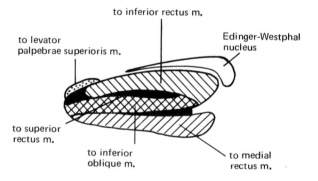

FIG. 8–2. Warwick's schema for the organization of the oculomotor nucleus (lateral view of the right oculomotor nucleus). (From Warwick R: J Comp Neurol 98:449–504, 1953)

ferior rectus, inferior oblique, and medial rectus muscles. On the medial side of these there is a subnucleus for the superior rectus muscle. The unpaired cell group, which is called the caudal central nucleus, supplies the levator palpebrae superioris muscle on either side. Medullated axons from the oculomotor nucleus curve ventrally through the tegmentum, many of them traversing the red nucleus. The fibers emerge as a series of roots along the side of the interpeduncular fossa, and these roots converge immediately to form the oculomotor nerve. Oculomotor fibers are partly crossed and partly uncrossed. Although full details are lacking for man, it appears that uncrossed fibers only supply the medial rectus, inferior rectus, and inferior oblique muscles. The superior rectus muscle receives crossed fibers only, and the levator palpebrae superioris muscle has an essentially bilateral innervation from the unpaired caudal central nucleus. (Smooth muscle fibers of the levator are supplied by sympathetic nerves.) Earlier accounts included a midline nucleus in the caudal two-thirds of the oculomotor complex. It was known as the nucleus of Perlia and was considered as a center for ocular convergence; it is doubtful that such a nucleus and center exist. The small size of the motor unit, in which about six muscle fibers are supplied by a nerve fiber, attests to the delicate neuromuscular mechanisms required for coordinated movement of the eyes in binocular vision.

The *Edinger–Westphal nucleus* is situated in the median plane, dorsal to the rostral two-thirds of the main oculomotor nucleus (Fig. 8–2). The cells are small and tend to be spindle-shaped, like other preganglionic parasympathetic neurons. Fibers from the Edinger–Westphal nucleus accompany other oculomotor fibers into the orbit, where they terminate in the ciliary ganglion. Postganglionic fibers then pass through short ciliary nerves to the constrictor pupillae and ciliary muscles of the eye.

A lesion interrupting fibers of the oculomotor nerve causes paralysis of all extraocular muscles except the superior oblique and lateral rectus muscles. The constrictor muscle of the pupil and the ciliary muscle are likewise paralyzed. The consequences of such a lesion are external strabismus (unopposed action of the lateral rectus muscle), inability to move the eye inward or vertically, and closure of the eye through drooping of the upper lid (ptosis). Interruption of the parasympathetic fibers causes dilation of the pupil because of unopposed action of the dilator pupillae muscle of the iris, which has a sympathetic innervation. There is no longer pupillary constriction in response to an increase in light intensity or to accommodation for near objects. Neither does the ciliary muscle contract to allow the lens to increase in thickness for focusing on a near object.

TROCHLEAR NERVE

The *trochlear nucleus* for the superior oblique muscle is immediately caudal to the oculomotor nucleus, at the level of the inferior colliculus (Fig. 8–3). Trochlear nerve fibers have an unusual course, and this is the only nerve to emerge from the dorsum of the brain stem. Small bundles of fibers wind around the periaqueductal gray matter with a caudal slope and decussate in the superior medullary velum with fibers from the companion nucleus; the slender nerve emerges just behind the inferior colliculus. The superior oblique muscle, like the superior rectus, is therefore supplied by crossed fibers. Paralysis of the superior oblique muscle impairs ability to turn the eye downward and outward. The defect is difficult to detect on clinical examination,

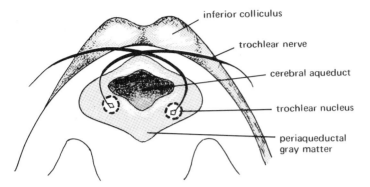

FIG. 8–3. The trochlear nerve in the midbrain.

but a person so affected may experience difficulty in walking downstairs.

ABDUCENS NERVE

The *abducens nucleus* for the lateral rectus muscle is situated beneath the facial colliculus in the floor of the fourth ventricle (Fig. 8–4). A bundle of facial nerve fibers curves over the nucleus, contributing to the facial colliculus. Fibers from the abducens nucleus pass through the pons in a ventrocaudal direction, emerging from the brain stem at the junction of the pons and the pyramid. Interruption of the abducens nerve causes internal strabismus and inability to direct the affected eye laterally. Functional impairment of any of the extraocular muscles causes diplopia (double vision).

AFFERENTS TO NUCLEI SUPPLYING EXTRAOCULAR MUSCLES

The main part of the oculomotor nucleus (i.e., all but the parasympathetic compo-

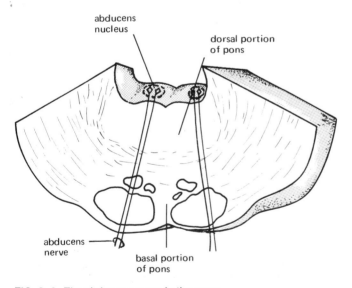

FIG. 8–4. The abducens nerve in the pons.

nent) and the trochlear and abducens nuclei receive fibers from the same sources, as is to be expected. *Tectobulbar fibers* from the superior colliculus function in connection with several ocular movements. These include scanning, reflex turning of the eyes toward the source of visual, auditory, or cutaneous stimuli, and probably ocular changes when accommodating to near objects. The *medial longitudinal fasciculus,* which lies adjacent to the three nuclei, carries impulses from the vestibular nuclei and provides for coordinated movements of the eyes and head. Included in the fasciculus are axons of cells within the nuclei for extraocular muscles (or cells situated close to the nuclei). These fibers, which are crossed and uncrossed, pass from one nucleus to another. They have the important function of coordinating the action of extraocular muscles, precise coordination being essential to avoid diplopia in binocular vision. Cells in the reticular formation adjacent to the abducens nucleus are thought to constitute a *parabducens nucleus*, which functions as a "center for lateral gaze." These cells send fibers to the ipsilateral abducens nucleus and, through the medial longitudinal fasciculus, to those cells of the contralateral oculomotor nucleus that supply the medial rectus muscle. The actions of the medial and lateral recti muscles are thereby coordinated in horizontal movements of the eyes.

Corticobulbar fibers for voluntary eye movements originate mainly in the primary motor area of the frontal lobe. It is a general rule that small internuncial neurons in the brain stem intervene between corticobulbar fibers and motor nuclei of cranial nerves. Although corticobulbar fibers to the oculomotor, trochlear, and abducens nuclei are predominantly crossed, there is a substantial number of uncrossed fibers. Voluntary paralysis of the extraocular muscles is not, therefore, a feature of upper motor neuron lesions.[*] However, anterior to the primary motor area there is a cortical area known as the "frontal eye field," which has a special role in voluntary scanning movements. The pathway from the frontal eye field to the third, fourth, and sixth nerve nuclei has not been determined with certainty. The fibers are no doubt closely associated with the corticobulbar fibers mentioned above, but whether there is a relay in the superior colliculus has not been resolved. In any event, damage to the frontal eye field causes paralysis of contralateral gaze and transient deviation of the eyes to the side of an acute lesion.

CONNECTIONS OF THE EDINGER–WESTPHAL NUCLEUS

Since the Edinger–Westphal nucleus is an autonomic nucleus, it receives fibers from the hypothalamus through the *dorsal longitudinal fasciculus.* However, the more important afferents from the clinical point of view are those concerned with reflex responses to light and accommodation. An increase in the intensity of light falling on the retina causes constriction of the pupil.

[*] In the discussion of lesions of the spinal cord in Chapter 5, it was pointed out that voluntary movements involving the axial and limb musculature are mediated through both the corticospinal tract and extrapyramidal pathways. By extrapolation, extrapyramidal pathways, in addition to the corticobulbar tract, may function in the voluntary control of muscles that are supplied by cranial nerves. Of several possible pathways that may be involved and which would be of interest in connection with an upper motor neuron lesion, there are corticorubral and corticoreticular connections, together with projections from the red nucleus and reticular formation to motor nuclei of cranial nerves. However, there are no experimental or clinical data that shed light on this matter. The neural mechanisms for voluntary contraction of some head muscles, in particular muscles lacking skeletal attachments, may differ from those for the muscles generally.

The afferent limb of the reflex arc consists of fibers in the optic nerve and tract reaching the *pretectal nucleus* by way of the superior brachium. The pretectal nucleus projects to the Edinger–Westphal nucleus, from which fibers traverse the oculomotor nerve to the ciliary ganglion in the orbital cavity. Postganglionic fibers travel through the short ciliary nerves to the constrictor pupillae muscle of the iris.

The reflex response to accommodation accompanies ocular convergence produced by voluntary fixation on a near object. The efferent limb of the reflex arc consists of pre- and postganglionic fibers from the Edinger–Westphal nucleus and ciliary ganglion, respectively. The postganglionic fibers supply the ciliary muscle which, on contraction, allows the lens to increase in thickness, thereby increasing refractive power for focusing on a near object. The constrictor pupillae muscle contracts at the same time, sharpening the image by decreasing the diameter of the pupil and reducing spherical aberration in the refractive media. The afferent side of the reflex pathway for accommodation is not entirely clear. The impulses appear to be cortical in origin, and the most probable source is cortex of the occipital lobe in which the visual area receiving data from the retina is located. The pathway may be from cortex of the occipital lobe to the superior colliculus and then to the oculomotor nucleus, or from occipital cortex to the motor cortex of the frontal lobe and then to the oculomotor nucleus through corticobulbar fibers. The pathways for pupillary responses to light and accommodation are obviously different because the reflexes may be disassociated by disease. For example, in the Argyll Robertson pupil there is constriction of the pupil when attention is directed to a near object, although pupillary constriction in response to light is absent. The Argyll Robertson pupil is characteristically seen in patients with tabes dorsalis, a syphilitic disease of the central nervous system.

TRIGEMINAL NERVE

The *trigeminal nerve* is the principal sensory nerve for the head and the motor nerve for the muscles of mastication.

SENSORY COMPONENTS

The cell bodies of most of the primary sensory neurons are in the *semilunar* or *gasserian ganglion*, the remainder being in the mesencephalic nucleus. The peripheral processes of semilunar ganglion cells constitute the ophthalmic and maxillary nerves and the sensory component of the mandibular nerve. (The mandibular nerve in particular includes sensory fibers from the mesencephalic nucleus, as will be discussed presently.) The trigeminal nerve is responsible for general sensation from the skin of the face and forehead, the scalp as far back as the vertex of the head, the mucosa of the oral and nasal cavities and the sinuses, and the teeth (Fig. 8–5). The trigeminal nerve also contributes sensory fibers to most of the dura mater. The scalp of the back of the head and an area of skin at the angle of the jaw are supplied by the second and third cervical nerves. The external ear has a complicated and overlapping innervation. The anterior border of the ear, anterior wall of the auditory canal, and anterior part of the tympanic membrane receive trigeminal fibers. The external ear in general, most of the auditory canal and tympanic membrane, and a cutaneous area behind the ear are supplied by the facial and vagus nerves—in some instances by the glossopharyngeal nerve, and by the second and third cervical nerves.

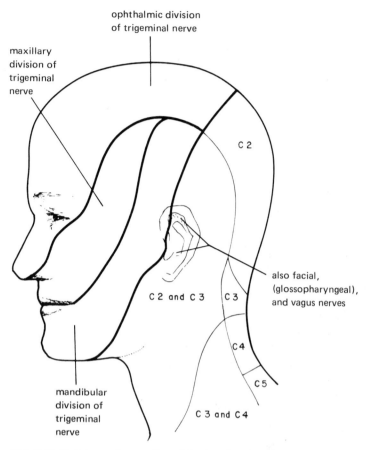

ophthalmic division
of trigeminal nerve

maxillary
division of
trigeminal
nerve

C 2

also facial,
(glossopharyngeal),
and vagus nerves

C 2 and C 3   C 3

C 4

C 5

mandibular
division of
trigeminal
nerve

C 3 and C 4

FIG. 8–5. Cutaneous innervation of the head and neck.

Chief Sensory Nucleus

The central processes of semilunar ganglion cells make up the large sensory root of the trigeminal nerve; these fibers enter the pons and terminate in the chief sensory nucleus and the nucleus of the trigeminal spinal tract. The chief sensory nucleus, also called the principal or superior nucleus, is in the dorsolateral area of the pontine tegmentum at the level of entry of the sensory fibers (Fig. 8–6). Fibers of large diameter for discriminative touch terminate in the chief sensory nucleus. Other fibers of medium caliber divide on nearing the chief sensory nucleus; one branch enters this nucleus and

the other branch turns caudally in the spinal tract to end in the nucleus of the spinal tract. These afferents are for simple touch and pressure, and both nuclei must therefore participate in these modalities of sensation. The chief sensory nucleus is essentially a mammalian nucleus, developing along with encapsulated tactile endings.

Trigeminal Spinal Tract and Nucleus of the Spinal Tract

Large numbers of sensory root fibers of intermediate size and many fine, unmyelinated fibers turn caudally on entering the pons. These fibers, which conduct impulses for pain and temperature, combine with descending branches of afferents mentioned above to form the trigeminal spinal tract (Fig. 8–6). (As will be described

later, the spinal tract includes a relatively small complement of fibers from the facial, glossopharyngeal, and vagus nerves. The latter fibers conduct general sensory data from the external ear and the mucosa of the

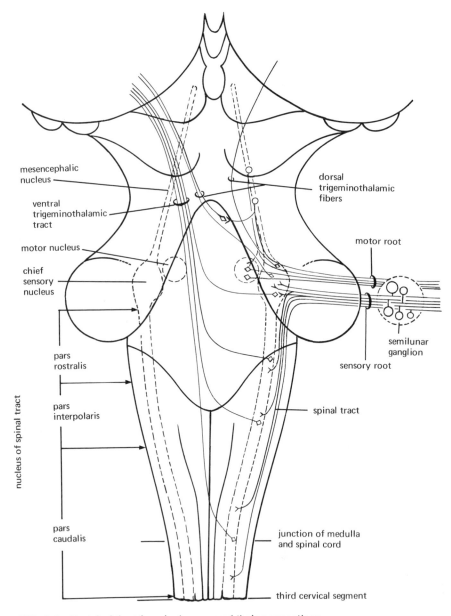

FIG. 8–6. Nuclei of the trigeminal nerve and their connections.

posterior third of the tongue, the pharynx, and the larynx.) Some of the spinal tract fibers descend as far as the upper three segments of the cord, where they inter-mingle with fibers of the dorsolateral fas-ciculus or Lissauer's zone. There is a spatial arrangement of fibers in the sensory root and spinal tract, corresponding to the three divisions of the trigeminal nerve. In the sensory root, ophthalmic fibers are dorsal, mandibular fibers ventral, and max-illary fibers in between. There is a rotation of the fibers as they approach the brain stem, with the result that the mandibular fibers are dorsal and the ophthalmic fibers ventral in the trigeminal spinal tract.

Fibers of the spinal tract terminate in the subjacent nucleus of the spinal tract (Fig. 8–6). This nucleus extends from the chief sensory nucleus to the caudal limit of the medulla; the nucleus of the spinal tract and the apical portion of the dorsal gray horn are indistinguishable from one another in the upper three cervical segments of the spinal cord. Based on cytoarchitecture, the nucleus of the spinal tract is divided into three regions or subnuclei. In the *pars caudalis*, a layer of small cells identical with the substantia gelatinosa lies external to a zone containing larger neurons, the latter zone being similar cytologically to the chief nucleus of the dorsal horn. The pars caudalis receives fibers for pain, tempera-ture, touch, and pressure, those for pain and temperature predominating. As in the substantia gelatinosa, there is integration, modification, and screening of incoming data by means of the small association-type neurons. It will be apparent that the pars caudalis is essentially a rostral extension of the apical region of the dorsal gray horn of the cord. Similarly, the trigeminal spinal tract in the region of the pars caudalis is comparable to the dorsolateral fasciculus of Lissauer. In the first three cervical segments these structures are concerned with pain

and temperature in both the trigeminal area of distribution and that of the upper four cervical nerves (neck and back of head).

Of the remaining two regions of the nucleus of the spinal tract (Fig. 8–6), the *pars interpolaris* is characterized by the presence of rather large cells scattered among diffusely arranged small and medium-sized neurons. In the *pars rostralis* there is a more dense arrangement of cells of small and medium size. Fibers of the spinal tract terminating in these regions appear to be concerned in the main with touch and pressure sensibilities. Some of the fibers are descending branches of affer-ents that also send a branch to the chief sensory nucleus. There is still much to be learned about the functional properties of the pars interpolaris and pars rostralis and, indeed, the whole of the nucleus of the tri-geminal spinal tract.

Efferent fibers from the sensory trigemi-nal nuclei proceed in various directions. Some of them connect with motor nuclei of the trigeminal and facial nerves, the nu-cleus ambiguus, and the hypoglossal nu-cleus for reflex responses to stimuli arising in the area of distribution of the trigeminal nerve. For example, touching the cornea causes the eyelids to close reflexly; the afferent fibers are in the ophthalmic nerve and the efferent fibers of the reflex arc are in the facial nerve. As a further example, irritation of the nasal mucosa causes sneez-ing. For this reflex, afferent impulses in the maxillary nerve are relayed to motor nuclei of the trigeminal and facial nerves, the nucleus ambiguus, the hypoglossal nucleus, and (through a reticulospinal relay) to the phrenic nucleus and motor cells in the cord supplying the intercostals and other respi-ratory muscles.

Fibers from the sensory nuclei are also distributed to the reticular formation; they are an important source of cutaneous stimuli for the ascending reticular activating system. Other fibers enter the cerebellum through the inferior peduncle. The principal pathway from the chief sensory and spinal nuclei to the thalamus (ventral posterior nucleus) is the crossed *ventral trigeminothalamic tract* (Fig. 8–6), which ascends close to the medial lemniscus. Fewer crossed and uncrossed fibers proceed from the chief sensory nucleus to the thalamus in the *dorsal trigeminothalamic tract.*

Mesencephalic Nucleus

The mesencephalic nucleus consists of a slender strand of cells extending from the chief sensory nucleus through the midbrain (Fig. 8–6). The nucleus is located beneath the lateral edge of the floor of the fourth ventricle in the pons and in the lateral region of the periaqueductal gray matter in the midbrain. The unipolar cells are primary sensory neurons in an unusual location; they are the only such cells that are incorporated in the neuraxis, rather than being in cerebrospinal ganglia. Fibers from the nucleus constitute the slender *mesencephalic root* of the trigeminal nerve which runs alongside the mesencephalic nucleus. The single process of each cell divides into a peripheral and a central branch. Most of the peripheral branches (dendrites) enter the motor root of the trigeminal nerve and are distributed with the mandibular division (Fig. 8–6). These fibers end in deep receptors of proprioceptive type in the region of the temporomandibular joint and adjacent to the teeth of the lower jaw, and also in neuromuscular spindles in the muscles of mastication. Some dendrites from the mesencephalic nucleus traverse the sensory root and semilunar ganglion for distribution by way of the maxillary division to endings in the hard palate and adjacent to the teeth of the upper jaw. Central branches (axons) of the single processes terminate in the trigeminal motor

nuclei of both sides, with or without a relay in the reticular formation. This connection establishes the stretch reflex originating in neuromuscular spindles in the masticatory muscles, together with a reflex for control of the force of the bite. Other central branches synapse with cells of the reticular formation, from which fibers proceed to the ventral posterior thalamic nucleus along with dorsal trigeminothalamic fibers. In addition, fibers from the mesencephalic nucleus enter the cerebellum through the superior peduncle.

MOTOR COMPONENT

The *motor nucleus* of the trigeminal nerve, consisting of typical multipolar neurons, is situated medial to the chief sensory nucleus (Fig. 8–6). Fibers from the motor nucleus constitute the bulk of the motor root, which joins sensory fibers just distal to the semilunar ganglion to form the mandibular nerve. This nerve supplies the muscles of mastication (masseter, temporal, and lateral and medial pterygoid muscles) and several small muscles. The latter consist of the tensor tympani, tensor veli palatini, digastric (anterior belly), and mylohyoid muscles. The motor nucleus receives afferents from the corticobulbar tract; most of these are crossed, but there is a significant proportion of uncrossed fibers. Afferents for reflexes come mainly from the sensory trigeminal nuclei, including the mesencephalic nucleus. Cells supplying the tensor tympani muscle receive acoustic fibers from the superior olivary nucleus. By reflex contraction, the tensor tympani muscle checks excessive movement of the tympanic membrane in response to loud sounds.

SOME CLINICAL COMMENTS

Of pathologic conditions affecting the trigeminal complex, major trigeminal neuralgia or *tic douloureux* is of special importance because of the excruciating pain. Tic douloureux is characterized by paroxysms of pain in the area of distribution of one of the trigeminal divisions, usually with periods of remission and exacerbation. The maxillary nerve is most frequently involved, then the mandibular, and least frequently, the ophthalmic nerve. The paroxysm, which is of sudden onset, may be set off by mild stimulation of the face, such as touching the skin; there is often an especially sensitive "trigger zone." The cause of tic douloureux is not known. A pathologic process affecting the cells of the semilunar ganglion has been suggested, while some feel that the disorder has a central basis, perhaps in the nucleus of the spinal tract.

Surgical intervention may be necessary if the paroxysms of pain cannot be controlled medically. The simplest surgical procedure is avulsion of the cutaneous branch to the affected area. Another method practiced is section of the sensory root of the trigeminal nerve. The corneal reflex is retained if the portion of the sensory root consisting of ophthalmic fibers is spared. This is important because anesthesia of the cornea, with loss of the blink reflex, may lead to corneal damage and ulceration. The same end is attained by section of the spinal tract at about the level of the obex. Although this procedure sections pain fibers and leaves most of the touch fibers intact (thus preserving the corneal reflex), the higher mortality risk attending trigeminal tractotomy discourages its use except in special cases. An effective procedure in favor at the present time consists of removal of the dura mater over the semilunar ganglion, which is then disturbed mechanically in various ways. When used in the younger patient especially, this "decompression" procedure often results in freedom from pain for several years, with retention of sensation in the peripheral territory of the trigeminal nerve. It should be pointed out, however, that surgical intervention in tic douloureux is becoming less frequent as medical management increases in effectiveness.

The sensory and motor nuclei of the trigeminal nerve may be included in areas of degeneration in the brain stem, or the intracranial portion of the nerve may be affected by trauma, tumor growth, or other lesion. Interruption of the motor fibers causes paralysis and eventual atrophy of the muscles of mastication. The mandible deviates to the affected side because of the unopposed action of the normal external pterygoid muscle, the function of this muscle being to protrude the jaw. Interruption of corticobulbar fibers causes voluntary paresis of the masticatory muscles on the side opposite the lesion. Complete paralysis is lacking because the motor nucleus receives some uncrossed fibers from the motor cortex.

FACIAL NERVE

The facial nerve has two sensory components: One supplies taste buds and the other contributes cutaneous fibers to the external ear. There are also two motor or efferent components, one for the facial muscles of expression and one for the submandibular and sublingual salivary glands and the lacrimal gland.

SENSORY COMPONENTS

The cell bodies of primary sensory neurons are in the geniculate ganglion, which is situated at the bend of the nerve as it traverses the facial canal of the petrous temporal bone. The peripheral processes of cells for *taste*, these cells composing most of the ganglion, enter the chorda tympani branch of the facial nerve which joins the lingual branch of the mandibular nerve. The fibers are distributed to taste buds on the anterior two-thirds of the tongue, most of them being on its lateral border. Fibers for palatal taste buds follow a complicated route and, as is true also of parasympathetic fibers in the facial and glossopharyngeal nerves, an understanding of the gross anatomy of the head is necessary in order to visualize their course. In brief, the sensory fibers in question leave the facial nerve in the greater petrosal branch at the level of the geniculate ganglion; this branch proceeds into the pterygopalatine fossa above the palate, where the fibers join palatine branches of the maxillary division of the trigeminal nerve. The trigeminal fibers of the palatine nerves provide for general sensation in the palate and inner surface of the gums, while the fibers from the facial nerve terminate in taste buds on the hard and soft palates.

Turning to the central processes of geniculate ganglion cells subserving taste, the fibers enter the brain stem in the sensory root of the facial nerve (nervus intermedius) and turn caudally in the solitary fasciculus (Fig. 8–7). The facial fibers of the fasciculus are joined more caudally by gustatory fibers from the glossopharyngeal and vagus nerves. Fibers from these three sources terminate in the *nucleus of the solitary fasciculus,* consisting of a column of cells adjacent to, and partly surrounding, the fasciculus. From the latter nucleus, connections are established with efferent nuclei of the brain stem, especially the salivatory nuclei and the dorsal motor nucleus of the vagus nerve. There is also a discharge to the intermediolateral cell col-

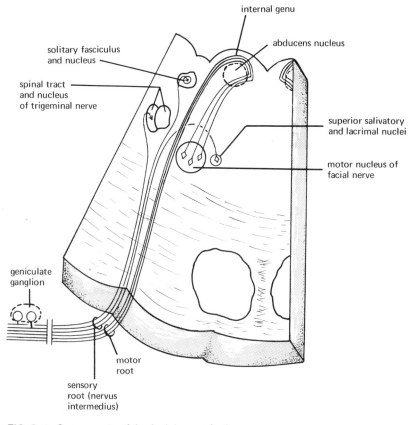

FIG. 8–7. Components of the facial nerve in the pons.

umn of the cord through reticulospinal connections. Ascending fibers from the nucleus of the solitary tract reach the hypothalamus and the ventral posterior thalamic nucleus by running close to the medial lemniscus. There is a further projection from the thalamus to the cortical area for awareness of taste which is located at the lower end of the general sensory strip in the parietal lobe.

With respect to the *cutaneous* sensory component, the fibers leave the facial nerve just after the latter exits from the facial canal. These fibers are distributed to the skin of the external ear, a small area behind the ear, the wall of the auditory canal, and the outer surface of the tympanic membrane. The central processes of the geniculate ganglion cells for cutaneous sensation enter the brain stem through the nervus intermedius and continue into the spinal tract of the trigeminal nerve (Fig. 8–7). They are joined in the tract by similar fibers for pain and other general sensations from the glossopharyngeal and vagus nerves. The combined fibers form a small bundle in the dorsal part of the spinal tract and terminate in the subjacent nucleus.

MOTOR COMPONENTS

For Supply of Striated Muscles

The motor component of the facial nerve for muscles of expression and certain additional small muscles is the most important part of the nerve from the clinical point of view. The *motor nucleus* is situated in the ventrolateral area of the pontine tegmentum, in its caudal one-third (Fig. 8–7). Efferent fibers of the nucleus pursue an aberrant course. Directed initially toward the floor of the fourth ventricle, the fibers form a compact bundle which runs forward along the medial side, and then over the rostral end, of the abducens nucleus. The

fibers then proceed to the point of emergence of the motor root by passing between the nucleus of origin and the nucleus of the trigeminal spinal tract. The configuration of the fiber bundle around the abducens nucleus is called the *internal genu,* the external genu of the facial nerve being in the facial canal at the level of the geniculate ganglion. The explanation given for the unusual course of facial motor fibers in the pons is based on a migration of cells in the embryo. It has been suggested that neurons destined to form the abducens and facial nuclei are intermingled at an early embryonic stage. The facial neurons move subsequently in a ventrolateral direction under the influence of the trigeminal spinal tract and its nucleus. Concurrently the abducens neurons move toward the medial longitudinal fasciculus. The fibers extending from the facial nucleus to the region of the abducens nucleus indicate the direction and extent of the change in position of the nuclei during embryonic development. Such shifts in position of groups of nerve cells during development are said to be the result of neurobiotaxis, i.e., the tendency of neurons to move toward major sources of stimuli.

The motor root of the facial nerve consists entirely of fibers from the motor nucleus. They supply the muscles of expression (mimetic muscles), the platysma and stylohyoid muscles, and the posterior belly of the digastric muscle. The facial nerve also supplies the stapedius muscle of the middle ear; this small muscle is inserted on the stapes and, by reflex contraction in response to loud sounds, prevents excessive movement of the stapes.

The motor nucleus receives afferents from several sources, including important connections for reflexes. Tectobulbar fibers from the superior colliculus complete a reflex pathway through which there is squinting in response to bright light or protective closure of the eyelids in response to a sudden visual stimulus. Fibers from trigeminal sensory nuclei function in the corneal reflex and in chewing or sucking responses on placing food in the mouth. Fibers from the superior olivary nucleus on the auditory pathway permit reflex contraction of the stapedius muscle. Corticobulbar afferents are crossed except for those terminating on cells that supply the frontalis and orbicularis oculi muscles which receive both crossed and uncrossed fibers. Contralateral voluntary paralysis of the *lower facial muscles* is therefore a feature of upper motor neuron lesions. However, under such circumstances the facial muscles continue to respond involuntarily to changing moods and emotions. The central connections for spontaneous changes of facial expression are not known; fibers from the hypothalamus or the corpus striatum may relay impulses to the facial motor nucleus from the thalamus and other higher centers concerned with the emotions. Emotional changes of facial expression are typically lost in Parkinson's disease (mask-like facies), although voluntary use of the facial muscles is retained.

Parasympathetic Nuclei

The *superior salivatory* and *lacrimal nuclei* consist of indefinite clusters of small cells, partly intermingled, medial to the motor nucleus (Fig. 8–7). These parasympathetic nuclei supply the submandibular and sublingual salivary glands and the lacrimal gland. Fibers from the nuclei leave the brain stem in the nervus intermedius and continue in the facial nerve until branches are given off in the facial canal. The fibers follow a devious route to their destination, running part of the way in branches of the trigeminal nerve. Briefly stated, fibers from the superior salivatory nucleus leave the facial nerve in the chorda tympani branch and join the lingual branch of the mandibu-

lar nerve to reach the floor of the buccal cavity. There they terminate in the submandibular ganglion and on scattered nerve cells in the submandibular gland. Short postganglionic fibers are distributed to the parenchyma of the sublingual and submandibular glands, where they stimulate secretion and cause vasodilation. Fibers from the lacrimal nucleus leave the facial nerve in the greater petrosal branch and terminate in the pterygopalatine ganglion located in the fossa of the same name. Postganglionic fibers for stimulation of secretion and vasodilation reach the lacrimal gland through the zygomatic branch of the maxillary nerve. Other postganglionic fibers are distributed to glands of the nasal mucosa and the mucosa of nasal sinuses.

The superior salivatory nucleus comes under the influence of the hypothalamus through the dorsal longitudinal fasciculus, and of the olfactory system through relays in the reticular formation. Data from taste buds and the mucosa of the buccal cavity are received by way of the nucleus of the solitary tract and the sensory trigeminal nuclei, respectively. The chief sources of impulses to the lacrimal nucleus are the hypothalamus for emotional responses and the trigeminal spinal nucleus for lacrimation caused by irritation of the cornea and conjunctiva.

SOME CLINICAL COMMENTS

The facial nuclei and associated fiber bundles may be included in degenerative or other lesions of the brain stem, with facial paralysis and other signs. However, the facial nerve is most commonly affected as it traverses the facial canal in the petrous temporal bone. The usual condition, known as *Bell's palsy*, consists of weakness (paresis) or paralysis of the facial muscles on the affected side. The symptoms develop rapidly and the etiology is thought to be a viral infection, with edema of connective tissue lining the facial canal and pressure on the facial nerve. The signs of Bell's palsy depend not only on the severity of the viral infection (assuming this to be the cause), but also on where the facial nerve is affected in its passage through the facial canal. All functions of the nerve are lost if the damage is proximal to the geniculate ganglion. In addition to the paralysis of facial muscles, there is loss of taste sensation on the anterior two-thirds of the tongue and the palate of the affected side, together with impairment of secretion by the submandibular, sublingual, and lacrimal glands. In addition, sounds are abnormally loud because of paralysis of the stapedius muscle.

In mild cases, most of the nerve fibers are not so severely damaged as to result in wallerian degeneration and the outlook for recovery is good. Recovery is slow and frequently incomplete when it must rely on nerve fiber regeneration. Sensory fibers do not regenerate if the lesion is proximal to the geniculate ganglion. Also, in the case of a lesion in the proximal part of the nerve, some regenerating salivary fibers may find their way into the greater petrosal nerve and reach the pterygopalatine ganglion. This results in lacrimation (crocodile tears) when aromas and taste sensations cause stimulation of cells in the superior salivatory nucleus. When the nerve is affected in the distal part of the facial canal after the greater petrosal and chorda tympani branches are given off, the condition is limited to paresis or paralysis involving both the upper and lower facial muscles on the side of the lesion. The prospect for recovery is generally good.

GLOSSOPHARYNGEAL, VAGUS, AND ACCESSORY NERVES

The ninth, tenth, and eleventh cranial nerves have much in common functionally and share certain nuclei of the medulla. While it is customary to discuss these nerves individually, repetition can be avoided by considering them as a group.

AFFERENT COMPONENTS

The glossopharyngeal and vagus nerves include sensory fibers for the special visceral sense of taste from the posterior third of the tongue, the pharynx, and the epiglottis together with general visceral afferents from the carotid sinus, carotid body, and viscera of the thorax and abdomen. There are also sensory fibers for pain, temperature, and touch from the mucosa of the back of the tongue, the pharynx and nearby regions, and from the skin of the ear. The cell bodies of primary sensory neurons are located in the superior and inferior ganglia of each of the nerves.

Visceral Afferents

The cell bodies of the *gustatory fibers* are in the inferior ganglia of the glossopharyngeal and vagus nerves. The fibers are distributed through the glossopharyngeal nerve to taste buds in the back of the tongue and, in few numbers, the pharyngeal mucosa. Vagal fibers supply taste buds on the epiglottis; these are unimportant since few persist into adult life. Central processes of the ganglion cells join the solitary fasciculus and terminate in the nucleus of this fasciculus (Figs. 8–8 and 8–9). The rostral portion of the nucleus of the solitary fasciculus is concerned with taste, impulses being received by way of the facial, glossopharyngeal, and vagus nerves; it is frequently referred to as the *gustatory nucleus*. Projections from the nucleus for reflexes and for awareness of taste are as described for the facial nerve.

The cell bodies of afferent neurons for *general visceral reflexes* are also in the inferior ganglia of the glossopharyngeal and

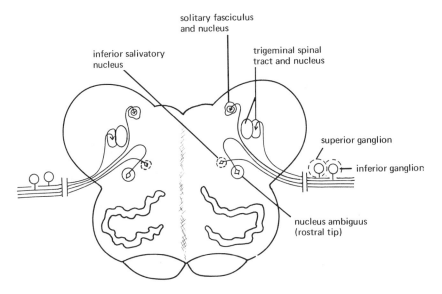

FIG. 8–8. Components of the glossopharyngeal nerve in the medulla.

vagus nerves. These fibers in the glosso-pharyngeal nerve supply the carotid sinus at the bifurcation of the common carotid artery and the adjacent carotid body. Nerve endings in the wall of the carotid sinus function as baroreceptors, which monitor arterial blood pressure, while the carotid body contains chemoreceptors that monitor oxygen tension in the circulating blood. Vagal fibers similarly supply baro-receptors in the aortic arch and chemo-receptors in the small aortic bodies adja-cent to the arch. The vagus nerve also contains many afferent fibers that are dis-tributed to the viscera of the thorax and abdomen; impulses conveyed centrally are of importance in reflex control of cardiovas-cular, respiratory, and alimentary func-tions. The central processes of the primary sensory neurons for the above reflexes de-scend in the solitary tract and end in the more caudal part of its nucleus (Figs. 8–8 and 8–9). From the latter site, connections are established with the dorsal motor nu-cleus of the vagus nerve, visceral centers in the reticular formation, and cells of the

reticular formation that project to the inter-mediolateral cell column of the cord. Data of visceral origin are also relayed to the hypothalamus.

Other Afferent Fibers

The glossopharyngeal nerve includes fibers for the general sensations of pain, tempera-ture, and touch in the mucosa of the poste-rior third of the tongue, upper part of the pharynx (including the tonsillar area), eustachian tube, and middle ear. The vagus nerve carries fibers having the same func-tions to the lower part of the pharynx, the larynx, and the esophagus. The areas thus supplied are of entodermal origin and in this respect the sensory neurons are visceral in nature. However, the sensations aroused are similar to those of cutaneous or somatic origin. There is some uncertainty, there-fore, with respect to the central connections of these particular sensory fibers. The ques-tion has been resolved for pain afferents (and probably for temperature). Since the pathway for pain from the areas indicated

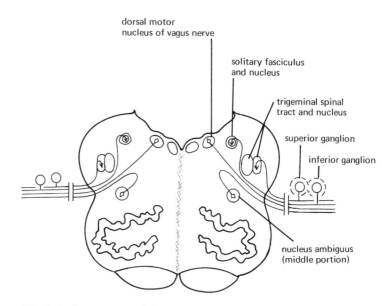

dorsal motor
nucleus of vagus nerve

solitary fasciculus
and nucleus

trigeminal spinal
tract and nucleus

superior ganglion

inferior ganglion

nucleus ambiguus
(middle portion)

FIG. 8–9. Components of the vagus nerve in the medulla.

is interrupted by trigeminal tractotomy, it may be concluded that pain fibers in the glossopharyngeal and vagus nerves descend in the trigeminal spinal tract and end in its nucleus (Figs. 8–8 and 8–9). This being the case, the cell bodies are probably in the small superior ganglia of the glossopharyngeal and vagus nerves. Fibers carrying data for touch from the posterior part of the tongue, pharynx, and adjacent areas may accompany visceral afferents to the nucleus of the solitary tract or they may terminate with somatic afferents in the nucleus of the trigeminal spinal tract. In either event, such afferents are important in the "gag reflex" through a reflex pathway that includes the nucleus ambiguus and the hypoglossal nucleus.

Finally, the vagus nerve, through its auricular branch, contributes sensory fibers to the external ear, a cutaneous area behind the ear, the wall of the auditory canal, and the tympanic membrane. The glossopharyngeal nerve contains a few such fibers, although inconstantly. The cell bodies are in the superior ganglia of the nerves and the central processes join other somatic afferent fibers in the trigeminal spinal tract.

EFFERENT COMPONENTS

The ninth, tenth, and eleventh cranial nerves all include motor fibers for striated muscles, and the ninth and tenth nerves also contain parasympathetic efferents.

For Supply of Striated Muscles

The *nucleus ambiguus* is a column of typical motor neurons situated dorsal to the inferior olivary nucleus (Figs. 8–8 through 8–10). Fibers from the nucleus ambiguus are directed dorsally at first. They then turn sharply to mingle with other fibers in the glossopharyngeal and vagus nerves, and constitute the entire cranial root of the accessory nerve. The nucleus ambiguus supplies muscles of the soft palate, pharynx, and larynx, together with striated muscle fibers in the upper part of the esophagus. The only muscle in the foregoing regions not supplied by this nucleus is the tensor veli palatini muscle, which is innervated by the trigeminal nerve.

A small group of cells in the rostral end of the nucleus ambiguus supplies the stylopharyngeus muscle through the glossopharyngeal nerve (Fig. 8–8). A large region of the nucleus supplies the remaining pharyngeal muscles, the cricothyroid muscle (an external muscle of the larynx), and the striated muscle of the esophagus through the vagus nerve (Fig. 8–9). Fibers from the caudal part of the nucleus leave the brain stem in the cranial portion of the accessory nerve (Fig. 8–10). The latter fibers join the spinal accessory root temporarily, then pass over to the vagus nerve in the region of the jugular foramen. These fibers are for innervation of the muscles of the soft palate and the intrinsic muscles of the larynx. It would be much simpler, although contrary to convention, to consider the cranial root of the accessory nerve as part of the vagus, leaving the spinal root as the definitive accessory nerve.

The nucleus ambiguus receives afferents from sensory nuclei of the brain stem, most importantly the nucleus of the trigeminal spinal tract and the nucleus of the solitary tract. These connections establish reflexes for coughing, gagging, and vomiting, the stimuli arising in the mucosa of the respiratory and alimentary passages. Corticobulbar afferents are both crossed and uncrossed; muscles supplied by the nucleus ambiguus are not paralyzed therefore in the event of a unilateral lesion of the upper motor neuron type.

Motor neurons for the sternocleidomastoid and trapezius muscles differentiate in the embryo near cells that are destined to form the nucleus ambiguus. The former cells subsequently migrate into the spinal cord (segments C1 through C6) and take up a position in the lateral part of the ventral gray horn. Arising as a series of rootlets along the side of the cord just behind the denticulate ligament, the *spinal root of the accessory nerve* ascends alongside the spinal cord, thus retracing the migration of cells of origin. On reaching the side of the medulla by passing through the foramen magnum, the spinal and cranial roots unite and continue as the accessory nerve as far as the jugular foramen. Fibers from the nucleus ambiguus then join the vagus nerve as noted above, and those of spinal

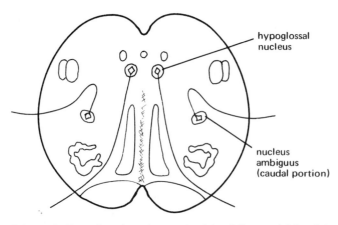

FIG. 8–10. Hypoglossal nucleus and origin of the cranial (medullary) root of the accessory nerve.

origin proceed to the sternocleidomastoid and trapezius muscles. Corticospinal fibers to the spinal accessory neurons are almost all crossed. There is therefore contralateral weakness (paresis) of the sternocleidomastoid and trapezius muscles as a result of an upper motor neuron lesion.

Parasympathetic Nuclei

There are parasympathetic fibers in the glossopharyngeal nerve, and these are especially numerous in the vagus nerve. The *inferior salivatory nucleus* for the parotid gland is a small collection of cells caudal to the superior salivatory nucleus and near the rostral tip of the nucleus ambiguus (Fig. 8–8). Fibers from the inferior salivatory nucleus are included in the glossopharyngeal nerve, enter its tympanic branch, and reach the otic ganglion by way of the tympanic plexus and the lesser petrosal nerve. Postganglionic fibers join the auriculotemporal branch of the mandibular nerve and thus reach the parotid gland. The parasympathetic supply to the parotid gland is secretomotor and vasodilator. The inferior salivatory nucleus is influenced by stimuli from the hypothalamus, olfactory system, nucleus of the solitary fasciculus, and sensory trigeminal nuclei.

The main parasympathetic nucleus is the *dorsal motor nucleus of the vagus nerve.* This column of cells, which are mainly of medium size and spindle-shaped, extends through most of the medulla in the gray matter around the central canal and beneath the vagal triangle of the rhomboid fossa (Fig. 8–9). The portion of the nucleus supplying the heart and respiratory system lies beneath the floor of the fourth ventricle, while the caudal portion of the nucleus sends fibers to abdominal viscera. Preganglionic fibers in the vagus nerve are distributed to parasympathetic ganglia and

plexuses in or near viscera, from where short postganglionic fibers continue to smooth and cardiac muscle and to secretory cells of glands. The dorsal motor nucleus receives afferents from several sources; the more important are the hypothalamus, the olfactory system, autonomic centers in the reticular formation, and the nucleus of the solitary fasciculus.

Isolated lesions involving the ninth, tenth, or eleventh cranial nerves separately are uncommon. However, several pathologic events, most frequently of vascular origin, cause destruction of the central nuclei. A unilateral lesion of the nucleus ambiguus, for example, results in ipsilateral paralysis of the soft palate, pharynx, and larynx, with the expected signs of hoarseness and difficulty in breathing and swallowing. Extensive lesions, especially if bilateral, carry a poor prognosis. Complete laryngeal paralysis leads to asphyxia unless immediate precautions are taken to restore the airway. Interruption of the parasympathetic outflow causes visceral dysfunction, including cardiac acceleration.

HYPOGLOSSAL NERVE

The *hypoglossal nucleus*, consisting of motor cells like those of the ventral horn of the cord, lies between the dorsal motor nucleus of the vagus nerve and the midline of the medulla (Fig. 8–10). The hypoglossal triangle of the rhomboid fossa marks the position of the rostral part of the nucleus. Fibers from the hypoglossal nucleus course ventrally on the lateral side of the medial lemniscus and emerge along the sulcus between the pyramid and the olive. The hypoglossal nerve supplies the intrinsic muscles of the tongue and the three extrinsic muscles (genioglossus, styloglossus, and hyoglossus). The nucleus receives afferents from the nucleus of the solitary tract and sensory trigeminal nuclei for reflex movements of the tongue in swallowing, chewing, and sucking in response to gustatory and other stimuli from the buccal and pharyngeal mucosae. Corticobulbar afferents are predominantly crossed; a unilateral upper motor neuron lesion therefore causes paresis of the opposite side of the tongue, although demonstration of the muscle weakness may be difficult. Paralysis and eventual atrophy of the affected muscles follow destruction of the hypoglossal nucleus or interruption of the nerve. The tongue deviates to the weak side on protrusion because of the unopposed protrusor action of the healthy genioglossus muscle.

AFFERENT NERVE SUPPLY OF MUSCLE SPINDLES

Neuromuscular spindles in the muscles of mastication are supplied with afferent fibers by the mesencephalic nucleus of the trigeminal nerve. The afferent supply of spindles in muscles that receive their motor innervation through cranial nerves other than the trigeminal has been a perplexing question which is not yet resolved for all the muscles supplied by cranial nerves.

The extraocular muscles contain spindles of a special type. It has been shown in experimental animals that these spindles are supplied by neurons with cell bodies in the trigeminal semilunar ganglion. The peripheral processes of these cells reach the orbit by way of the ophthalmic nerve while the central processes enter the brain stem through the trigeminal sensory root, turn caudally in the spinal tract, and end in the rostral part of the nucleus of the spinal tract. Afferent fibers supplying spindles in the muscles of the larynx have been identified in the vagus nerve; their cell bodies must be in the ganglia of the vagus nerve, because the fibers persist when the nerve is

sectioned proximal to the ganglia. Proprioceptive endings in the sternocleidomastoid and trapezius muscles receive afferent fibers through the second, third, and fourth cervical spinal nerves. The main uncertainty surrounds muscle spindles in lingual and facial muscles. Spindles have been described in muscles of the tongue; fibers supplying them have been identified in the hypoglossal nerve, but the location of their cell bodies is uncertain. The situation regarding facial muscles is still more obscure, since even the presence of spindles in these muscles has not been established conclusively. From what is presently known, it appears that the peripheral distribution of fibers from the mesencephalic nucleus may be limited to proprioceptors associated with the muscles of mastication and the temporomandibular joint, together with proprioceptive-like endings adjacent to the teeth and in the hard palate.

CLASSIFICATION OF COMPONENTS OF CRANIAL AND SPINAL NERVES

The spinal nerves and most of the cranial nerves have now been discussed and their components can be classified under seven headings. Of these, four are present in both spinal and cranial nerves; three more are added in the latter to include the special senses and to take cognizance of different embryologic origins of the muscles of the head. Cranial nerve nuclei in the brain stem are shown in Figure 8–11 according to the following classification.

AFFERENT COMPONENTS

General somatic afferent nuclei receive impulses from general sensory endings and are therefore concerned with pain, temperature, touch, pressure, proprioception,

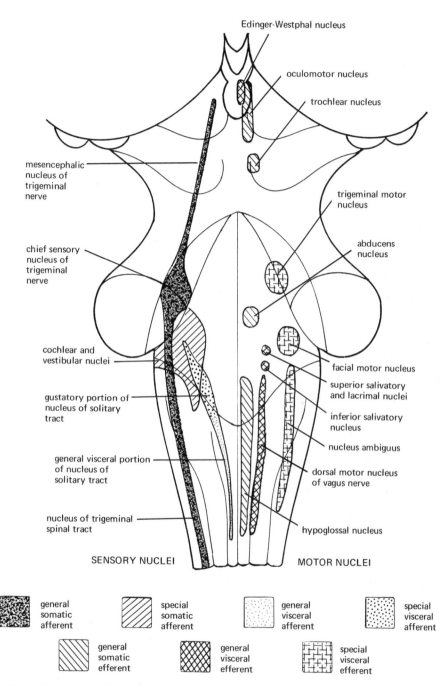

FIG. 8–11. Classification of the nuclei of cranial nerves.

and vibration. The cells are in the dorsal gray horn of the spinal cord, the gracile and cuneate nuclei, and the sensory trigeminal nuclei. The *special somatic afferent* group consists of nuclei for those special senses that relate the body to the external environment. This group consists of the visual system (optic nerve) and the cochlear and vestibular divisions of the eighth cranial nerve. *General visceral afferent* components are for visceral reflexes and for sensations such as fullness of hollow organs and pain of visceral origin. The cells of second order neurons are in the dorsal gray horn of the spinal cord and the nucleus of the solitary tract (caudal portion). *Special visceral afferents* are for taste, with second order neurons located in the rostral part of the nucleus of the solitary tract (gustatory nucleus). The olfactory nerves are considered conventionally as visceral because of the important influence of smell on visceral functions; they are therefore included under the heading of special visceral afferents.

EFFERENT COMPONENTS

Lower motor neurons included under the heading of *general somatic efferent* supply muscles that are derived from myotomes of the embryonic somites. They are the oculo-motor, trochlear, abducens, and hypoglossal nuclei and ventral horn cells of the spinal cord. *General visceral efferents* are the preganglionic neurons of the autonomic nervous system. In the brain stem, they include the Edinger–Westphal nucleus, lacrimal nucleus, superior and inferior salivatory nuclei, and the dorsal motor nucleus of the vagus nerve. In the spinal cord, this category consists of the intermediolateral cell column in the thoracic and upper lumbar segments and parasympathetic cells in the sacral cord. *Special visceral efferents* supply muscles derived from the branchial or gill arches of the embryo. They are classified as "visceral" because of the respiratory function of the gill arches in aquatic forms. The distinction between general somatic and special visceral efferents is academic, because the striated muscles they supply are indistinguishable histologically. There are three special visceral efferent nuclei: 1) the trigeminal motor nucleus for the muscles of mastication, which develop from the first branchial arch; 2) the facial motor nucleus for the muscles of expression, of second branchial arch derivation; and 3) the nucleus ambiguus for muscles of the palate, pharynx, larynx, and upper esophagus, these muscles being derived from the third, fourth, and fifth branchial arches.

SUGGESTIONS FOR ADDITIONAL READING

Adata AK, Gehring EN: Proprioceptive innervation of the tongue. J Anat 110:215–220, 1971

Brodal A: The Cranial Nerves: Anatomy and Anatomicoclinical Correlations, 2nd ed. Oxford, Blackwell, 1965

Brodal A: Neurological Anatomy, 2nd ed. London, Oxford University Press, 1969

Carpenter MB, Strominger NL: The medial longitudinal fasciculus and disturbances of conjugate horizontal eye movements in the monkey. J Comp Neurol 125:41–65, 1965

Courville J: The nucleus of the facial nerve: The relation between cellular groups and peripheral branches of the nerve. Brain Res 1:338–354, 1966

Crosby EC, Humphrey T, Lauer EW: Correlative Anatomy of the Nervous System. New York, Macmillan, 1962

Eisenman J, Landgren S, Novin D: Functional organization in the main sensory trigeminal nucleus and in the rostral subdivision of the nucleus of the spinal trigeminal tract in the cat. Acta Physiol Scand 59 (Suppl 214):1–44, 1963

Henkin RI, Graziadei PPG, Bradley DF: The molecular basis of taste and its disorders. Ann Intern Med 71:791–821, 1969

Kerr FWL: The divisional organization of afferent fibers of the trigeminal nerve. Brain 86:721–733, 1963

Kerr FWL: The etiology of trigeminal neuralgia. Arch Neurol 8:15–25, 1963

Kugelberg E, Lindblom U: The mechanism of the pain in trigeminal neuralgia. J Neurol Neurosurg Psychiatry 22:36–43, 1959

Kunc Z: Treatment of essential neuralgia of the 9th nerve by selected tractotomy. J Neurosurg 23:494–500, 1965

Manni E, Palmieri G, Marini R: Peripheral pathway of the proprioceptive afferents from the lateral rectus muscle of the eye. Exp Neurol 30:46–53, 1971

Manni E, Palmieri G, Marini R: Pontine trigeminal termination of proprioceptive afferents from the eye muscles. Exp Neurol 36:310–318, 1972

Morest DH: Experimental study of the projections of the nucleus of the tractus solitarius and the area postrema in the cat. J Comp Neurol 130:277–299, 1967

Olszewski J: On the anatomical and functional organization of the spinal trigeminal nucleus. J Comp Neurol 92:401–413, 1950

Rhoton AL, Jr, O'Leary JL, Ferguson JP: The trigeminal, facial, vagal, and glossopharyngeal nerves in the monkey. Arch Neurol 14:530–540, 1966

Schwartz HG, Roulhac GE, Lam RL, O'Leary JL: Organization of the fasciculus solitarius in man. J Comp Neurol 94:221–237, 1951

Wall PD, Taub A: Four aspects of trigeminal nucleus and a paradox. J Neurophysiol 25:110–126, 1962

Warwick R: Representation of the extra-ocular muscles in the oculomotor nuclei of the monkey. J Comp Neurol 98:449–503, 1953

Warwick R: The ocular parasympathetic nerve supply and its mesencephalic sources. J Anat 88:71–93, 1954

Warwick R: The so-called nucleus of convergence. Brain 78:92–114, 1955

9

Reticular Formation

The reticular formation of the brain stem has a long phylogenetic history. The brains of primitive vertebrates consist in large part of neural tissue that is not well organized as nuclei and tracts; this diffuse arrangement of neurons is said to be "reticular" (forming a network). In the evolution of the mammalian brain, the rostral part developed preferentially, with additions to the thalamus and the appearance of neocortex. Fiber tracts were acquired to connect the spinal cord and the forebrain, and the tracts of necessity traverse the brain stem. Large nuclei including the red nucleus, substantia nigra, and inferior olivary nucleus also appeared or increased in size in the mammalian brain stem. The primitive reticular formation did not disappear; on the contrary, it persisted as an important component of the mammalian brain stem in those regions not completely occupied by tracts and nuclei.

The reticular formation is the recipient of data from most of the sensory systems and has efferent connections, direct or indirect, with all levels of the neuraxis. Constituting, in a sense, a central core of the brain, the reticular formation makes a significant contribution to several aspects of brain function, including a role in the arousal-sleep cycle. The reticular system of neurons is integrated into the motor system of the brain and spinal cord, and includes centers that regulate visceral functions. The primitive "reticular" characteristic is retained in the multineuronal or polysynaptic nature of intrinsic pathways.

CYTOARCHITECTURE

Histologic analysis of the reticular formation is difficult because the constituent neurons are not, for the most part, assembled in compact groups. Nevertheless a number of regions or nuclei are recognized on the basis of cellular characteristics and connections. Five such nuclei are present in the

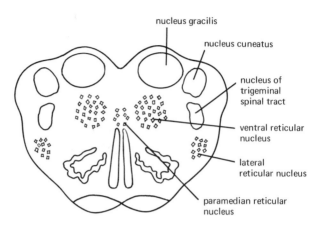

FIG. 9–1. Reticular nuclei at the level of the caudal portion of the inferior olivary nucleus.

medulla (Figs. 9–1 and 9–2). The *lateral reticular nucleus,* which is sufficiently discrete to permit its identification in Weigert-stained sections (Figs. 7–4 through 7–6), is situated near the surface of the medulla and extends from a point caudal to the inferior olivary nucleus to the midolivary level. The *paramedian nucleus* is adjacent to the midline of the medulla. The lateral and paramedian nuclei have connections with the cerebellum.

The remaining three reticular nuclei of the medulla are in the region bounded ventrally by the inferior olivary nucleus, dorsally by the nuclei gracilis and cuneatus and the vestibular nuclear complex, and laterally by the nucleus of the trigeminal spinal tract. Cells of the *ventral reticular nucleus* are scattered through the medial two-thirds of this area at the level of the caudal half of the inferior olivary nucleus (Fig. 9–1). Rostral to the ventral reticular

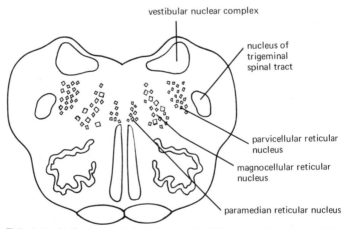

FIG. 9–2. Reticular nuclei at the level of the rostral portion of the inferior olivary nucleus.

nucleus, the reticular formation in the medial portion of the area outlined above consists of large neurons mingled with smaller cells and is known as the *magnocellular nucleus* (Fig. 9–2). The *parvicellular nucleus,* in which the nerve cells are small, occupies an area bounded by the magnocellular nucleus, the trigeminal spinal nucleus, and the vestibular nuclear complex, extending from the midolivary level to the rostral limit of the medulla (Fig. 9–2). As will be noted presently the parvicellular nucleus receives afferents from the spinal cord and trigeminal sensory nuclei, and projects to more medial reticular nuclei. It is consequently regarded as a "sensory" or "association" region of the reticular formation.

Reticular nuclei in the *tegmentum of the pons* are, by convention, described separately from those of the medulla, but two of them are in fact rostral extensions of medullary nuclei. The *caudal pontine reticular nucleus* (Fig. 9–3) is similar cytologically to the magnocellular nucleus of the medulla, of which it is essentially a forward extension. Further forward in the pons, the *rostral pontine reticular nucleus* in the medial area of the tegmentum is lacking in the large neurons. The *parvicellular reticular nucleus,* situated in the lateral tegmentum of the pons (Fig. 9–3), is an extension of the same nucleus in the medulla and part of the sensory or association region of the reticular formation.

The reticular formation of the pons continues into the *midbrain,* where the *mesencephalic reticular nucleus* consists of scattered cells in an area bounded by the tectum, red nucleus, and ascending lemnisci (Fig. 9–4). The reticular formation extends rostrally into the subthalamic region of the diencephalon, where it constitutes the zona incerta of the subthalamus (Chapter 11).

It is helpful from the functional point of view to consider the reticular system as comprising three regions or nuclear groups. *Group 1* consists of the lateral and paramedian nuclei of the medulla, both of

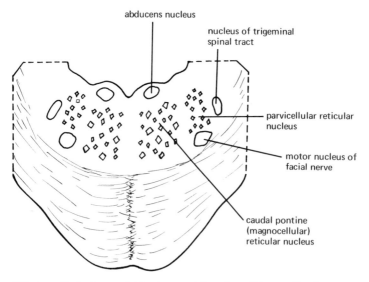

FIG. 9–3. Reticular nuclei in the caudal region of the pontine tegmentum.

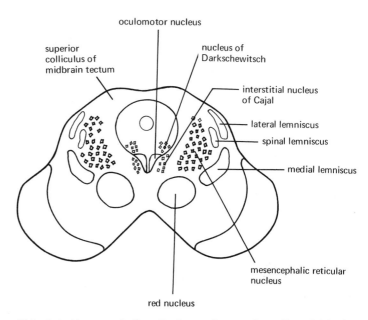

FIG. 9–4. Mesencephalic reticular nucleus and small nuclei in the rostral part of the midbrain.

which have cerebellar connections. *Group 2* includes the parvicellular nuclei of the medulla and pons, constituting essentially a single nucleus in the lateral area of the brain stem. With afferents from several sensory systems, the parvicellular nuclei send fibers to the medial part of the reticular formation. *Group 3* consists of nuclei in the medial part of the medulla and pons, extending into the midbrain. This group therefore includes the ventral and magnocellular nuclei of the medulla, the caudal and rostral pontine nuclei, and the mesencephalic reticular nucleus, to which may be added the zona incerta of the subthalamus. These nuclei receive afferents from the lateral or "sensory" part of the reticular formation (parvicellular nuclei) and from other sources. Axons of cells of group 3 nuclei run longitudinally in the brain stem and give off numerous collateral branches as they ascend or descend; the branches synapse with other reticular cells. The

many collateral branches make possible a great deal of interaction among neurons and form the basis of the polysynaptic pathways which are characteristic of impulse transmission through the reticular formation.

FUNCTIONAL ORGANIZATION

CONNECTIONS WITH THE CEREBELLUM

The lateral reticular nucleus receives spinoreticular fibers and collaterals from the spinal lemniscus; efferent fibers enter the cerebellum through the inferior peduncle. There is thus established an auxiliary pathway for transmission of general sensory data to the cerebellum. The lateral reticular nucleus also receives fibers from the red nucleus and is therefore a cell station on a feedback circuit, the circuit being completed by fibers proceeding from cerebellar nuclei to the red nucleus. The paramedian reticular nucleus is on a simpler feedback circuit, receiving fibers from, and sending fibers to, the cerebellum.

ASCENDING RETICULAR ACTIVATING SYSTEM

The ascending activating system consists of the sensory input to the reticular formation and rostral transmission through polysynaptic pathways to certain thalamic nuclei, from which the impulses spread to the cerebral cortex. The system has an important bearing on the sleep-arousal cycle and on attention.

All nuclei of the reticular formation, with the exception of the lateral and paramedian nuclei of the medulla, participate in the ascending activating system. Discussion of connections is simplified if the nuclei so involved are considered as forming two regions or areas. The *lateral area,* corresponding to group 2 nuclei, consists of the parvicellular nuclei of the medulla and pons. The *medial area* corresponds to group 3 nuclei, i.e., the ventral and magnocellular nuclei of the medulla, the caudal and rostral pontine nuclei, and the mesencephalic reticular nucleus.

Sensory Input

The sensory input for the reticular activating system is as follows. The lateral reticular area receives collateral branches from the spinal lemniscus, fibers from the trigeminal spinal nucleus, and fibers from the nucleus of the solitary fasciculus. The reticular formation therefore receives impulses originating in receptors for pain, temperature, touch, and pressure throughout the entire body, and also impulses from sensory endings in the viscera. The medial lemniscus, which transmits data for the more discriminative aspects of general sensation, does not contribute afferents to the reticular formation. The lateral area

also receives afferents from vestibular nuclei and nuclei on the central auditory pathway. Axons from the lateral reticular area proceed to various parts of the medial area. The connections just described account for the expression "sensory or association part of the reticular formation," with respect to the parvicellular nuclei of the medulla and pons.

Other afferents to the reticular formation are not related specifically to the lateral area. Spinoreticular fibers terminate mainly in the magnocellular part of the medial area, the remainder ending in the rostral pontine reticular nucleus and in the lateral area. The spinoreticular fibers represent a phylogenetically old system, compared with the more recent spinothalamic tracts. Impulses of retinal origin reach various parts of the reticular formation through a relay in the superior colliculus. Olfactory impulses reach the reticular formation through several routes, including olfactotegmental fibers ending in the mesencephalic reticular nucleus. The reticular formation has an input therefore from all sensory systems, somatic and visceral, with the exception of the dorsal column system for discriminative touch and proprioception. Finally, corticoreticular fibers originate in widespread areas of cortex, including the general sensory area. Corticoreticular fibers end in various regions of the reticular formation and function in the well known effect of psychic stimuli on attention.

Projections to Higher Centers

As mentioned previously, ascending axons of cells in the medial reticular area give off collateral branches which synapse with other reticular cells. By repetition of relays, there is polysynaptic, adrenergic transmission of nerve impulses into the diencephalon. Many of the ascending fibers run in the central tegmental tract, and the last axons in the relay terminate in thalamic nuclei and the hypothalamus.

The particular thalamic nuclei receiving fibers from the reticular formation are the intralaminar nuclei and the nucleus of the midline (see also Chapter 11). A thin sheet of myelinated fibers (the internal medullary lamina) extends vertically through the thalamus in an anteroposterior plane. The lamina encloses several *intralaminar nuclei,* one of which, the *centromedian nucleus,* is especially well developed in man (Fig. 9–5). The intralaminar nuclei have few, if any, direct connections with the cerebral cortex. However, they send fibers to other thalamic nuclei that do project to the cortex, and through the latter nuclei the polysynaptic nature of the reticular activating system is preserved. The general sensory nucleus of the thalamus (ventral posterior nucleus), which is the destination of the medial lemniscus, spinothalamic tracts, and trigeminothalamic tracts, projects to the somesthetic area of the parietal lobe. In contrast the intralaminar nuclei, through relays in other thalamic nuclei, project to widespread cortical areas, including nonspecific association areas and areas that are important with respect to the emotions. The intralaminar nuclei have still other connections, notably with thalamic nuclei that participate in emotional aspects of brain function and with the corpus striatum, a motor center of the extrapyramidal system.

The *nucleus of the midline,* which consists of groups of nerve cells in the medial part of the thalamus adjacent to the third ventricle (Fig. 9–5), represents the oldest part of the thalamus phylogenetically. The midline nucleus is immediately dorsal to the *hypothalamus.* Fibers from the reticular formation terminate in the hypothalamus, and impulses from the reticular formation also reach the hypothalamus through a relay in the nucleus of the midline. These

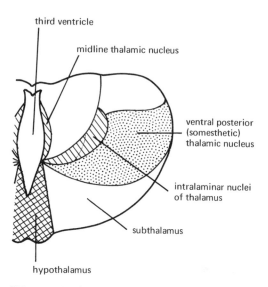

FIG. 9–5. Regions of the diencephalon receiving fibers of the lemniscal and extralemniscal systems.

connections contribute to the emotional and visceral responses that are associated with sensory stimuli reaching higher centers by way of the reticular formation.

Functions of the Reticular Activating System

The role of the reticular activating system is best understood when compared with that of the lemniscal system. Sensory information conveyed by the latter system, when projected from the ventral posterior nucleus of the thalamus to the somesthetic cortical area, is interpreted in a highly specific manner with respect to the nature of the sensory stimulus and its quantitative and discriminative aspects. The ascending reticular system is relatively nonspecific; the sensory modalities are merged in the polysynaptic pathway through the reticular formation and the thalamus, giving at best a vague awareness of any particular sensory function. The cortex in general is stimulated, with a profound effect on the waking state and on alerting reactions to sensory stimuli. When cortical stimulation by way of the reticular formation occurs during sleep, either under natural circumstances or in the experimental animal, the electrical activity of the cortex (as seen on the electroencephalogram) changes from the large-wave random pattern of sleep to the small-wave pattern of the waking state. When one is awake, stimuli reaching the cortex through the activating system sharpen attentiveness and create optimal conditions for perception of sensory data conveyed through more direct pathways. Cutaneous stimuli appear to be especially important in maintaining the awake or conscious state while visual, auditory, and psychic stimuli have a special bearing on alertness and attention. Impulses from the trigeminal area of distribution have a significant influence on consciousness. This is the basis of methods found by experience to be useful in restoring a person from a "fainting spell." To cite a once popular example, smelling salts contain ammonia or other substances that stimulate trigeminal sensory endings in the nasal mucosa.

The reticular activating system is of considerable pharmacologic interest. Under the influence of barbiturates and general anesthetics, transmission through the reticular formation is suppressed, although it continues by the lemniscal route. Many drugs have a tranquilizing effect or produce unconsciousness by impeding transmission in the polysynaptic pathway through the brain stem. Prolonged coma results from serious damage to the reticular formation. There is additional interest in the system because its malfunction, perhaps on a biochemical basis, may be an etiological factor in certain types of mental illness.

MOTOR FUNCTIONS

Descending fibers from the reticular formation constitute the diffuse *reticulospinal system,* and similar fibers functionally end in motor nuclei of cranial nerves. The fibers originate in the medial area, especially its magnocellular portion, and terminate on both alpha and gamma motor neurons. In addition to reflexes involving the sensory input and reticulospinal connections, the medial area of the reticular formation relays impulses from the red nucleus, substantia nigra, corpus striatum, and cerebellum. Impulses from motor areas of the cerebral cortex in the frontal lobe also reach lower motor neurons after a synaptic relay in the reticular formation. The gamma reflex loop has a significant role in producing the motor responses arising from activity in the reticular formation.

VISCERAL CENTERS

Groups of neurons in the reticular formation regulate visceral functions through connections with nuclei of the autonomic outflow and, in the case of respiration, with motor neurons in the phrenic nucleus and the thoracic cord. Respiratory and cardiovascular centers have been identified by electrical stimulation within the brain stem in experimental animals. Maximal inspiratory responses are obtained from the magnocellular nucleus of the medulla, while expiratory responses are evoked by stimulation of the parvicellular nucleus of the medulla. A pneumotaxic center in the pontine reticular formation controls normal respiratory rhythm. Stimulation of the ventral and magnocellular reticular nuclei of the medulla has a depressor effect on the circulatory system, with slowing of the heart rate and lowering of blood pressure. The opposite or pressor effect is produced by stimulation in the lateral reticular area of the medulla. Damage to the brain stem is hazardous to life because of the presence of these centers controlling vital functions.

MISCELLANEOUS NUCLEI OF THE BRAIN STEM

Several small nuclei in the brain stem may conveniently be considered at this time, although not all of them are strictly components of the reticular formation.

The *area postrema* is a narrow strip of neural tissue in the caudal part of the rhomboid fossa between the vagal triangle and the margin of the fossa (Fig. 6–3). The most characteristic cell in the area postrema resembles astroblasts of the newborn; there are also astrocytes, a few oligodendrocytes, and a moderate number of nerve cells. The area is richly vascular and contains many large sinusoids; the "blood-brain barrier," which prevents certain substances from entering nervous tissue from capillary blood elsewhere, is lacking. The area postrema receives a few ascending visceral fibers from the spinal cord, and there are reciprocal connections with the nucleus of the solitary tract. It is thought to play a role in the physiology of vomiting and to send fibers to a "vomiting center" in the lateral area of the reticular formation. The area postrema has been shown in dogs to be an emetic trigger zone, serving as a chemoreceptor region for emetic drugs such as apomorphine and digitalis.

The *locus ceruleus*, at the rostral end of the floor of the fourth ventricle on either side, marks the position of a nucleus consisting of neurons that contain melanin pigment. The cells synthesize catecholamines like the melanin-containing cells of the substantia nigra which presumably act as neurotransmitters at the axon terminals of these cells. The nucleus is thought to have a role in the ascending reticular activating system and may have other functions that have not yet been clarified.

There are several small nuclei worthy of brief mention in the midbrain. The *nucleus of Darkschewitsch* is situated in the central gray matter just dorsal to the oculomotor nucleus, while the *interstitial nucleus of Cajal* lies lateral to the oculomotor nucleus (Fig. 9–4). The connections of the foregoing nuclei have not been fully worked out. They appear to receive afferents from the superior colliculus and the corpus striatum as well as from vestibular nuclei through the medial longitudinal fasciculus. They relay impulses to the oculomotor nucleus and other motor nuclei of cranial nerves. In addition, fibers from these nuclei descend in the medial longitudinal fasciculus and enter the sulcomarginal fasciculus of the spinal cord.

Two additional midbrain nuclei are incorporated in a pathway originating in the olfactory and limbic systems. The *interpeduncular nucleus*, which is small in man, lies just above the interpeduncular fossa in the midline of the rostral end of the midbrain. The *dorsal tegmental nucleus* is located in the central gray matter, caudal to the nucleus of Darkschewitsch. The connections of the interpeduncular and dorsal tegmental nuclei are rather complicated. One pathway in which they participate begins in forebrain regions associated with the olfactory and limbic systems from which fibers travel to the habenular nucleus of the diencephalon. Habenulointerpeduncular fibers constitute the next link in this pathway. The interpeduncular nucleus then sends fibers to the dorsal tegmental nucleus, which in turn contributes descending fibers to the reticular formation via the dorsal longitudinal fasciculus. Through synaptic relays in the reticular formation, data related to the sense of smell and the emotions reach autonomic nuclei in the brain stem and spinal cord—notably the salivatory nuclei, the dorsal motor nucleus of the vagus nerve, and the intermediolateral cell column of the cord. (The habenular nucleus and its connections are described with the epithalamus in Chapter 11.)

The *ventral tegmental nucleus* occupies the same position as the interstitial nucleus of Cajal (Fig. 9–4), but is caudal to the latter and at the same level as the dorsal tegmental nucleus. The ventral tegmental nucleus is a component of the midbrain reticular formation and its principal connections are with the hypothalamus. Finally, the *nucleus of the posterior commissure* lies dorsal to the periaqueductal gray matter at the rostral limit of the midbrain. This nucleus adjoins the posterior commissure and is a relay nucleus on connections utilizing this commissure.

SUGGESTIONS FOR ADDITIONAL READING

Borison HL, Wang SC: Physiology and pharmacology of vomiting. Pharmacol Rev 5:193–230, 1953

Brodal A: The Reticular Formation of the Brain Stem: Anatomical Aspects and Functional Correlations. Edinburgh, Oliver & Boyd, 1957

Brodal A: Neurological Anatomy, 2nd ed. London, Oxford University Press, 1969

Jasper HH, Proctor LD, Knighton RS, Noshay WC, Costello RT: (eds.). Reticular Formation of the Brain. Boston, Little, Brown, 1958

Magoun HW: The Waking Brain, 2nd ed. Springfield, Ill., Thomas, 1969

Merrill EG: The lateral respiratory neurones of the medulla: Their associations with nucleus ambiguus, nucleus retroambigualis, the spinal accessory nucleus and the spinal cord. Brain Res 24:11–28, 1970

Morest DK: A study of the structure of the area postrema with Golgi methods. Am J Anat 107: 291–303, 1960

Moruzzi G: Active processes in the brain stem during sleep. Harvey Lect 58:233–297, 1963

Moruzzi G, Magoun HW: Brain stem recticular formation and activation of the EEG. Electroencephalogr Clin Neurophysiol 1:455–473, 1949

Olson L, Fuxe K: On the projections from the locus coeruleus noradrenaline neurons: The cerebellar innervation. Brain Res 28:165–171, 1971

Ramón–Moliner E, Nauta WJH: The isodendritic core of the brain stem. J Comp Neurol 126:311–335, 1966

Rossi GF, Zanchetti A: The brain stem reticular formation: Anatomy and physiology. Arch Ital Biol 95:199–435, 1957

10
Cerebellum

Although the cerebellum has an abundant input from sensory receptors it is essentially a motor part of the brain, functioning in the maintenance of equilibrium and coordination of muscle action in both stereotyped and nonstereotyped movements. The cerebellum makes a special contribution to synergy of muscle action, i.e., to the synchronization of muscles that make up a functional group, ensuring that there is contraction of the right muscles at the right time. This synergistic influence on muscles is especially important in voluntary movements, although the cerebellum does not seem to initiate such movements. It follows that cerebellar lesions become manifest as disturbances of motor function without voluntary paralysis. The cerebellum increased in size in the course of vertebrate phylogeny. Maximal development is found in the human brain, man having a particular need for synergy of muscles in learned activities that require precision.

The cerebellum consists of 1) a *cortex* or surface layer of gray matter, which has a very irregular contour because of numerous transverse folds or folia; 2) a *medullary center* of white matter, consisting of incoming fibers proceeding to the cortex, fibers running from the cortex to cerebellar nuclei, and fewer fibers connecting different parts of the cortex; and 3) four pairs of *central nuclei* embedded in the medullary center. As described in the context of the brain stem, three pairs of *peduncles* containing afferent and efferent fibers attach the cerebellum to the brain stem. They are the inferior, middle, and superior peduncles, which connect the cerebellum with the medulla, pons, and midbrain, respectively.

GROSS ANATOMY

The superior cerebellar surface is elevated in the midline, conforming to the dural reflexion or tentorium that forms a roof for the posterior cranial fossa. The inferior surface is grooved deeply in the midline; the remainder of this surface is convex on either side and rests on the floor of the posterior cranial fossa (Fig. 10–1).

Certain terms are useful for identifying regions of the cerebellar surface. The region in and near the midline is known as the *vermis* and the remainder as the *hemispheres*. The superior vermis is not demarcated from the hemispheres, but the inferior vermis lies in a deep depression (the vallecula) and is well delineated.

Three major regions, called the flocculonodular, anterior, and posterior lobes, are recognized in the horizontal plane (Fig.

10–1). The *flocculonodular lobe* (or lobule) is a small component, and the oldest phylogenetically, at the rostral edge of the inferior surface. The nodule is the rostral portion of the inferior vermis. The flocculi are irregular-shaped masses on either side. The cerebellum is deeply indented by several transverse fissures. The *posterolateral fissure* along the caudal border of the flocculonodular lobe is the first of these to appear during embryologic development. The main mass of the cerebellum, i.e., all but the flocculonodular lobe, is called the *corpus cerebelli* and consists of anterior

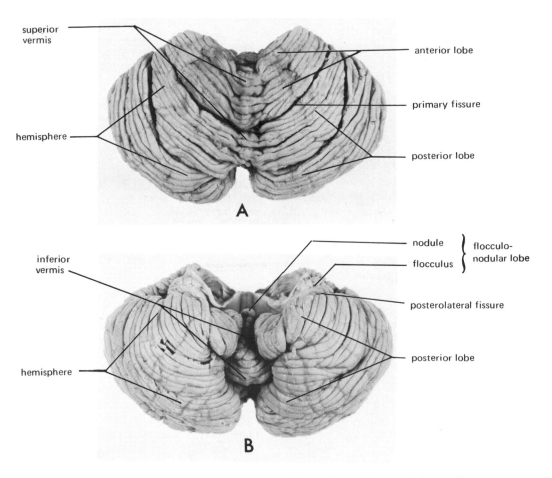

FIG. 10–1. A. Superior surface of the cerebellum. **B.** Inferior surface of the cerebellum. ×⅔

and posterior lobes. The *anterior lobe* is that part of the superior surface rostral to the *primary fissure*, this being the second fissure to appear during embryologic development. The remainder of the cerebellum on both surfaces constitutes the *posterior lobe*.

The roof of the forward part of the fourth ventricle is formed by the superior cerebellar peduncles and the superior medullary velum (Fig. 10–2). The remainder of the roof consists of the thin inferior medullary velum, formed by pia mater and ependyma. This membrane, in which a deficiency constitutes the foramen of Magendie (Fig. 6–4), frequently adheres to the inferior vermis. The three pairs of peduncles are attached to the cerebellum in the interval between the flocculonodular and anterior lobes.

Fissures that need not be identified by name outline further subdivisions or lobules, especially in the posterior lobe. The names given to these lobules by early anatomists have no functional significance; neither is there common acceptance of a single system of nomenclature. Figure 10–3 is inserted for reference in the event that it is necessary to identify smaller subdivisions of the cerebellum. The lingula, not seen in Figure 10–3, is a small, flattened portion of the superior vermis beneath the central lobule and adherent to the superior medullary velum (Fig. 10–2).

The functional anatomy of the cerebellum is based primarily on the destination of afferent fiber bundles. Viewed in this way, there is a *vestibulocerebellum*, a *spinocerebellum*, and a *pontocerebellum*. Since the foregoing divisions appeared progressively later in vertebrate phylogeny, they are also known as the *archicerebellum, paleocerebellum*, and *neocerebellum*, respectively. The functional divisions are not reflected in corresponding differences in the cytoarchitecture of the cortex which, in fact, is the

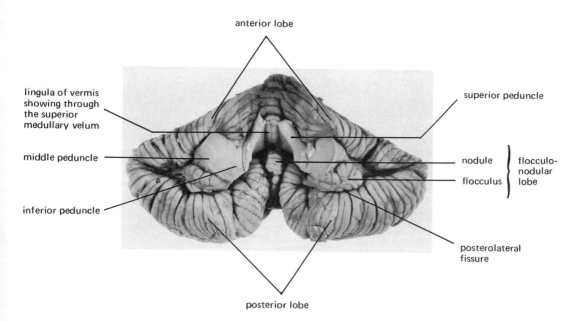

anterior lobe

lingula of vermis showing through the superior medullary velum

middle peduncle

inferior peduncle

superior peduncle

nodule } flocculo-
flocculus } nodular lobe

posterolateral fissure

posterior lobe

FIG. 10–2. Cerebellum viewed from in front and below, showing the cut surfaces of the cerebellar peduncles. ×⅔

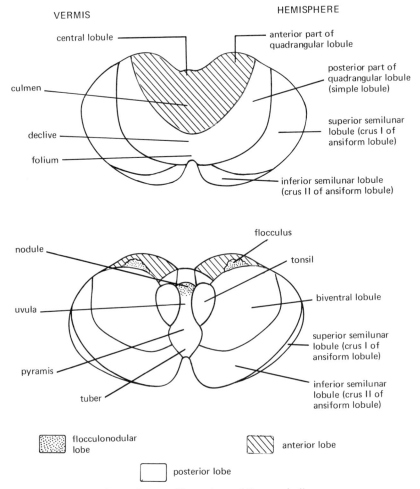

FIG. 10–3. Nomenclature for specific regions of the cerebellum.

same in all parts of the cerebellum. The four central nuclei are likewise similar at the cellular level. The cortex and nuclei are therefore described at this point, after which the functional divisions will be considered.

CEREBELLAR CORTEX

Because of the extensive folding of the cerebellar surface in the form of thin transverse *folia,* 85 percent of the cortical surface is concealed. There is therefore a large cortical area, which is about three-quarters as extensive as that of the much larger cerebrum.

CORTICAL LAYERS

Three layers are evident in histologic sections. From the surface to the white matter of the folium, these are the molecular layer, the layer of Purkinje cells, and the granule cell layer (Figs. 10–4 and 10–5). The *Purkinje cell layer* consists of

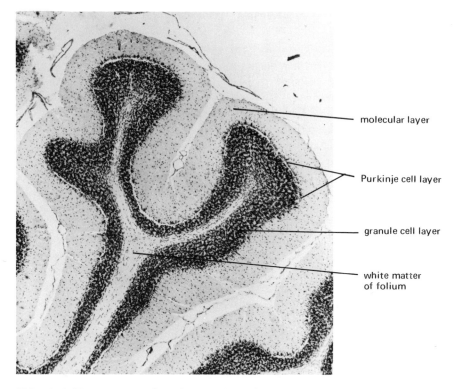

molecular layer

Purkinje cell layer

granule cell layer

white matter
of folium

FIG. 10–4. Transverse section of cerebellar folia, showing the three layers of cortex and the white matter of the folia. Cresyl violet stain. ×35

FIG. 10–5. Transverse section of cerebellar folia, showing the three layers of cortex and the white matter of the folia. Cajal silver nitrate method. ×35

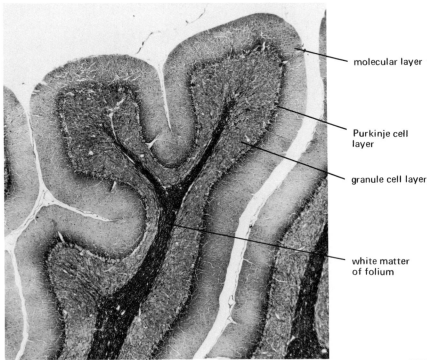

molecular layer

Purkinje cell
layer

granule cell layer

white matter
of folium

a single row (in sections) of bodies of Purkinje cells. The *molecular layer* contains relatively few nerve cells; it is largely a synaptic layer, made up of profusely branching dendrites of Purkinje cells and axons of the granule cells in the deepest layer. The term "molecular" is derived from the punctate appearance of this layer in sections stained for nerve fibers. The molecular layer includes scattered stellate cells near the surface and modified stellate cells, known as basket cells, at a deeper level. The *granule cell layer* consists of closely packed small neurons, from which axons extend into the molecular layer. There are scattered neurons known as Golgi cells in the outer zone of the granule cell layer.

There are two types of afferent fibers to the cortex. *Mossy fibers* terminate in synaptic contact with granule cells of the innermost layer, while *climbing fibers* enter the molecular layer and wind among the dendrites of Purkinje cells. The only fibers leaving the cortex are axons of Purkinje

cells. These fibers terminate in central nuclei of the cerebellum, with the exception that some from the cortex of the flocculonodular lobe leave the cerebellum and end in brain stem nuclei.

CYTOARCHITECTURE

The five types of neurons in the cerebellar cortex establish a complex but remarkably regular pattern of intracortical circuits. The precise three-dimensional orientation of dendrites and axons, as shown by the Golgi staining method, has encouraged the study of cortical physiology at the cellular level by means of recording microelectrodes. The basic pattern of the neurons is indicated in Figure 10–6.

Granule Cells and Mossy Fibers

The granule cells are small and closely packed together. Each cell has a spherical nucleus with a coarse chromatin pattern

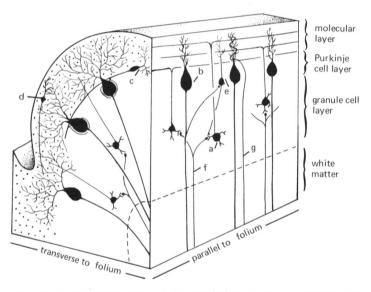

FIG. 10–6. Cytoarchitecture of the cerebellar cortex. *a*, granule cell; *b*, Purkinje cell; *c*, basket cell; *d*, stellate cell; *e*, Gogi cell; *f*, mossy fiber; *g*, climbing fiber.

and the scanty cytoplasm lacks clumps of Nissl substance. The short dendrites have claw-like endings which make synaptic contact with mossy fibers. The unmyelinated axon enters the molecular layer, where it bifurcates and runs parallel with the folium. Because of the density of the granule cell population, the whole of the molecular layer contains closely arranged parallel fibers. Each granule cell axon traverses the dendritic trees of some 450 Purkinje cells, with which it makes synaptic contacts. These axons also synapse with dendrites of stellate, basket, and Golgi cells in the molecular layer.

A large proportion of the afferent fibers to the cerebellum are mossy fibers terminating in synaptic relation with dendrites of granule cells. While still in the white matter, a mossy fiber divides into several branches which may enter the cortex of adjacent folia. On entering the granular layer, the fiber loses its myelin sheath and there is further terminal branching. Along the terminal portion of the fiber and at its

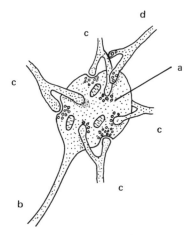

FIG. 10–7. A glomerulus in the granule cell layer. *a,* rosette; *b,* branch of a mossy fiber; *c,* dendrites of granule cells; *d,* axon of a Golgi cell.

end, there are swellings known as *rosettes,* with which the dendrites of several granule cells make synaptic contact (Fig. 10–7). The synaptic configuration that includes the rosette of a mossy fiber, dendrites of granule cells, and the axon of a Golgi cell (see below) is known as a *glomerulus.*

Purkinje Cells and Climbing Fibers

The Purkinje cells, or efferent cortical neurons, were described in Chapter 2 as an example of large Golgi type I neurons. The number of Purkinje cells is on the order of 15 million. Their most remarkable characteristic is the profuse dendritic branching in the molecular layer, in a plane transverse to the folium. The primary and secondary branches are smooth, while the finer branches bear regularly spaced projections or spines, of which there are some 100,000 on each Purkinje cell dendrite. Electron micrographs show the spines indenting parallel fibers (granule cell axons) to form synaptic junctions. The parallel arrangement of granule cell axons and the transverse orientation of Purkinje cell dendrites, with respect to a folium, provide maximal opportunity for a Purkinje cell to receive stimuli from a very large number of granule cells, and also allow a granule cell to contact about 450 Purkinje cells. The molecular layer is therefore a rich synaptic field, to which stellate, basket, and Golgi cells also contribute.

Axons of Purkinje cells traverse the granule cell layer, acquire myelin sheaths on entering the white matter, and terminate in central cerebellar nuclei. Collateral branches given off by the axons synapse with adjacent Purkinje cells or, more frequently, with Golgi cells in the outer part of the granule cell layer.

As the mossy fibers have a special relationship with granule cells, so the climbing fibers have a special relation to Purkinje cells. Climbing fibers enter the cortex from the medullary center, traverse the granule cell layer, and wind among the dendritic branches of Purkinje cells like a vine growing on a tree. Each climbing fiber makes synaptic contact with the smooth surface of the larger branches of a Purkinje cell dendrite. The synapse is excitatory, but the function of climbing fibers in a broader sense is still unknown. In addition, branches of climbing fibers synapse with stellate, basket, and Golgi cells. The source of climbing fibers has been controversial for many years; the current view is that they come from the inferior olivary complex of the medulla.

Basket Cells

The basket cells are scattered in the molecular layer near the bodies of Purkinje cells. The dendrite of a basket cell branches in the transverse plane of the folium, making contact with many granule cell axons and also receiving stimuli from branches of climbing fibers. The axon is directed across the folium, and collateral branches form characteristic synapses with about 250 Purkinje cells. Each collateral forms a basket-like arrangement around the perikaryon of a Purkinje cell, the fibers concentrating around the origin of the Purkinje cell axon (Fig. 10–8). Because of an overlapping arrangement, collateral branches of several basket cell axons contribute to the synapse with a single Purkinje cell.

Stellate and Golgi Cells

The granule, Purkinje, and basket cells have special features, while the stellate and Golgi cells are similar to small neurons elsewhere in the nervous system.

There are scattered stellate cells in the superficial part of the molecular layer. Their dendrites are in contact with parallel

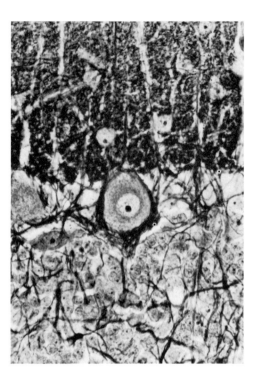

FIG. 10–8. Cell body of a Purkinje cell situated between the molecular layer and granule cell layer of cerebellar cortex. The fibers surrounding the Purkinje cell body consist mainly of terminal branches of basket cell axons. Cajal silver nitrate method. ×450

fibers from granule cells and, to a lesser extent, with branches of climbing fibers. The axons synapse mainly with Purkinje cell dendrites, but a few enter the innermost cortical layer and establish a feedback circuit by synapsing with granule cells. The Golgi cells are situated in the outer portion of the granule cell layer; their dendrites extend into the molecular layer, where they make contact with parallel fibers. Other afferents to Golgi cells consist of collateral branches of Purkinje cell axons and branches of climbing fibers. Axons of Golgi cells enter glomeruli, where they synapse with the dendrites of granule cells (Fig. 10–7). In the main, therefore, Golgi cells form reverberating circuits with granule cells.

Intracortical Circuits

Recordings from microelectrodes inserted in the cerebellar cortex have yielded information about whether synapses between specific types of neurons produce an excitatory postsynaptic potential (EPSP) or an inhibitory postsynaptic potential (IPSP). Studies of this kind indicate that synapses between mossy fibers and granule cells, granule cells and Purkinje cells, and climbing fibers and Purkinje cells are all excitatory. The input to the cortex is therefore excitatory. However, this is modified by intracortical circuits that inhibit Purkinje cells and therefore suppress transmission from cortex to central nuclei. For example, parallel fibers produce an EPSP in stellate and basket cells, but synapses between these and Purkinje cells produce an IPSP. Also, parallel fibers excite Golgi cells, which inhibit granule cells. The inhibitory circuits involve more synapses than the excitatory relays. Therefore, afferent volleys to the cortex first produce an EPSP in Purkinje cells, followed after 1–2 msec by an IPSP. The inhibitory circuits tend to limit the area of cortex excited and the degree of excitation resulting from an incoming volley.

CENTRAL NUCLEI

Four pairs of nuclei are embedded deep in the medullary center; in a medial to lateral direction, they are the fastigial, globose, emboliform, and dentate nuclei (Fig. 10–9). The phylogenetic development of these nuclei was in the same order.

The *fastigial nucleus* is nearly spherical, close to the midline, and almost in contact with the roof of the fourth ventricle. The *globose nucleus* consists of two or three small cellular masses, and the larger *emboliform nucleus* is oval or plug-shaped. In mammals as high in the phylogenetic scale as the monkey, a single nucleus (the nucleus interpositus) is situated between the fastigial and dentate nuclei. In the highest primates, including man, the nucleus interpositus is represented by the globose and emboliform nuclei. The *dentate nucleus* is the most prominent of the central nuclei; this mammalian nucleus is largest in primates, especially in man. The dentate nucleus has the irregular shape of a crumpled purse, like that of the inferior olivary nucleus, with the hilus facing medially. Its efferent fibers occupy the interior of the nucleus and leave through the hilus.

The input to the cerebellar nuclei is from two sources, the first being extracerebellar and the second from the Purkinje cells of the cerebellar cortex. The extrinsic input is still under investigation. Pontocerebellar and spinocerebellar fibers appear to be im-

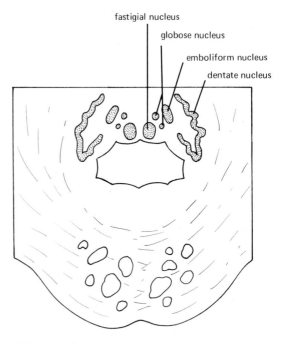

fastigial nucleus

globose nucleus

emboliform nucleus

dentate nucleus

FIG. 10–9. Central nuclei of the cerebellum.

portant, together with reticulocerebellar fibers from the lateral reticular nucleus of the medulla; a few olivocerebellar fibers also enter the cerebellar nuclei. Some of the above afferents are collateral branches of fibers proceeding to the cerebellar cortex. The fastigial nucleus also receives afferents from the vestibular nerve and nuclei. A few rubrocerebellar fibers end in the globose and emboliform nuclei. The fastigial nucleus discharges to the brain stem through the juxtarestiform body of the inferior peduncle; efferents from the remaining nuclei leave the cerebellum in the brachium conjunctivum, most of them terminating in the red nucleus and thalamus.

Physiologic studies indicate that Purkinje cells inhibit neurons of the central nuclei and that the input from outside the cerebellum is excitatory. Crudely processed information in the central nuclei is infinitely refined by the feedback from the cortex. The combination of the two inputs maintains a tonic discharge of impulses from the central nuclei to the brain stem and thalamus. This discharge changes continually according to the afferent input to the cerebellum at any given time.

MEDULLARY CENTER AND CEREBELLAR PEDUNCLES

The white matter is scanty in the region of the vermis, where it produces a branching, tree-like pattern in a sagittal section (Fig. 10–10). Each hemisphere, however, contains a large *medullary center*, in which the dentate nucleus is embedded (Fig. 10–11). Most of the constituent fibers belong to afferent tracts proceeding to the cortex or are Purkinje cell axons going from the cortex to central nuclei. The white matter also includes Purkinje cell axons joining different areas of cortex, some of these fibers being commissural.

The afferent and efferent systems are discussed in connection with the functional divisions of the cerebellum. They are identified at this point only as components of the cerebellar peduncles.

The *inferior cerebellar peduncle* consists of two parts: The larger part is called the *restiform body,* on the medial side of which lies the *juxtarestiform body* (Fig. 7–8). The restiform body consists of the following afferent tracts or fiber systems: olivocerebellar, dorsal spinocerebellar, cuneocerebellar, reticulocerebellar, and trigeminocerebellar (from the chief sensory and spinal tract nuclei of the trigeminal nerve). The juxtarestiform body contains afferents from the vestibular nuclear complex and the vestibular nerve, together with the only efferent fibers in the inferior peduncle. These are fibers proceeding from the cortex of the flocculonodular lobe and the fastigial nucleus to vestibular nuclei and the reticular formation of the brain stem.

The *middle cerebellar peduncle* or *brachium pontis* consists entirely of pontocerebellar fibers. The *superior cerebellar peduncle* consists mainly of the *brachium conjunctivum,* which is made up of efferent fibers from the globose, emboliform, and dentate nuclei. The other components of the superior peduncle are afferent to the cerebellum. They include the ventral spinocerebellar tract on the dorsolateral surface of the brachium conjunctivum (Fig. 7–11), a small contingent of rubrocerebellar fibers, and fibers from the trigeminal mesencephalic nucleus. There are also tectocerebellar fibers from the inferior colliculi, but most of these reach the cerebellum by running in the superior medullary velum.

FUNCTIONAL ANATOMY

Three functional divisions are recognized based on the termination of afferent sys-

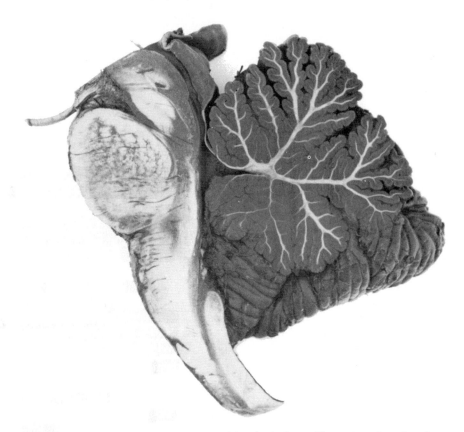

FIG. 10–10. Cerebellar surface in the midsagittal plane. The cut surface has been stained by a method which differentiates gray matter and white matter. ×1½

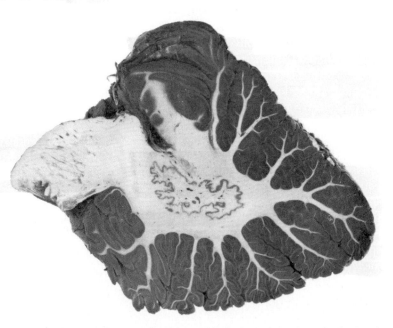

FIG. 10–11. Cerebellar surface in a parasagittal plane through the hemisphere, stained to differentiate gray matter and white matter. The dentate nucleus is shown embedded in the medullary center of white matter. ×1½

tems in the cortex and the sequence of phylogenetic development. The *vestibulocerebellum* or *archicerebellum* is the oldest part, constituting the entire cerebellum of fishes; it is concerned with maintenance of equilibrium. The *spinocerebellum* or *paleocerebellum* appeared next and is present in submammalian terrestrial vertebrates. In general, the paleocerebellum influences muscle tonus and synergy of muscles during movements inherent in postural changes and locomotion. A *pontocerebellum* or *neocerebellum* was added in mammals and is the largest part of the human cerebellum. Neocerebellar activity ensures the synergy and delicate adjustments of muscle tonus that are necessary for accuracy of nonstereotyped movements, especially those based on learning experience. The three divisions overlap to a considerable degree in both the cortex and the central nuclei; they are also connected with one another by means of association fibers in the medullary center.

The following generalizations are helpful as a background for the discussion of functional divisions. First, olivocerebellar fibers are distributed to all parts of the cortex; the accessory olivary nuclei project to the flocculonodular lobe and vermis, and the inferior olivary nuclei to the hemispheres. The second generalization is concerned with the termination of Purkinje cells in the central nuclei. The cortex of the vermis sends fibers to the fastigial nucleus; the cortex of the medial portion of the hemisphere (paravermal or intermediate zone) projects on the globose and emboliform nuclei; and the large lateral region of hemispheral cortex sends fibers to the dentate nucleus.

ARCHICEREBELLUM

The *archicerebellum* consists of the flocculonodular lobe, together with a region of the inferior vermis adjacent to the nodule and known as the uvula (Figs. 10–3 and 10–12). A few vestibular fibers end in other parts of the vermis, so that archicerebellar and paleocerebellar areas partially overlap. Afferent impulses originate in the vestibular portion of the inner ear and are conveyed centrally in the vestibular nerve. Some fibers of the nerve enter the cerebellum, but these are outnumbered by indirect vestibular afferents from vestibular nuclei. The afferent fibers, which are included in the juxtarestiform body of the inferior peduncle, terminate in the archicerebellar cortex and the fastigial nucleus.

A proportion of Purkinje cell axons from archicerebellar cortex proceed to the brain stem (an exception to the general rule that such fibers end in central nuclei), and the remainder terminate in the fastigial nucleus. Fibers from the cortex and fastigial nucleus traverse the juxtarestiform body to their termination in the vestibular nuclear complex and reticular formation of the medulla and pons. A bundle of fastigiobulbar fibers, known as the *uncinate fasciculus* (of Russell), has an aberrant course; the fasciculus curves over the root of the superior peduncle and then joins the other efferents in the juxtarestiform body.

The archicerebellum influences lower motor neurons through the vestibulospinal tract, the medial longitudinal fasciculus, and reticulospinal fibers. It is concerned, as previously stated, with adjustment of muscle tonus in response to vestibular stimuli, and hence functions in maintaining equilibrium and in other motor responses to vestibular stimulation (see Chapter 22).

PALEOCEREBELLUM

The *paleocerebellum* is defined as the portion receiving data from general sensory receptors, mainly through ascending fasciculi of the spinal cord. The area has been

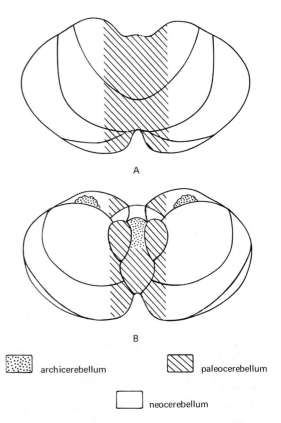

archicerebellum   paleocerebellum

neocerebellum

FIG. 10–12. Functional regions of the cerebellum.
A. Superior surface. **B.** Inferior surface.

delineated in experimental animals, including the monkey, by establishing the course and termination of afferent fibers by neuroanatomical methods and by recording evoked potentials in the cortex during peripheral nerve stimulation. From the above studies, with some supporting evidence for man, the paleocerebellum is considered to consist of the superior vermis, most of the inferior vermis, and the paravermal or intermediate zones on the superior and inferior surfaces of the hemispheres (Fig. 10–12).

The following afferent systems project specifically to paleocerebellar cortex. The dorsal and ventral spinocerebellar tracts convey data from proprioceptive endings and from touch and pressure receptors. The dorsal tract carries information from the arm, trunk, and leg while the ventral tract is involved mainly in conduction from the leg. Cuneocerebellar fibers from the lateral cuneate nucleus reinforce the dorsal spinocerebellar tract for conduction from the arm, and they constitute the main pathway for impulses originating in deep and cutaneous receptors of the neck. Data from cutaneous receptors are also carried by spinoreticular fibers to the lateral reticular nucleus from which fibers project to the paleocerebellar cortex. Finally, the paleocerebellum receives fibers from the three sensory trigeminal nuclei.

Each half of the body is represented in

the ipsilateral cortex; if fibers cross the midline from cells of origin at lower levels, they cross again in the medullary center of the cerebellum. Studies in the monkey show a dual somatotopic representation with the feet forward; one area is on the superior surface and the other on the inferior surface. The paleocerebellum also receives pontocerebellar fibers, so that in this respect there is an overlap between paleocerebellum and neocerebellum. The principle underlying cerebellar cortical localization is not so much punctate topography as in some areas of the cerebral cortex, but rather a localization that is in line with the computing function of the cerebellar cortex. Consistent with this there is an overlap of different inputs so that their influences are brought to bear on the same Purkinje cells.

The paleocerebellar cortex projects on the fastigial nucleus (from the vermis) and on the globose and emboliform nuclei (from the paravermal zone or medial portion of the hemisphere). Synergy of muscle action and control of muscle tonus are effected in part through fastigiobulbar connections, as described for the archicerebellum. Fibers from the globose and emboliform nuclei traverse the brachium conjunctivum and terminate in the red nucleus, especially its magnocellular portion. Through this connection, paleocerebellar activity is brought to bear on lower motor neurons by means of the rubrospinal tract, rubroreticular and reticulospinal fibers, and rubrobulbar fibers to motor nuclei of cranial nerves. The influence of the paleocerebellum on skeletal musculature is ipsilateral. For example, the right half of the paleocerebellar cortical area, which receives sensory data from the right side of the body, influences lower motor neurons for right-sided muscles through compensating decussations, that of the brachium

conjunctivum and the decussation of rubrospinal and rubroreticular fibers. Alpha and gamma motor neurons are both involved in the cerebellar control of muscle function.

Before reaching the red nucleus, some cerebellorubral fibers give off collateral branches which run caudally in the brain stem and end in the reticular formation, including the paramedian reticular nucleus of the medulla. These collaterals participate in feedback circuits between the brain stem and the cerebellum, and in a projection to lower motor neurons through reticulospinal connections.

In summary, the paleocerebellum receives information from proprioceptive endings and from exteroceptors for touch and pressure. Data thus received are processed by the computer-like circuitry of the cerebellar cortex and further modified in the central nuclei. Lower motor neurons, especially the gamma efferents, are influenced through relays in the vestibular nuclei, the red nucleus, and the reticular formation. The end result is control of muscle tonus and synergy of collaborating muscles, as appropriate at any moment according to changes of posture and in many types of movement, including those of locomotion.

NEOCEREBELLUM

Pontocerebellar fibers constitute the whole of the middle cerebellar peduncle or brachium pontis. Originating in the nuclei pontis of the opposite side, these fibers are distributed throughout the cortex of the corpus cerebelli, i.e., to all of the cortex except the flocculonodular lobe. However, the greatest concentration of input from the pons is to the lateral portions of the hemispheres that make up the *neocerebellum* (Fig. 10–12). Through the nuclei pontis, the afferent input originates in widespread areas of the contralateral cerebral cortex, with input from the frontal and parietal lobes predominating. In common with the cerebellar cortex generally, the neocerebellum receives large numbers of olivocerebellar fibers.

Cortical efferents of the neocerebellum terminate in the dentate nucleus, the efferent fibers of which make up most of the brachium conjunctivum. After traversing the decussation of the brachium conjunctivum, some of the fibers terminate in the parvicellular portion of the red nucleus. The majority, however, pass through or around the red nucleus, continuing forward to a thalamic relay nucleus (ventral lateral nucleus) which in turn projects to motor areas of cortex in the frontal lobe. The latter areas are the source of a large proportion of the fibers of the pyramidal motor system; they also send extrapyramidal fibers to several motor nuclei, including the corpus striatum and substantia nigra.

The neocerebellum may be thought of as a computer that is especially well developed in man and designed for the refinement of voluntary movements. Data received from association areas of the cerebral cortex and from other sources are subjected to a complex computerization in the neocerebellar cortex. The output from the dentate nuclei, which reaches motor areas of the cerebral cortex via the thalamus, constantly fluctuates according to the excitatory input to the dentate nuclei from extracerebellar sources and the all important refinement of discharge of the neurons comprising these nuclei by the inhibitory influence of Purkinje cells. A cerebellar hemisphere influences the musculature of the same side of the body because of two decussations, the decussation of the brachia conjunctiva and that of the pyramids. Through the above circuit, the neocerebel-

lum ensures a smooth and orderly sequence of muscular contraction and the intended precision in the force, direction, and extent of volitional movements.

OTHER CEREBELLAR CONNECTIONS

Laboratory studies, including research using monkeys, show that impulses of auditory and visual origin reach the cerebellar cortex. The area concerned is in the posterior part of the superior and inferior surfaces, including paleocerebellar cortex and the medial part of the neocerebellar cortex. There are two projections from the midbrain tectum to the cerebellum: tectocerebellar fibers in the superior medullary velum, and tectopontine and pontocerebellar fibers. The relay for the latter pathway is in the dorsolateral region of the nuclei pontis. There is evidence that the tectocerebellar fibers originate in the inferior colliculus and therefore convey auditory data, while the tectopontine fibers carry visual data from the superior colliculus. Although corticopontine fibers originate mainly in association areas of cerebral cortex, there is a significant contribution from primary cortical areas. It has been shown, again experimentally, that impulses from the visual and auditory areas reach the visuoauditory area of cerebellar cortex, and that impulses from the somesthetic and motor areas reach paleocerebellar cortex.

Animal experiments also indicate that the cerebellum has a role in visceral functions. Under certain conditions, electrical stimulation of paleocerebellar cortex produces respiratory, cardiovascular, pupillary, and urinary bladder responses. The responses are sympathetic in nature when the anterior lobe is stimulated and parasympathetic when the tonsils (Fig. 10–3) of the posterior lobe are stimulated. The pathways have not been identified with certainty, but it has been suggested that impulses are relayed to the hypothalamus through the reticular formation.

SIGNS OF CEREBELLAR DYSFUNCTION

Cerebellar disorders resulting from vascular occlusion, tumor growth, or other pathologic conditions are classified broadly into those affecting the vestibulocerebellum (flocculonodular lobe) and those affecting the main mass of the cerebellum (corpus cerebelli).

The vestibular portion of the cerebellum may be invaded by a tumor, typically a medulloblastoma occurring in childhood, and the resulting disorder of cerebellar function is known as the archicerebellar syndrome. The patient is unsteady on his feet, walks on a wide base, and sways from side to side. The signs are limited at first to a disturbance of equilibrium; reflexes and voluntary movements are not otherwise affected. However, cerebellar signs described below soon appear as the tumor invades other parts of the cerebellum.

With respect to the corpus cerebelli, signs of cerebellar dysfunction accompany lesions that interrupt afferent pathways, cause destruction of the cortex and medullary center, or involve the central nuclei and efferent pathways in the brachium conjunctivum. There is considerable recovery with time because of compensation by intact regions and other motor systems. The motor disorder is more severe and more enduring when a lesion involves the central nuclei and brachium conjunctivum. The signs of destructive lesions of the corpus

cerebelli or the major afferent and efferent pathways are commonly referred to as the neocerebellar syndrome, although in many instances the paleocerebellum is also involved. When the lesion is unilateral, which is most frequently the case, the signs of motor dysfunction are on the same side of the body as the lesion. This follows from the compensating decussations that were pointed out above.

The following signs, in varying degrees of severity, are characteristic of the neocerebellar syndrome. Movements tend to be ataxic (intermittent or jerky). There is also dysmetria; for example, when reaching out with the finger to an object, the finger overshoots the mark or deviates from it (past-pointing). Rapidly alternating movements such as flexion and extension of the fingers or pronation and supination of the forearms are performed in a clumsy manner (adiadochokinesia). Asynergy is reflected in separation of voluntary movements that normally flow smoothly in sequence into a succession of mechanical or puppet-like movements (decomposition of movements). There may be hypotonia of muscles, and the muscles tend to tire easily. Cerebellar tremor is characteristically terminal, occurring at the end of a particular movement (intention tremor). Asynergy may involve muscles used in speech, which is then thick and monotonous. There may be nystagmus, especially if the lesion encroaches on the vermis, because of involvement of projections to the oculomotor, trochlear, and abducens nuclei via the vestibular nuclei and the red nucleus. The deficits noted above are entirely motor and superimposed on volitional movements which are themselves basically intact.

SUGGESTIONS FOR ADDITIONAL READING

Bloomfield S, Marr D: How the cerebellum may be used. Nature (London) 227:1224–1228, 1970

Braitenberg V, Atwood RP: Morphological observations on the cerebellar cortex. J Comp Neurol 109:1–33, 1958

Carpenter MB, Stevens GH: Structural and functional relationships between the deep cerebellar nuclei and the brachium conjunctivum in the rhesus monkey. J Comp Neurol 107:109–163, 1957

Courville J, Cooper CW: The cerebellar nuclei of Macaca mulatta: A morphological study. J Comp Neurol 140:241–254, 1970

Eccles JC: The Dynamic Loop Hypothesis of Movement Control. In Leibovic KN (ed.): Information Processing in the Nervous System, pp. 245–269. New York, Springer–Verlag, 1969

Eccles JC, Ito M, Szentágothai J: The Cerebellum as a Neuronal Machine. New York, Springer, 1967

Evarts EV, Thach WT: Motor mechanisms of the CNS: Cerebrocerebellar interrelations. Ann Rev Physiol 31:451–498, 1969

Flumerfelt BA, Otabe S, Courville J: Distinct projections to the red nucleus from the dentate and interposed nuclei in the monkey. Brain Res 50: 408–414, 1973

Fox CA, Barnard JW: A quantitative study of the Purkinje cell dendritic branchlets and their relationship to afferent fibers. J Anat 91:299–313, 1957

Fox CA, Snider RS (eds.): The cerebellum. Progr Brain Res 25, 1967

Gray EG: The granule cells, mossy synapses and Purkinje spine synapses of the cerebellum: Light and electron microscope observations. J Anat 95: 345–356, 1961

Holmes G: The cerebellum of man. Brain 62:1–30, 1939

Koella WP: Some functional properties of optically evoked potentials in the cerebellar cortex of cats. J Neurophysiol 22:61–77, 1959

Oscarsson O: Functional organization of the spino- and cuneocerebellar tracts. Physiol Rev 45:495–522, 1965

Snider RS: The cerebellum. Sci Am 199/2:84–90, 1958

Snider RS, Eldred E: Cerebro-cerebellar relationships in the monkey. J Neurophysiol 15:27–40, 1952

Truex RC, Carpenter MB: Human Neuroanatomy, 6th ed. Baltimore, Williams & Wilkins, 1969

11
Diencephalon

The diencephalon and telencephalon together constitute the cerebrum, of which
the diencephalon forms the central core
and the telencephalon the cerebral hemispheres. Being almost entirely surrounded
by the hemispheres, only the basal surface
of the diencephalon is exposed to view in a
diamond-shaped area containing hypothalamic structures (Fig. 11–1). This area
is bounded in front by the optic chiasma,
and on either side by the optic tract and
the region of continuity between the internal capsule and the basis pedunculi of the
midbrain. The diencephalon is divided into
symmetrical halves by the slit-like third
ventricle. As seen in midsagittal section
(Fig. 11–2), the junction of the midbrain
and diencephalon is represented by a line
passing through the posterior commissure
and immediately caudal to the mammillary
body. The boundary between the diencephalon and telencephalon is represented
by a line traversing the foramen of Monro
and the optic chiasma.

GROSS FEATURES

SURFACES

The surfaces of each half of the diencephalon have the following landmarks and relations. The *medial surface* forms the wall of
the third ventricle (Fig. 11–2). A bundle of
nerve fibers called the stria medullaris
thalami forms an elevation along the junction of the medial and dorsal surfaces. The
ependymal lining of the third ventricle is
reflected from one side to the other along
the striae medullares, forming the roof of
the ventricle from which a small choroid
plexus is suspended.

The *dorsal surface* of the diencephalon is
largely concealed by the fornix (Fig.
11–3); this is a robust bundle of fibers
which originates in the hippocampus of the
temporal lobe, curves over the thalamus,
and ends mainly in the mammillary body.
The fornices outline a triangular interval
which constitutes a forward extension of

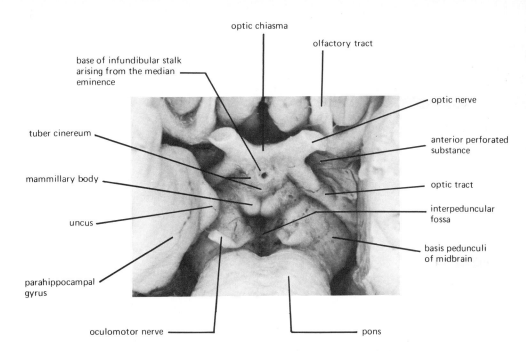

FIG. 11–1. An area of the basal surface of the brain, in which the diencephalon (hypothalamus) presents to the surface. ×1½

FIG. 11–2. Central region of the brain in midsagittal section. ×1¼

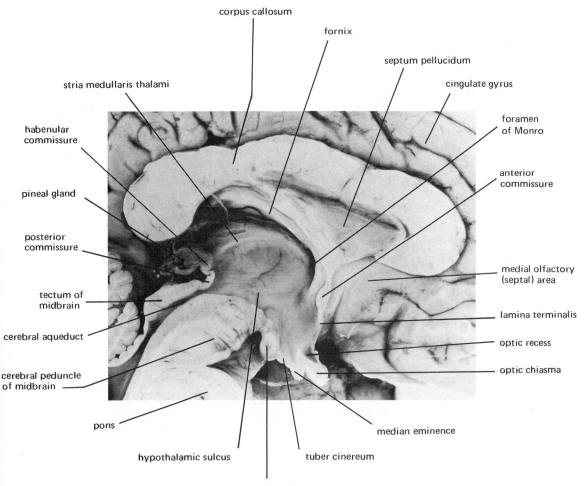

the *transverse cerebral fissure* into the cerebrum, the remaining part of the fissure intervening between the cerebellum and the cerebral hemispheres. Between the fornices, the transverse fissure is roofed over by the corpus callosum, while its floor is formed by a small area of the diencephalon and the roof of the third ventricle. The vascular connective tissue occupying the space just delineated is known as the *tela choroidea* and is continuous under the fornices with the vascular core of the choroid plexuses of the lateral ventricles. Lateral to the fornix, the dorsal surface of the thalamus forms the floor of the lateral ventricle, much of which is concealed by the choroid plexus (Fig. 11–3).

The *lateral surface* of the diencephalon is bounded by the thick internal capsule of white matter, consisting of fibers connecting the cerebral cortex with the thalamus and other parts of the neuraxis. The medial part of the *basal surface* presents to the surface of the brain, as noted above, while the lateral part is bounded by the internal capsule in the region of its continuity with the basis pedunculi of the midbrain.

MAJOR DIVISIONS

The diencephalon consists of four parts, each represented bilaterally, which differ in structure and function. The following general statements simply record the nature of the four divisions; their components are discussed in some detail further on.

The *thalamus* (dorsal thalamus) is the largest portion; this mass of gray matter is

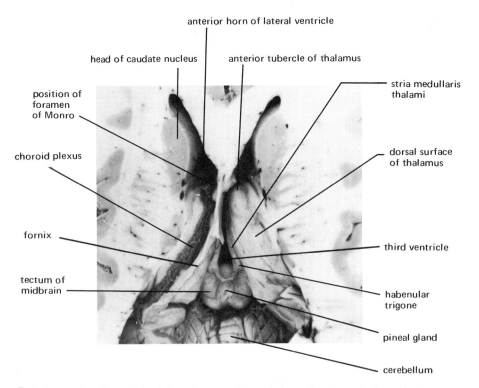

anterior horn of lateral ventricle

head of caudate nucleus   anterior tubercle of thalamus

position of
foramen
of Monro

stria medullaris
thalami

choroid plexus

dorsal surface
of thalamus

fornix

third ventricle

tectum of
midbrain

habenular
trigone

pineal gland

cerebellum

FIG. 11–3. Dorsal aspect of the diencephalon, with the fornix and choroid plexus removed on the right side. ×1

subdivided into several nuclei on the basis of fiber connections and sequence of phylogenetic development. Certain thalamic nuclei receive specific sensory input for the general senses, taste, vision, and hearing; these nuclei project to sensory areas of the cerebral cortex. Other thalamic nuclei participate in emotional aspects of brain function, are functionally related to association areas of cortex, or have a role in the ascending reticular activating system. The *subthalamus* (ventral thalamus) is a complex region bounded by the thalamus above and the internal capsule below. The subthalamus includes a motor nucleus (the subthalamic nucleus), sensory fiber tracts terminating in the thalamus, and bundles of fibers originating in the cerebellum and corpus striatum. The reticular formation, red nucleus, and substantia nigra extend from the midbrain into the subthalamus. The *epithalamus*, situated dorsomedial to the thalamus and adjacent to the roof of the third ventricle, is a particularly old part of the diencephalon phylogenetically. The epithalamus includes an endocrine organ (the pineal gland) and structures concerned with affective and olfactory reflex responses. The *hypothalamus* occupies the region between the ventral part of the third ventricle and the subthalamus; it is the main cerebral center for integrative control of the autonomic nervous system.

THALAMUS

The thalamus, measuring about 3 cm anteroposteriorly and 1.5 cm in the other two directions, makes up four-fifths of the diencephalon. Thin laminae of white matter outline the thalamus; the *stratum zonale* on the dorsal surface, best developed anteriorly (Fig. 11–11), is one such sheet of nerve fibers. The *external medullary lamina* is a thin layer of nerve fibers covering the

lateral surface of the thalamus (Fig. 11–8). It consists mainly of thalamocortical and corticothalamic fibers running along the surface of the thalamus briefly before entering or leaving the internal capsule. The external medullary lamina and internal capsule are separated by an attenuated layer of nerve cells constituting the thalamic reticular nucleus.

The *internal medullary lamina* (Figs. 11–4 and 11–8), consisting mainly of fibers passing from one thalamic nucleus to another, divides the thalamus into three gray masses. These are the lateral nuclear mass, the medial nucleus, and the anterior nucleus, the last named being enclosed by a bifurcation of the lamina. The lateral nuclear mass consists of ventral and dorsal tiers of nuclei which have been identified because of differing fiber connections (Fig. 11–4). Five nuclei are recognized in the ventral tier—the medial and lateral geniculate nuclei, and the ventral posterior, ventral lateral, and ventral anterior nuclei. (Alternatively, the geniculate nuclei are described as composing the metathalamus.) The dorsal tier consists of the pulvinar, lateral posterior nucleus, and lateral dorsal nucleus. In the central part of the thalamus, the internal medullary lamina partially encloses several collections of nerve cells (intralaminar nuclei), including the well-developed centromedian nucleus (Fig. 11–4). The midline nucleus lies between the medial nucleus and the third ventricle.

On the basis of phylogeny, connections with other parts of the brain, and function, the thalamic nuclei may be classified according to the following scheme.

1. Reticular nucleus, a thalamic portion of the reticular formation of the brain.
2. Midline and intralaminer nuclei, which receive afferents from the reticular formation of the brain stem and project to

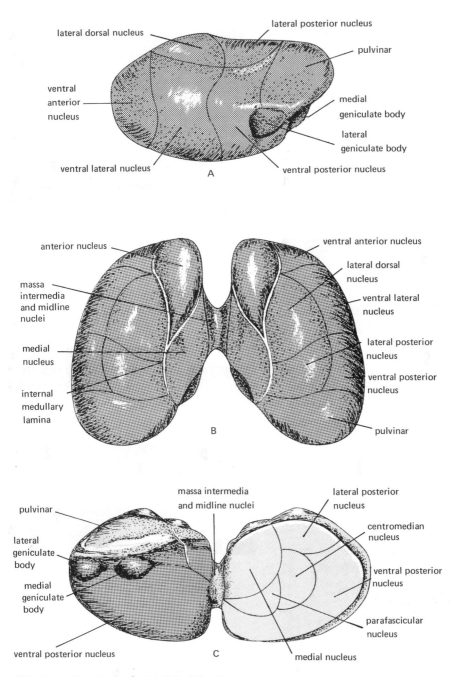

FIG. 11–4. Drawings of a model of the thalami. **A.** Lateral view. **B.** Dorsal view. **C.** Posterior view with the posterior part of the right thalamus cut away. (Model prepared by Dr. D. G. Montemurro)

other parts of the diencephalon. These nuclei have no direct cortical connections.

3. Specific thalamic nuclei projecting to sensory and motor areas of cortex. The medial geniculate nucleus (hearing), lateral geniculate nucleus (vision), and ventral posterior nucleus (general sensations and taste) are specific sensory nuclei. The ventral lateral nucleus and ventral anterior nucleus are specific motor nuclei; receiving data from the cerebellum, corpus striatum, and possibly the substantia nigra, they project to motor areas of cortex in the frontal lobe.

4. Nonspecific thalamic nuclei, which have reciprocal connections with association areas of cortex. This group includes the medial and anterior nuclei and the dorsal tier of the lateral nuclear mass, i.e., the pulvinar, lateral posterior nucleus, and lateral dorsal nucleus.

RETICULAR NUCLEUS

As noted above, the *reticular nucleus* consists of a thin sheet of nerve cells intervening between the external medullary lamina and the internal capsule. The reticular formation of the brain stem extends forward into the subthalamus, where it is known as the zona incerta (Fig. 11–8), and the latter is continuous with the thalamic reticular nucleus. The reticular nucleus receives data through the polysynaptic relays of the reticular formation and also has cortical afferents, as does the reticular formation generally. Fibers project from the thalamic reticular nucleus to widespread areas of cortex. Through the latter projection, suppplemented by an indirect route that involves other thalamic nuclei, this portion of the reticular formation participates in the ascending activating system. The thalamic reticular nucleus is probably involved as well in synaptic relays between various thalamic nuclei and the cerebral cortex.

MIDLINE AND INTRALAMINAR NUCLEI

Midline Nucleus

The *hypothalamic sulcus,* running from the foramen of Monro to the opening of the cerebral aqueduct (Fig. 11–2), divides the wall of the third ventricle into a thalamic region above and a hypothalamic region below. The midline nucleus consists of clusters of nerve cells adjacent to the third ventricle, above the hypothalamic sulcus. The midline nucleus is prominent in lower vertebrates, but a minor part of the human thalamus. In 70 percent of brains, the *massa intermedia* forms a bridge of gray matter across the third ventricle and constitutes part of this primitive nuclear complex (Fig. 11–9).

The polysynaptic pathway of the brain stem reticular formation is the principal source of afferents to the midline nucleus. Data of visceral origin, including those for taste, are of special importance. The hypothalamus receives unmyelinated and thinly myelinated fibers from the midline nucleus, and this nucleus is therefore involved in autonomic responses at the diencephalic level. The midline nucleus also has connections with the medial thalamic nucleus, which has a role in affective reactions, and with the intralaminar nuclei, the latter being of special significance with respect to the reticular activating system.

Intralaminar Nuclei

There are several nuclei, known collectively as the intralaminar nuclei, in the region of the internal medullary lamina and partly surrounded by the lamina. Of these the *centromedian nucleus* is especially well represented in anthropoid apes and man (Figs. 11–4 and 11–6). A smaller *parafascicular nucleus* lies adjacent to the habenulointerpeduncular fasciculus; other intralaminar nuclei are too small in man to merit consideration.

The intralaminar nuclei receive afferents from the reticular formation of the brain stem, through which data from most of the sensory systems are relayed. Some spino-thalamic and trigeminothalamic fibers also terminate in the intralaminar nuclei, although most of these fibers have the ventral posterior nucleus as their destination. The intralaminar nuclei project to surrounding parts of the thalamus, i.e., to the lateral nuclear mass and the medial and anterior nuclei, which in turn project to widespread areas of cortex. This is the anatomic basis for the important effect of the reticular system on levels of consciousness and degrees of alertness. It is also the basis for vague awareness of sensory stimulation without specificity or discriminative qualities, but with emotional responses, especially to painful stimuli. The intralaminar nuclei, through thalamic nuclei having cortical projections, constitute the key generator of much of the synchronized activity of the cerebral cortex, as shown in the rhythmic brain wave activity of the electroencephalogram. The intralaminar nuclei also send fibers to the corpus striatum and therefore have a role in motor responses at a subcortical level.

Destruction of the intralaminar nuclei results in lethargy, somnolence, and diminished response to sensory stimulation. An electrolytic lesion placed in the nuclei is reported to be effective in relief of intractable pain.

SPECIFIC THALAMIC NUCLEI

Medial Geniculate Nucleus

This nucleus on the auditory pathway forms a swelling (the medial geniculate body) on the posterior surface of the thalamus beneath the pulvinar (Figs. 7–14, 7–15, and 11–4). Afferent fibers to the medial geniculate nucleus constitute the inferior brachium coming from the inferior colliculus, which is the terminus of the lateral lemniscus. The nucleus receives data from the organ of Corti of both sides, but predominantly from the opposite ear. This bilateral projection stems from the presence of a few ipsilateral fibers in the lateral lemniscus and decussating fibers in the commissure of the inferior colliculus. There is a topographic pattern in the medial geniculate nucleus with respect to pitch; the pattern simulates a spiral, corresponding to the spiral-shaped organ of Corti.

Efferents from the medial geniculate nucleus constitute the auditory radiation, which terminates in the auditory area of the temporal lobe (Fig. 11–12). Experimental evidence suggests that there is a general awareness of sounds at the thalamic level in subprimates and perhaps minimally in primates. With this possible exception, the integrity of the auditory cortex and adjacent areas of the temporal lobe is necessary for appreciation of sounds, including discriminative aspects of hearing and recognition on the basis of memory recall.

Lateral Geniculate Nucleus

The lateral geniculate body beneath the pulvinar marks the position of the lateral geniculate nucleus on the visual pathway to the cerebral cortex (Figs. 11–4 and 11–6). The nucleus consists of six layers of nerve cells, numbered consecutively from its ventral surface. Layers 1 and 2 consist of large neurons, while layers 3 through 6 are made up of small cells. The lateral geniculate nucleus is the terminus of all but a few of the fibers of the optic tract. The fibers originate in the ganglion cell layer of the retina; they are divided equally between those coming from the lateral half of the ipsilateral eye and from the medial half of the contralateral eye, the latter fibers having crossed the midline in the optic chiasma. Each nucleus therefore receives data relative to the opposite field of vision. The crossed fibers terminate in layers 1, 4, and 6, while the uncrossed fibers end in layers 2, 3, and 5.

There is a detailed point-to-point projection of the retina on the lateral geniculate nucleus. In a more general way the superior retinal quadrants project to the medial portion of the nucleus, the inferior quadrants to the lateral portion, and the macular region for central vision projects to the posterior part of the nucleus. Axons of cells in the lateral geniculate nucleus constitute the geniculocalcarine tract, which terminates in the visual area of the occipital lobe adjacent to the calcarine sulcus (Fig. 11–12). At the latter site, and in the surrounding association cortex, there is awareness of visual stimuli, together with discriminative and mnemonic analysis of these stimuli.

Ventral Posterior Nucleus

The ventral posterior nucleus (Figs. 11–4, 11–6, and 11–7) functions as a thalamic center for the general senses and for the sense of taste. The lateral and ventral spinothalamic tracts, the medial lemniscus, and the trigeminothalamic tracts all terminate in this nucleus. Fibers are also received from the gustatory nucleus in the brain stem, consisting of the rostral part of the nucleus of the solitary fasciculus.

There is a detailed topographic projection of the opposite half of the body on the ventral posterior nucleus. The lower extremity is represented in the dorsolateral part of the nucleus, the upper extremity in an intermediate position, and the head most medially. The medial region receiving sensory data from the head conforms to the shape of the centromedian and parafascicular nuclei (Fig. 11–4) and is known as the semilunar or arcuate nucleus. The image of the body is distorted, the more important parts of the body with respect to sensory function, such as the hand and face, being disproportionately large. In addition, the more discriminative senses of fine touch and proprioception are represented further forward than the nociceptive senses of pain and temperature. Nevertheless, the topographic projection of the body on the ventral posterior nucleus (and on the somesthetic area of cortex) is the basis for precise recognition of the source of stimuli. Fibers conducting data from taste buds terminate in the arcuate nucleus along with other afferents for the head. The ventral posterior nucleus also receives general visceral information through the poorly defined ascending visceral pathways of the spinal cord and brain stem.

Nerve fibers leave the lateral surface of the nucleus in large numbers, traverse the internal capsule and medullary center, and end in the general sensory area of the parietal lobe (Fig. 11–12). The opposite side of the body has an inverted representation in the somesthetic cortex, and the area for taste is at the lower end of the sensory strip in the region of the head area. Fibers from the ventral posterior nucleus also project to other thalamic nuclei—notably nuclei of the dorsal tier of the lateral thalamus and the medial nucleus.

Experimental and clinical evidence show that there is awareness of general sensory stimulation at the thalamic level. This is certainly true for pain and probably for temperature, simple touch, and vibration. In addition to poor localization of the source of stimuli, quantitative assessment is lacking and stimuli are not interpreted in the context of previous experience. Cortical participation is essential for refinement of the above modalities of sensation and for

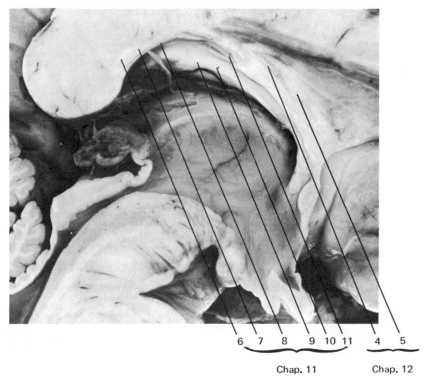

6 7 8 9 10 11 4 5

Chap. 11   Chap. 12

FIG. 11–5. Key to levels of Figures 11–6 through 11–11 and Figures 12–4 and 12–5. (See also Figure 11–2.)

FIG. 11–6. Transverse section at the transition between the midbrain and the diencephalon, immediately caudal to the mammillary bodies. Weigert stain. ×1⅘

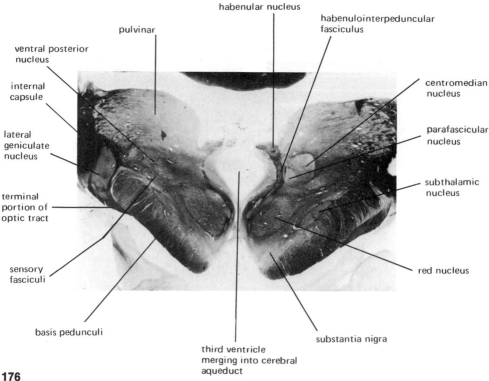

habenular nucleus

pulvinar

habenulointerpeduncular fasciculus

ventral posterior nucleus

centromedian nucleus

internal capsule

parafascicular nucleus

lateral geniculate nucleus

subthalamic nucleus

terminal portion of optic tract

sensory fasciculi

red nucleus

basis pedunculi

substantia nigra

third ventricle merging into cerebral aqueduct

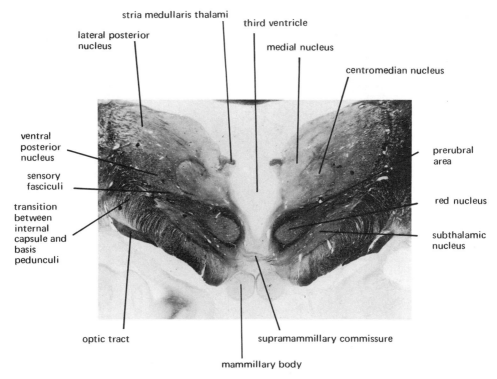

FIG. 11-7. Diencephalon at the level of the mammillary bodies. Weigert stain. ×1⅘

FIG. 11-8. Diencephalon at the level of the infundibular stalk of the neurohypophysis. Weigert stain. ×1⅘

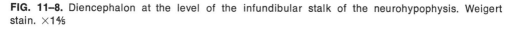

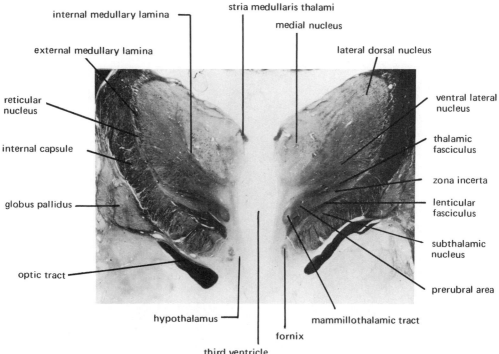

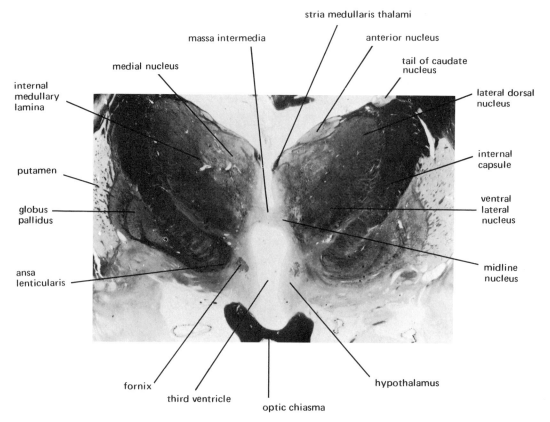

FIG. 11–9. Diencephalon at the level of the optic chiasma. Weigert stain. ×1⅘

FIG. 11–10. Diencephalon rostral to the level of the optic chiasma. Weigert stain. ×1⅘

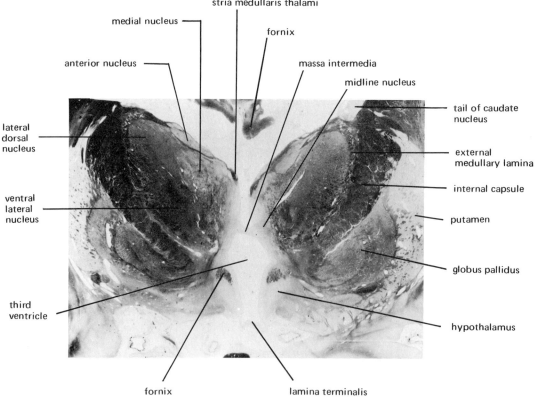

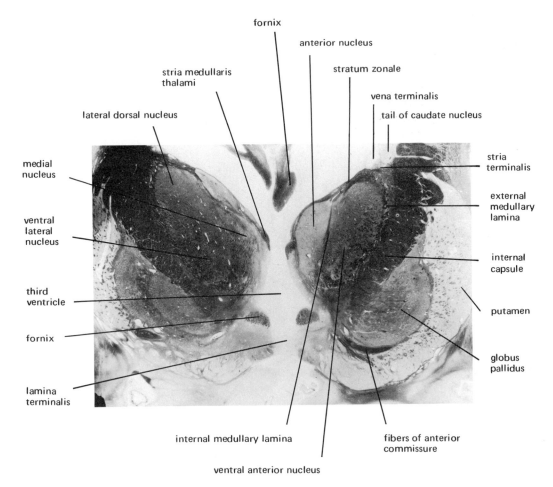

FIG. 11–11. Rostral region of the diencephalon. Weigert stain. ×2

any awareness of discriminative touch and the proprioceptive senses of position and movement of body parts.

Ventral Lateral and Ventral Anterior Nuclei

These nuclei are motor components of the thalamus and the boundary between them is arbitrary because of overlapping connections. The input to the ventral lateral nucleus (Figs. 11–4 and 11–8 through 11–10) is mainly from the dentate nucleus of the cerebellum through the brachium conjunctivum. Additional afferents come from the globus pallidus, and possibly the substantia nigra. Efferent fibers of the ventral lateral nucleus enter the internal capsule for distribution to the motor and premotor areas of the frontal lobe (Fig. 11–12). These areas include large numbers of neurons giving rise to pyramidal and extrapyramidal motor fibers. The connections thus established influence voluntary motor action in such a way that withdrawal or disturbance of their function contributes to the motor abnormalities coming under the general heading of the dyskinesias.

The connections of the ventral anterior nucleus (Figs. 11–4 and 11–11, *right*) are rather diverse and not fully known. The globus pallidus and perhaps the substantia nigra are sources of afferent fibers, and the nucleus projects to the premotor and motor areas of the frontal lobe. The connections of the ventral lateral and ventral anterior nuclei therefore partially overlap. Both nuclei are on a pathway through which motor areas of the frontal lobe are influenced by the corpus striatum, and also by the substantia nigra which has definite connections with the corpus striatum. As noted above, the thalamic nuclei apparently discharge abnormally when there are degenerative changes in these extrapyramidal motor nuclei, giving rise to one or another form of dyskinesia. In the case of Parkinson's disease (paralysis agitans), in which the substantia nigra and to a lesser degree the corpus striatum are affected by degenerative changes, the motor disturbances may become more tolerable if a lesion is placed in the thalamic nuclei. In practice, the lesion is placed in the ventral lateral nucleus or, alternatively, in the subthalamic region with the object of interrupting the afferent fibers to the ventral lateral and ventral anterior nuclei. (Surgical forms of treatment in Parkinson's disease have been used less frequently since the introduction of L-dopa therapy.)

Among other connections that have been described, the ventral anterior nucleus sends fibers to the corpus striatum. The ventral anterior nucleus also appears to have a special role in the alerting system of the brain. While various thalamic nuclei relay activity from the intralaminar nuclei to the cerebral cortex, electrical stimulation of the ventral anterior nucleus is said to be especially effective in evoking cortical responses that are characteristic of the activating system.

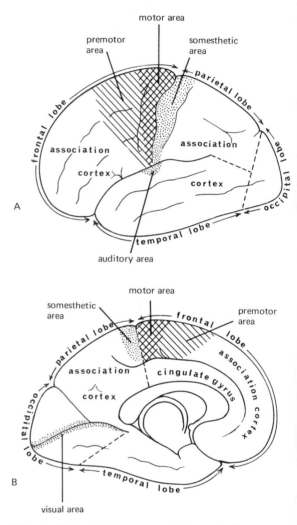

FIG. 11–12. Cortical areas receiving projections from specific thalamic nuclei. **A.** Dorsolateral surface of a cerebral hemisphere. **B.** Medial surface of a cerebral hemisphere.

NONSPECIFIC THALAMIC NUCLEI

The dorsal tier of nuclei in the lateral thalamus, the medial nucleus, and the anterior nucleus constitute the nonspecific nuclei, which are connected with association areas of cortex.

Dorsal Tier of Lateral Nuclei

The *pulvinar, lateral posterior nucleus,* and *lateral dorsal nucleus,* all situated in the dorsal part of the lateral nuclear mass (Figs. 11–4 and 11–6 through 11–8), have similar connections and functions. As noted above, they receive fibers from other thalamic nuclei, including intralaminar nuclei and the ventral posterior nucleus. The three nuclei of the dorsal tier have reciprocal connections with association cortex of the parietal and occipital lobes and the posterior part of the temporal lobe (Fig. 11–12). The parieto-occipito-temporal association cortex is responsible for analysis of sensory input at the highest level and contributes to the neural substrate of the intellect. The activity of the cortex with respect to these exceedingly important functions is apparently reinforced by the nonspecific nuclei of the lateral thalamus.

Medial Nucleus

The medial thalamic nucleus (Figs. 11–4 and 11–9) includes several subnuclei; one of these, the *dorsomedial nucleus,* is well developed in man and occupies most of the medial nuclear complex.

The connections of the dorsomedial nucleus are varied and complex. Fibers enter the nucleus from other parts of the thalamus including the lateral nuclear mass, intralaminar nuclei, and midline nucleus. It is conceivable that sensory data, both somatic and visceral, are made available in modified form to the dorsomedial nucleus from the above sources. There is a large reciprocal connection between the dorsomedial nucleus and association cortex of the frontal lobe (prefrontal cortex) (Figs. 11–12). In addition, a bundle of fibers known as the *inferior thalamic peduncle* passes downward to the base of the

hemisphere. This bundle provides reciprocal connections between the medial thalamic nucleus and various gray areas, including orbital cortex of the frontal lobe, gray matter underlying the anterior perforated substance, and the amygdaloid nucleus. Through the above connections the dorsomedial nucleus constitutes part of a system which contributes to those aspects of the emotions generally thought of as "moods" or "feeling tone." Depending on the nature of the present sensory input and past experience, the mood may be pleasant or unpleasant, of well-being or malaise, or of euphoria or mild depression. Visceral changes may accompany changes in mood through reciprocal connections between the medial thalamic nucleus and the hypothalamus. Motor responses arising from a projection from the medial nucleus to the corpus striatum may include changes in facial expression and gesticulations.

Severe anxiety states are ameliorated by interfering with the above system through placing lesions in the dorsomedial nuclei, or more commonly, by severing the connections between these nuclei and the prefrontal cortices (leukotomy or prefrontal lobotomy). However, there are usually undesirable side-effects of a behavioral nature, since the prefrontal cortex is also concerned with foresight and judgment. This form of psychosurgery has now been largely replaced by medical therapy.

The dorsomedial thalamic nucleus appears to play a role in memory. In Korsakoff's syndrome, in which amnesia is a particularly characteristic symptom, the degenerative changes in the brain follow a variable pattern. However, the lesions are typically in regions surrounding the third ventricle, and the dorsomedial nucleus is reported as being affected most consistently. In addition, memory deficits have been reported following surgical destruction of the dorsomedial thalamic nuclei.

Anterior Nucleus

The anterior thalamic nucleus (Figs. 11–4 and 11–11) is responsible for the anterior tubercle of the thalamus which, with the fornix, bounds the foramen of Monro (Fig. 11–3). This nucleus is included in the limbic system of the brain, only the components of which need be identified here. The cortical areas of the limbic system consist of the hippocampus, dentate gyrus, and parahippocampal gyrus (all in the temporal lobe), and the cingulate gyrus on the medial surface of the hemisphere above the corpus callosum. The diencephalic components are the hypothalamus (especially the mammillary bodies) and the anterior nucleus of the thalamus. The principal fiber bundles of the limbic system are the fornix, which projects from the hippocampus to the hypothalamus, and the mammillothalamic tract (bundle of Vicq d'Azyr), through which reciprocal connections are established between the mammillary body and the anterior thalamic nucleus. This nucleus also has reciprocal connections with the cortex of the cingulate gyrus. (Additional components of the limbic system, e.g., the amygdaloid nucleus and its connections, are discussed in Chapter 18.)

Since the principal connections of the anterior thalamic nucleus are with the mammillary body and the cingulate gyrus, the function of the nucleus must be in part that of the limbic system. This system is concerned with basic emotional drives of importance to preservation of the individual and the species. It also has a significant role in memory mechanisms of the brain.

THALAMIC SYNDROME

Aside from the motor function of the ventral lateral and ventral anterior nuclei, the thalamus is a sensory center of the brain and an integral part of the neural mechanism for emotional responses to sensory experience. The thalamic syndrome is essentially a disturbance of these aspects of thalamic function, subsequent to a lesion (usually vascular in origin) involving the thalamus or its connections. The symptoms vary according to the location and extent of the lesion. The threshold for touch, pain, and temperature sensibilities is usually raised on the opposite side of the body, but when the threshold is reached the sensations are exaggerated, perverted, and exceptionally disagreeable. For example, the prick of a pin may be felt as a severe burning type of pain, and music that is ordinarily pleasing may provoke unpleasant responses. There is spontaneous pain in some instances of the disorder, and the pain may become intractable to analgesics. There may also be emotional instability, with spontaneous or forced laughing and crying.

SUBTHALAMUS

The subthalamus contains several structures requiring brief description; these include sensory fasciculi, rostral extensions of midbrain nuclei, fiber bundles from the dentate nucleus of the cerebellum and the globus pallidus, and the subthalamic nucleus.

The *sensory fasciculi* are the medial lemniscus, the spinothalamic tracts, and the trigeminothalamic tracts. They are spread out immediately beneath the ventral posterior nucleus, in which the fibers terminate (Figs. 11–6 and 11–7).

The *substantia nigra* and the *red nucleus* extend from the midbrain part way into the subthalamus (Figs. 11–6 and 11–7). Dentatothalamic fibers of the brachium conjunctivum both surround and traverse the red nucleus. These fibers continue forward in the *prerubral area* or *field H of Forel* (*H, Haube*, a cap) (Figs. 11–7 and 11–8). The dentatothalamic fibers contribute to the thalamic fasciculus (see below) and enter the ventral lateral nucleus of the thalamus.

Efferent fibers of the globus pallidus are contained in two distinct bundles, the lenticular fasciculus and the ansa lenticularis. The *lenticular fasciculus* (Fig. 11–8) consists of fibers which cut across the internal capsule to reach the subthalamus, where they form a band of white matter known alternatively as *field H₂ of Forel*. The majority of the constituent fibers reverse direction in the prerubral area, enter the *thalamic fasciculus* (*field H₁ of Forel*), and terminate in the ventral lateral and ventral anterior thalamic nuclei. At a more rostral level, the *ansa lenticularis* forms a sharp bend around the medial edge of the internal capsule (Fig. 11–9). Some fibers of the ansa end in the ventral lateral and ventral anterior thalamic nuclei; others turn caudally and, along with some fibers of the lenticular fasciculus, proceed to the red nucleus, reticular formation, and inferior olivary complex. The mesencephalic reticular formation continues into the subthalamus, where it appears as the *zona incerta* between the lenticular and thalamic fasciculi (Fig. 11–8).

The *subthalamic nucleus* (of Luys) is a biconvex nucleus lying against the internal capsule (Figs. 11–6 through 11–8). It is one of the extrapyramidal motor nuclei and is best developed in primates. The connections of the subthalamic nucleus are varied, and not all of them have been established unequivocally. However, the major connection is with the globus pallidus; this consists of fibers running in both directions across the internal capsule and making up the *subthalamic fasciculus*. Fibers in the *supramammillary commissure* (Fig. 11–7)

connect one subthalamic nucleus with the other.

A lesion in the subthalamic nucleus causes a motor disturbance on the opposite side of the body known as *hemiballismus*. The condition is characterized by involuntary movements, coming on suddenly and of great force and rapidity. The movements are purposeless and generally of a throwing or flailing type, although they may be choreiform or jerky. The spontaneous movements affect the proximal portions of the extremities most severely, especially the arms, and the muscles of the face and neck are sometimes included.

EPITHALAMUS

The epithalamus consists of the habenular nuclei and their connections, and the pineal gland.

HABENULAR NUCLEUS (Habenula)

A slight swelling in the habenular trigone marks the position of the *habenular nucleus* (Figs. 11–3 and 11–6). Afferent fibers are received through the *stria medullaris thalami*, which runs along the dorsomedial border of the thalamus (Figs. 11–2, 11–3, and 11–8). Most of the cells of origin of the stria medullaris are situated in the medial olfactory (septal) area. This area is located on the medial surface of the frontal lobe beneath the rostral end of the corpus callosum (Fig. 11–2) and is part of both the olfactory and limbic systems of the brain. A few fibers of the stria terminalis (Fig. 11–11), originating in the amygdaloid nucleus in the temporal lobe, turn caudally in the region of the foramen of Monro and join the stria medullaris thalami.

The habenular nucleus gives rise to a well-defined bundle of fibers known as the *habenulointerpeduncular fasciculus* (fasciculus retroflexus of Meynert) (Fig. 11–6). The main destination of the fasciculus is the interpeduncular nucleus in the roof of the interpeduncular fossa of the midbrain. Fibers pass from the latter site to the dorsal tegmental nucleus, which in turn sends fibers to autonomic nuclei of the brain stem and the reticular formation by way of the dorsal longitudinal fasciculus. The stria medullaris thalami, habenular nucleus, and habenulointerpeduncular fasciculus constitute part of a pathway through which primitive aspects of brain function, namely, basic emotional drives and the sense of smell, influence the viscera.

PINEAL GLAND

The cone-shaped *pineal gland* (Figs. 11–2 and 11–3), which is about 7 by 5 mm in size, is attached to the diencephalon by the pineal stalk, into which the third ventricle extends as a pineal recess. The *habenular commissure* in the dorsal wall of the stalk (Fig. 11–2) includes fibers of the stria medullaris thalami that terminate in the opposite habenular ganglion. The ventral wall of the pineal stalk is attached to the *posterior commissure*. Although the pineal gland contains no nerve cells and is a proper subject for endocrinology, the close relationship of the pineal with the nervous system justifies further discussion in a neurologic context.

Few organs have undergone such remarkable structural and functional changes during phylogeny as the pineal gland. In fish, amphibians, and reptiles, the gland is located immediately beneath the dorsum of the head. It contains photoreceptors and nerve cells in these animals; the photoreceptors register changes in light intensity because of the translucence of the tissues overlying the pineal. Further, the output of the hormone melatonin (a tryptamine) by the gland is altered in response to changes in the level of illumination. Melatonin has the property of clumping melanin pigment granules in cutaneous melanocytes and thereby influences the lightness or darkness of the animal.

The pineal gland of mammals contains neither photoreceptors nor nerve cells, and the histophysiology of the gland has changed from that of submammalian vertebrates. Histologically, the parenchymatous cells (pinealocytes) are arranged as cords separated by connective tissue. These cells have a granular cytoplasm and processes ending in bulbous expansions; the latter are in close relationship to blood vessels at the surface of the cellular cords or in the intervening connective tissue septa. The cords contain a smaller population of neuroglial cells resembling astrocytes. After the age of about 16 years, granules of calcium and magnesium salts appear in the gland. These calcareous granules coalesce later to form larger particles (brain sand); the deposits may be a useful landmark in X-ray films for determining whether the pineal gland is displaced by a space-occupying lesion.

Clinical observations of long standing suggest an antigonadotropic function for the pineal gland in man, since a pineal tumor developing around the age of puberty may alter the age of onset of pubertal changes. Puberty may be precocious if the tumor is of a type that destroys parenchymatous cells, or delayed if the tumor is derived from the functional cells of the gland. It is only in recent years that experimental work has placed the antigonadotropic function of the pineal on a sounder basis, although many details remain for clarification.

Pinealectomy in experimental animals stimulates the genital system, with genital hypertrophy, precocious opening of the vagina in immature females, and changes in the estrous cycle. Administration of pineal extracts has the contrary effect through inhibition of the gonads. Chemical extraction of bovine pineal glands has produced several possible active principles, including melatonin and serotonin. Melatonin appears to be specific to the pineal because this is the only mammalian organ known to contain the enzyme required for the synthesis of melatonin. However, administration of pure melatonin does not produce all the effects of pineal extracts, and related compounds may also serve as pineal hormones.

In mammals, as in lower vertebrates, the activity of the pineal gland is influenced by light; its antigonadotropic activity is highest when the animal is in the dark and lowest when in a light environment. The pathway for the influence of light on the gland is known to originate in the retina; it is also known that perivascular sympathetic fibers from the superior cervical ganglion have an inhibitory effect on the gland. A connection between the retina and the intermediolateral cell column in the upper thoracic segments of the cord is therefore required. This connection has been shown in the rat to begin as fibers leaving the optic tract near the chiasma, these fibers terminating in the reticular formation of the midbrain tegmentum. Reticulospinal fibers presumably complete the pathway.

The site of action of the pineal hormone(s) is under continued investigation. The target cells may be in the gonads or in the pars distalis of the pituitary; alternatively, they may be hypothalamic cells that elaborate "releasing factors" for the gonadotropin-producing cells of the pituitary, or neurons that project to the hypothalamus. Recent work tends to implicate cells of the central nervous system, either hypothalamic cells or neurons in the midbrain reticular formation projecting to the hypothalamus. In addition to the antigonadotropic function, there is some evidence that pineal hormones influence pituitary cells producing the growth (somatotropic) hormone (STH), the thyroid-stimulating hormone (TSH), and the adrenocorticotropic hormone (ACTH). The importance of the pineal gland in human physiology has yet to be assessed.

HYPOTHALAMUS

The hypothalamus, occupying only a small part of the brain and weighing about 4 gm, has a functional importance that is quite out of proportion to its size. The hypothalamus is at a crossroads between the thalamus and cerebral cortex (especially that of the limbic system) on the one hand, and ascending fiber systems from the brain stem and spinal cord on the other. Input from the thalamus and limbic system has a special emotional significance and the ascending fibers carry information that is largely of visceral origin. However, the hypothalamus is not influenced solely by neuronal systems; the constituent nerve cells respond to properties of the circulating blood, including temperature, osmotic pressure, and the levels of various hormones. Hypothalamic function becomes manifest through efferent pathways to autonomic nuclei in the brain stem and spinal cord, and through an intimate relationship with the pituitary gland by means of neurosecretory cells. These cells elaborate the hormones of the neurohypophysis and produce "releasing factors" which control the hormonal output of the adenohypophysis. By the above means the hypothalamus has a major role in producing responses to emotional changes and to needs signaled by hunger and thirst, and is instrumental in maintaining a constant internal body environment (homeostasis).

The hypothalamus of either side is bounded by the wall of the third ventricle below the hypothalamic sulcus (Fig. 11–2) and occupies the interval between the third ventricle and the subthalamus (Figs. 11–8 through 11–10). The *mammillary bodies* are distinct swellings on the basal surface (Fig. 11–1). The region bounded by the mammillary bodies, optic chiasma, and beginning of the optic tracts is known as the *tuber cinereum.* The *infundibular stem* (pituitary stalk) arises from the *median eminence* just behind the optic chiasma and is continuous with the pars nervosa of the pituitary gland. The median eminence, infundibular stem, and pars nervosa have similar cytologic and functional characteristics; together they constitute the *neurohypophysis.*

The fornix traverses the hypothalamus to reach the mammillary body and serves as a point of reference for a sagittal plane dividing the hypothalamus into *medial* and *lateral zones.* The medial zone is further subdivided into three regions, *suprachiasmatic, tuberal,* and *mammillary,* with basal structures as landmarks. The medial zone consists of gray matter in which several nuclei are recognized on the basis of cellular characteristics and connections. It also includes a thin layer of fine myelinated and unmyelinated fibers beneath the ependymal lining of the third ventricle. The lateral zone or area contains fewer nerve cells, but there are many nerve fibers, most of them running in a longitudinal direction.

HYPOTHALAMIC NUCLEI

The lamina terminalis represents the rostral end of the embryonal neural tube and limits the third ventricle anteriorly (Fig. 11–13). The lamina extends from the optic chiasma to the anterior commissure, which consists of a bundle of fibers connecting areas of the right and left temporal lobes, and includes some commissural fibers connecting the olfactory bulbs. The lamina terminalis and anterior commissure are telencephalic structures. The gray matter immediately behind the lamina is also derived from the telencephalon of the embryo. However, it is included with the hypothalamus for convenience and is called the *preoptic area* of the hypothalamus.

Medial Zone

Within the medial zone (Fig. 11–13), the suprachiasmatic region contains the supraoptic, paraventricular, and anterior nuclei. The *supraoptic nucleus* consists of large cells and is best developed above the junction of the optic chiasma and optic tract. The *paraventricular nucleus* is characterized by large cells in a matrix of smaller neurons. These nuclei are conspicuous in Nissl-stained sections and have a plentiful supply of capillaries. The cells of the supraoptic and paraventricular nuclei elaborate neurohypophyseal hormones, and colloidal droplets in their cytoplasm are evidence of neurosecretory activity. Axons from the nuclei constitute the hypothalamohypophyseal tract, whose fibers terminate throughout the neurohypophysis where the hormones are released into capillary blood. The *anterior nucleus* is similar to the preoptic area cytologically, and they are not clearly demarcated from one another.

The tuberal region contains the *ventromedial, dorsomedial,* and *infundibular (arcuate) nuclei,* each nucleus consisting of small nerve cells. The mammillary region includes the *mammillary body* and the *posterior hypothalamic nucleus.* In man, the mammillary body is occupied almost entirely by a medial mammillary nucleus, the remainder consisting of an intermediate nucleus and a lateral nucleus. The cells of the lateral nucleus are large, while the bulk of the mammillary body is made up of

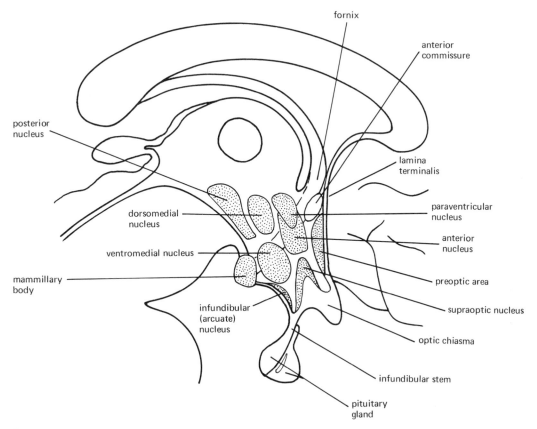

FIG. 11–13. Nuclei in the medial zone of the hypothalamus.

small neurons. The posterior hypothalamic nucleus consists of large neurons in a background of small nerve cells.

Lateral Zone

The large nerve cells throughout the lateral area are relatively sparse and collectively constitute the *lateral nucleus* of the hypothalamus. The cells are interspersed with longitudinally running nerve fibers passing to or from hypothalamic nuclei or through the area. This zone includes the *lateral tuberal nucleus,* which consists of several groups of nerve cells near the surface of the tuber cinereum. The hypothalamus of man

is characterized by the large size of the medial mammillary nucleus, the well defined lateral tuberal nucleus, and the presence of large neurons in the posterior and lateral nuclei.

AFFERENT CONNECTIONS OF THE HYPOTHALAMUS

As mentioned above, the hypothalamus receives information from diverse sources in order to serve as the main integrator of the autonomic nervous system.

Ascending visceral afferents convey data of visceral origin, among which the special visceral sense of taste is included. The pathways are not well defined, compared with somatic sensory tracts leading to the thalamus, and consist in part of relays through the reticular formation of the brain stem, tegmental nuclei of the midbrain, and the midline nucleus of the thalamus. Some of the ascending fibers are included in the dorsal longitudinal fasciculus, which also contains efferent fibers of the hypothalamus. Somatic sensory information, especially from erotogenic zones such as the nipples and genitalia, also reaches the hypothalamus.

The cells of origin of the *medial forebrain bundle* are chiefly in the septal or medial olfactory area, other fibers coming from the intermediate and lateral olfactory areas (Chapter 17). The medial forebrain bundle runs caudally in the lateral area of the hypothalamus, giving off fibers to hypothalamic nuclei. Other fibers of the bundle continue through the hypothalamus to the reticular formation of the midbrain. The afferents just described are related to basic emotional drives and the sense of smell. The medial forebrain bundle is small in the human brain, in comparison with the brains of animals that rely heavily on the sense of smell. A second input related to smell and emotional drives comes from the amygdaloid nucleus. This nucleus is situated in the temporal lobe in the region of the uncus, a small gyral configuration on the basal surface (Fig. 11–1). A slender strand of fibers known as the *stria terminalis* arises from the amygdaloid nucleus, arches over the thalamus along the inner side of the caudate nucleus (Fig. 11–11), and terminates in part in the preoptic area and anterior nucleus of the hypothalamus.

The *fornix,* originating in the hippocampus of the temporal lobe, is the largest of the various fiber bundles ending in the hypothalamus. As mentioned earlier, the fornix arches over the thalamus and into the hypothalamus, where the fibers terminate in several nuclei, but mainly in the mammillary body (Fig. 11–14). The mammillary body also receives fibers from the anterior thalamic nucleus through the mammillothalamic fasciculus, and is therefore in communication with the cortex of the cingulate gyrus. The hypothalamus is an integral part of the limbic system of the brain and essential to the intimate relationship between basic emotional drives and visceral function, which is an important aspect of the function of the limbic system.

The hypothalamus receives afferents from the *medial thalamic nucleus* and is thereby brought under the influence of the prefrontal cortex. These parts of the brain, it will be recalled, contribute to states of mind commonly referred to as moods, among other functions. There are direct *corticohypothalamic fibers,* especially from cortex on the orbital surface of the frontal lobe. *Pallidohypothalamic fibers* have been described as being included in the lenticular fasciculus, but the existence of a projection from the globus pallidus to the hypothalamus was later questioned.

EFFERENT CONNECTIONS OF THE HYPOTHALAMUS

There are two principal efferent pathways from the hypothalamus to the brain stem. The first of these begins as thinly myelinated and unmyelinated *periventricular fibers* beneath the ependyma of the third ventricle, continuing into the *dorsal longitudinal fasciculus* in the periaqueductal gray matter of the midbrain. Partly through relays in the reticular formation, impulses of hypothalamic origin reach parasympathetic nuclei of the brain stem, i.e., the salivatory and lacrimal nuclei and the dorsal motor nucleus of the vagus nerve. Reticulospinal fibers complete the pathway to autonomic nuclei in the spinal cord. Lower motor neurons supplying striated muscles are also recipients of impulses of hypothalamic origin. These include cells in the motor nuclei of the trigeminal and facial nerves, the nucleus ambiguus, and the hypoglossal nucleus, in connection with the role of the hypothalamus in feeding and drinking. Motor neurons of the spinal cord are influenced by the hypothalamus in temperature regulation, as in shivering to raise the body temperature.

The second major descending pathway, the *mammillotegmental tract,* arises from the mammillary body; the fibers accompany the mammillothalamic tract for a short distance, then turn caudally and end in the midbrain tegmentum. Further transmission to autonomic nuclei in the brain

stem and spinal cord is effected through relays in the reticular formation and tegmental nuclei of the midbrain. Finally, axons of some hypothalamic neurons enter the lateral zone and reach the midbrain along with fibers of the medial forebrain bundle.

Activity within the hypothalamus is transmitted to the thalamus and cerebral cortex, where it has an influence on affective states, both basic emotions of a primitive nature and those more closely related to mood. The large *mammillothalamic tract* (bundle of Vicq d'Azyr) connects the mammillary body with the anterior thalamic nucleus (Fig. 11–14), and the latter

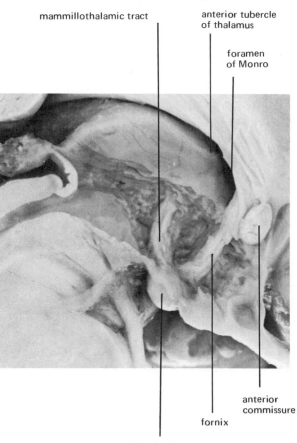

mammillothalamic tract

anterior tubercle of thalamus

foramen of Monro

anterior commissure

fornix

mammillary body

FIG. 11–14. Dissection demonstrating the fornix and the mammillothalamic tract (bundle of Vicq d'Azyr). ×2

nucleus has reciprocal connections with the cortex of the cingulate gyrus. As noted above, the anterior thalamic nucleus and cingulate cortex share with other components of the limbic system responsibility for those emotions and aspects of behavior that are related to preservation of the individual and the species. The hypothalamus contributes to the subjective experience of these emotions through projections to the thalamus and cortex, and to visceral manifestations of emotions through the autonomic nervous system. A supplementary contribution to the affect, in particular to an individual's feeling tone, derives from reciprocal connections between the hypothalamus and the medial thalamic nucleus, and between the latter and prefrontal cortex.

SOME FUNCTIONAL CONSIDERATIONS

Autonomic and Related Aspects

Electrical stimulation of the hypothalamus in experimental animals shows that some regions give parasympathetic, and others sympathetic, responses. Parasympathetic responses are most regularly elicited by stimulation of the anterior hypothalamus, notably the preoptic area and anterior nucleus. They include slowing of the heart rate, vasodilation, lowering of blood pressure, salivation, increased peristalsis in the gastrointestinal tract, contraction of the urinary bladder, and sweating. Sympathetic responses, most readily elicited by stimulation in the region of the posterior and lateral nuclei, include cardiac acceleration, elevation of blood pressure, cessation of peristalsis in the gastrointestinal tract, dilation of the pupils, and hyperglycemia.

The responses mentioned above are combined in maintaining homeostasis; regulation of body temperature is an instructive example. Certain hypothalamic cells act as a thermostat, monitoring the temperature of blood flowing through the capillaries and initiating the responses necessary to maintain a normal body temperature. Thermosensitive neurons in the parasympathetic region of the anterior hypothalamus respond to an increase in temperature of the blood. Mechanisms that promote heat loss, such as cutaneous vasodilation and sweating, are activated. A lesion in the anterior hypothalamus may therefore result in hyperthermia in a hot environment or under states of high metabolic rate. Cells in the sympathetic region, especially the posterior hypothalamic nucleus, respond to a lowering of blood temperature. Responses such as cutaneous vasoconstriction and shivering are triggered for conservation and production of heat, and a lesion in the posterior hypothalamus interferes with temperature regulation in a cold environment. A lesion in the posterior part of the hypothalamus may not only destroy cells involved in conservation and production of heat, but also interrupt fibers running caudally from the heat-dissipating region. This results in a serious impairment of temperature regulation in either a cold or a warm environment.

Hypothalamic regulation of food and water intake has also been demonstrated by electrical stimulation and by placing small electrolytic lesions in the hypothalamus. A hunger or feeding center has been located in the lateral zone, and a satiety center (inhibiting food intake) has been demonstrated in the region of the ventromedial nucleus. These centers are influenced by the glucose level of the blood, visceral afferent fibers, the olfactory system, and by thalamic and cortical regions concerned with the emotions. Destruction of the satiety center in an experimental animal, such as the rat, results in excessive food intake and obesity. Naturally occurring lesions affecting this center in man may also result in obesity, and hypothalamic cells that increase the output of gonadotropic hormones by the adenohypophysis may be destroyed at the same time. The combination of obesity and deficiency of secondary sex characteristics is known as the adiposogenital or Frölich's syndrome. Centers that inhibit or promote water intake have also been identified in the lateral and ventromedial nuclei, although not coinciding precisely with the centers for food intake.

Relations of the Hypothalamus with the Pituitary Gland (Hypophysis)

Neurohypophyseal hormones are elaborated in the hypothalamus, and hormone production by the adenohypophysis is controlled by chemical substances synthesized in hypothalamic cells. The nervous system, through the neurosecretory function of hypothalamic cells, has therefore an intimate relation with the entire endocrine system. With the exception of the special conditions inherent in the nervous control of the pineal gland, only the adrenal medulla is regulated by direct nervous connections. These are preganglionic sympathetic fibers, the cells of the adrenal medulla having the same embryologic origin as cells of sympathetic ganglia. Only the major points concerning hypothalamic-hypophyseal relationships are discussed here; the subject is a large one, comprising the specialty of neuroendocrinology.

Neurohypophysis. As noted above, the neurohypophysis consists of the median eminence, infundibular stem, and neural (posterior) lobe of the pituitary gland. All these structures are of diencephalic origin in the embryo. Although hormones enter the blood stream from the neurohypophysis, they are not elaborated there, but rather in the cells of the supraoptic and paraventricular nuclei. The two neurohypophyseal hormones are oxytocin and vasopressin. Oxytocin stimulates the smooth muscle of the uterus when the latter is sensitized by estrogen and not depressed by progesterone, and causes contraction of myoepithelial cells surrounding the secretory alveoli of the mammary gland. Vasopressin has two functional activities, pressor and antidiuretic, of which the pressor role through vasoconstriction is of comparatively little physiologic and clinical importance. The antidiuretic function results from the action of the hormone on the distal convoluted tubules of the kidney, with increased absorption of water from the glomerular filtrate. In experimental animals vasopressin is produced by the supraoptic nucleus and oxytocin by the paraventricular nucleus.

The precursors of vasopressin and oxytocin appear in the cytoplasm of cells of the supraoptic and paraventricular nuclei as neurosecretory droplets or granules. Axons from these nuclei constitute the *hypothalamohypophyseal tract* (also known as the supraopticohypophyseal tract) and terminate as bulbous expansions adjacent to capillaries throughout the neurohypophysis (Fig. 11–15). The neurosecretions are carried by axoplasmic flow from the cell bodies to the axon terminals, where they enter the blood passing through the capillary bed of the neurohypophysis. Tuberohypophyseal fibers from cells in the tuber cinereum have been described as contributing to the hypothalamohypophyseal tract. However, it is not certain whether they are part of the hypothalamohypophyseal system or fibers carrying releasing factors to the portal system for control of the pars distalis.

The supraoptic nucleus serves as an osmoreceptor, the secretory activity of its cells being influenced by the osmolarity of the blood flowing through this highly vascular nucleus. A slight elevation of osmotic

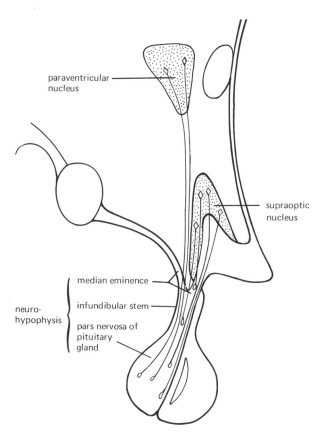

paraventricular
nucleus

supraoptic
nucleus

median eminence

neuro-
hypophysis

infundibular stem

pars nervosa of
pituitary
gland

FIG. 11–15. The hypothalamohypophyseal tract.

pressure causes the cells to synthesize anti-diuretic hormone (vasopressin) more rapidly, and an increased amount of the hormone enters the capillary blood of the neurohypophysis. Resorption of water from the distal convoluted tubules of the kidney is then accelerated and the osmolarity of the blood plasma returns to normal. A delicate mechanism is thereby provided to ensure homeostasis with respect to water balance. Destruction of the supraoptic nucleus or the neurohypophysis results in diabetes insipidus, which is characterized by excretion of large quantities of dilute urine (polyuria) and excessive thirst and water intake to compensate (polydipsia). A lesion restricted to the neural lobe of the

pituitary gland is not as a rule followed by diabetes insipidus, because adequate amounts of the antidiuretic hormone reach the blood stream from the median eminence and infundibular stem.

Pituitary Portal System. The following hormones are produced in the pars distalis of the adenohypophysis: 1) follicle-stimulating hormone (FSH), 2) luteinizing hormone (LH), 3) luteotropic hormone (LTH), 4) thyrotropic or thyroid-stimulating hormone (TSH), 5) adrenocorticotropic hormone (ACTH), and 6) growth or somatotropic hormone (STH). The first three mentioned are gonadotropic hormones. FSH promotes growth of ovarian follicles and spermatogenesis. LH promotes ovulation, converts the ruptured follicle into a corpus luteum, and stimulates interstitial cells of the testis. LTH stimulates the corpus luteum to secret progesterone and promotes secretion of milk in the lactating breast (hence also known as the lactogenic hormone or prolactin). Secretion of hormones by the pars distalis is under the control of the hypothalamus, but by a vascular route rather than nervous connections.

The pituitary portal system begins with the superior hypophyseal artery, which arises from the internal carotid artery at the base of the brain and breaks up into capillary tufts and loops in the median eminence (Fig. 11–16). The capillaries are drained by veins which enter the adenohypophysis, where they empty into the large capillaries or sinusoids of the pars distalis. The hypothalamus contains cells that produce tripeptide or polypeptide substances called "pituitary releasing factors," and at least one "inhibiting factor," specifically for prolactin. There is a separate releasing factor for each hormone of the pars distalis, and there is probably a topographic pattern of cells producing different factors (this is a subject of current research). The releasing factors pass by axoplasmic flow within the axons of the cells producing them and enter the capillaries of the portal system to reach the pars distalis, thus bringing the synthesis and release of hormones by the pars distalis under hypothalamic control. Cells producing releasing factors are influenced by the various afferent fiber connections of the hypothalamus. Their activity is also regulated by hor-

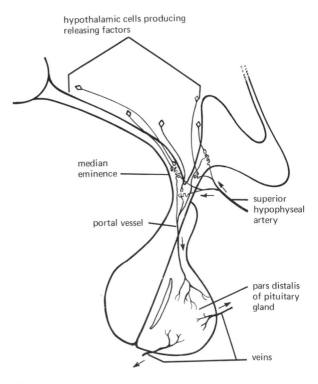

FIG. 11–16. The pituitary portal system.

mones of the target organs for pituitary hormones. For example, when the blood titer of sex hormones is high, hypothalamic cells producing the releasing factor for FSH are suppressed. Conversely, in hypogonadal conditions these hypothalamic cells produce an excess of the releasing factor and FSH secretion by the pituitary is elevated.

THIRD VENTRICLE

The diencephalic part of the ventricular system consists of the narrow third ventricle (Fig. 11–2). The anterior wall of this ventricle is formed by the lamina terminalis; the anterior commissure crosses the midline in the upper part of the lamina terminalis. The rather extensive lateral wall is marked by the hypothalamic sulcus, separating the thalamus from the hypothalamus. A massa intermedia bridges the ventricle in 70 percent of brains. The floor of the third ventricle is indented by the optic chiasma. There is an optic recess in front of the chiasma, and behind the chiasma the infundibular recess extends into the median eminence and the proximal part of the pituitary stalk. The floor then slopes upward to the aqueduct of the midbrain, the posterior commissure forming a slight prominence above the entrance to the aqueduct. A pineal recess extends into the stalk of the pineal gland, and the dorsal wall of the stalk accommodates the small habenular commissure. The membranous roof of the third ventricle is attached along the striae medullares thalami, and a small choroid plexus is suspended from the roof. Cerebrospinal fluid enters the third ventricle from each lateral ventricle through the foramen of Monro. The foramen is bounded by the fornix and the anterior tubercle of the thalamus and is closed posteriorly by a reflexion of ependyma between the fornix and the thalamus. The fluid leaves the third ventricle by way of the cerebral aqueduct of the midbrain, through which it reaches the fourth ventricle and then the subarachnoid space surrounding the brain and spinal cord.

SUGGESTIONS FOR ADDITIONAL READING

Ajmone Marsan C: The thalamus: Data on its functional anatomy and on some aspects of thalamo-cortical integration. Arch Ital Biol 103: 847–882, 1965

Axelrod J: The pineal gland. Endeavour 29:144–148, 1970

Bowsher D: Termination of the central pain pathway in man: The conscious appreciation of pain. Brain 80:606–622, 1957

Carpenter MB: Ventral Tier Thalamic Nuclei. In Williams D (ed.). Modern Trends in Neurology, pp. 1–20. London, Butterworth, 1967

Crosby EC, Humphrey T, Lauer EW: Correlative Anatomy of the Nervous System. New York, Macmillan, 1962

Harris GW: Neural Control of the Pituitary Gland. London, Arnold, 1955

Harris GW, Reed M, Fawcett CP: Hypothalamic releasing factors and the control of anterior pituitary function. Br Med Bull 22:266–272, 1966

Haymaker WE, Anderson E, Nauta WJH: The Hypothalamus. Springfield, Ill., Thomas, 1969

Kappers JA, Schadé JP (eds.): Structure and function of the epiphysis cerebri. Progr Brain Res 10, 1965

Kelly DE: Pineal organs: Photoreception, secretion, and development. Am Sci 50:597–625, 1962

Kuhlenbeck, H: The Human Diencephalon. Basel, Karger, 1954

Miller RA, Burack E: Atlas of the Central Nervous System in Man. Baltimore, Williams & Wilkins, 1968

Montemurro DG: Neural relationships in pituitary function. Can Cancer Conf 6:82–108, 1966

Purpura DP, Yahr MD: (eds.). The Thalamus. New York, Columbia University Press, 1966

Reiter RJ, Fraschini F: Endocrine aspects of the mammalian pineal gland: A review. Neuroendocrinology 5:219–255, 1969

Scharrer E, Scharrer B: Neuroendocrinology. New York, Columbia University Press, 1963

Spiegel EA, Wycis HT, Orchinik CW, Freed H: The thalamus and temporal orientation. Science 121:771–772, 1955

Tasker RR: Thalamotomy for pain: Lesion localization by detailed thalamic mapping. Can J Surg 12:62–74, 1969

Victor M: The amnesic syndrome and its anatomical basis. Can Med Assoc J 100:1115–1125, 1969

Von Euler C: Physiology and pharmacology of temperature regulation. Pharmacol Rev 13:361–398, 1961

Wurtman RJ, Axelrod J, Kelly DE: The Pineal. New York, Academic Press, 1968

12

Corpus Striatum

Several gray masses, collectively known as the basal ganglia of the telencephalon, are embedded in the white matter of each cerebral hemisphere. The largest of these is the *corpus striatum*, which consists of the *caudate nucleus* and the *lenticular nucleus*, the latter being further subdivided into the *putamen* and the *globus pallidus*. The *claustrum* and the *amygdaloid nucleus* are also telencephalic basal ganglia. The claustrum is a thin sheet of gray matter lateral to the putamen; its connections are not fully known and its function is obscure. The amygdaloid nucleus (amygdala) is situated in the temporal lobe, where the uncus (Fig. 11–1) is a landmark for the location of the nucleus. The amygdala is a component of the olfactory and limbic systems and is therefore described in Chapters 17 and 18.

The term "basal ganglia" is used more frequently to denote motor nuclei that are closely related functionally and therefore considered together in neuropathologic and clinical contexts. These are the corpus striatum, subthalamic nucleus, and substantia nigra. Lesions involving the above nuclei result in motor disturbances (dyskinesias), characterized by uncontrollable, purposeless movements and other signs.

The corpus striatum is a major center in the complex extrapyramidal motor system, as opposed to the corticobulbar and corticospinal tracts composing the pyramidal motor system. The motor components of the brain and spinal cord are reviewed in Chapter 23.

PHYLOGENETIC DEVELOPMENT

The corpus striatum of man is best understood against a phylogenetic background, even if stated in the most general terms. In fish and amphibians, the forerunner of the mammalian corpus striatum receives olfactory stimuli, a source which is of decreasing importance in higher animals and insignificant in man. This motor nucleus of fish and amphibians constitutes the *paleostriatum* (globus pallidus) in reptiles, birds, and mammals. A new component, the *neostriatum,* appeared on the lateral side of the paleostriatum in the reptilian stage of phylogeny and forms the largest part of the corpus striatum in mammals. The thalamus and corpus striatum constitute a sensorimotor integrating mechanism in submammalian animals and the corpus striatum is largely responsible for the stereotyped motor activity of these animals.

Further morphologic changes occurred with the development of neocortex (nonolfactory cortex), which is essentially a mammalian part of the cerebral hemisphere. Fibers connecting the neocortex with subcortical centers traverse the neostriatum and run along the medial side of

the smaller paleostriatum (globus pallidus) as the internal capsule. The neostriatum is thereby divided into the caudate nucleus on the medial side of the itinerant fibers, and the putamen lateral to the globus pallidus (Fig. 12–1). The globus pallidus and putamen make up the lenticular nucleus. As noted further on the two parts of the neostriatum remain connected at the base of the hemisphere, and by means of strands of gray matter running across the internal capsule. The gross division of the corpus striatum into caudate and lenticular nuclei is of secondary importance; the significant components remain the neostriatum and the paleostriatum.

The neostriatum is also called the *striatum,* and the globus pallidus is then referred to as the *pallidum.* These abbreviations are useful in naming afferent and

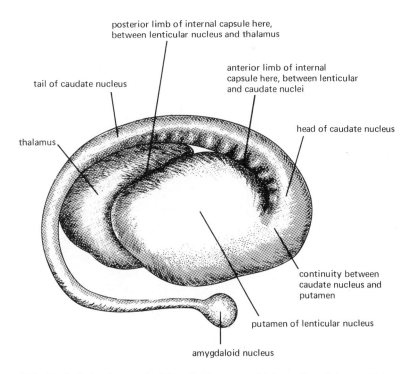

FIG. 12–1. Lateral aspect of the right corpus striatum. The globus pallidus of the lenticular nucleus is concealed by the larger putamen.

efferent connections (e.g., corticostriate and pallidothalamic fibers). The following correlations may be helpful in understanding the use of terms:

neostriatum = striatum = putamen + caudate nucleus

paleostriatum = pallidum = globus pallidus

lenticular nucleus = globus pallidus + putamen

LENTICULAR AND CAUDATE NUCLEI

As stated above, the division of the corpus striatum into lenticular and caudate nuclei

is of secondary importance with respect to the connections and functions of this motor nucleus. Nevertheless, it is necessary to understand the configuration and immediate relations of the lenticular and caudate nuclei.

LENTICULAR NUCLEUS

The *lenticular nucleus* (lentiform nucleus) is wedge-shaped and has been described as having the approximate size and shape of a Brazil nut. The narrow part of the wedge facing medially is occupied by the *globus pallidus,* which is further divided into medial and lateral parts by a *medial medullary lamina* (Figs. 11–8 through 11–11). The

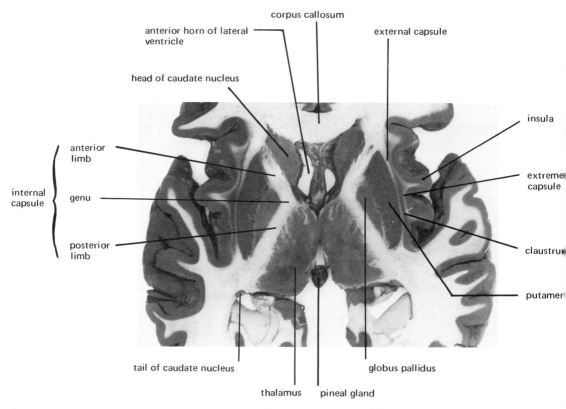

FIG. 12–2. Horizontal section of the cerebrum, stained by a method which differentiates gray matter and white matter, showing the components and relations of the corpus striatum. ×⁴⁄₅

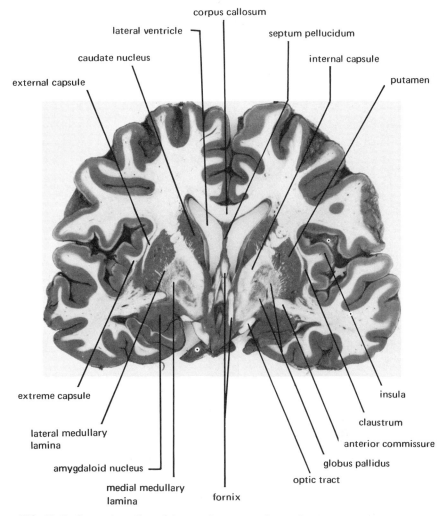

corpus callosum

lateral ventricle

septum pellucidum

caudate nucleus

internal capsule

external capsule

putamen

extreme capsule

insula

claustrum

lateral medullary
lamina

anterior commissure

amygdaloid nucleus

globus pallidus

optic tract

medial medullary
lamina

fornix

FIG. 12–3. Coronal section of the cerebrum, anterior to the thalamus, illustrating the relations of components of the corpus striatum with surrounding structures. ×⅘

globus pallidus of man occasionally has three divisions. The *putamen* forms the lateral portion of the lenticular nucleus and extends beyond the globus pallidus in all directions except at the base of the nucleus. The two components of the lenticular nucleus are separated by a *lateral medullary lamina* of nerve fibers.

The lenticular nucleus is bounded laterally by a thin layer of white matter constituting the *external capsule* (Figs. 12–2

and 12–3). This is followed by the *claustrum,* which consists of a thin sheet of gray matter coextensive with the putamen. The *extreme capsule* separates the claustrum from the *insula* (island of Reil), the latter consisting of an area of cortex buried in the depths of the lateral fissure of the cerebral hemisphere, also known as the fissure of Sylvius. The claustrum appears to be derived from the insula and has fiber connections with the cortex of the frontal, parietal,

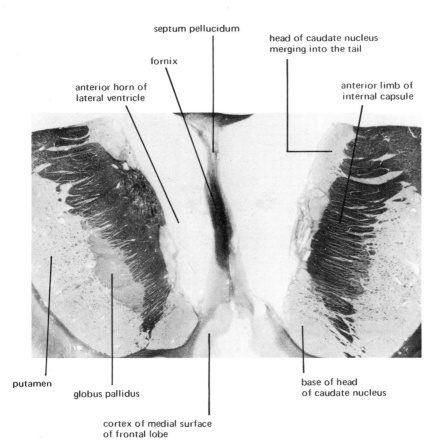

septum pellucidum

head of caudate nucleus
merging into the tail

fornix

anterior horn of
lateral ventricle

anterior limb of
internal capsule

putamen

globus pallidus

base of head
of caudate nucleus

cortex of medial surface
of frontal lobe

FIG. 12–4. Section through the corpus striatum anterior to the thalamus. Weigert stain. ×2 (See Figure 11–5 for the plane of the section illustrated here.)

and temporal lobes. The role of the claustrum is obscure; it has no demonstrable functional relationship with the corpus striatum. The medial surface of the lenticular nucleus lies against the internal capsule and the base of the nucleus is immediately above the anterior perforated substance (Fig. 11–1).

CAUDATE NUCLEUS

The *caudate nucleus* consists of an anterior portion or *head*, which tapers into a slender *tail* extending backward and then forward into the temporal lobe (Fig. 12–1). The ex-

tension of the caudate nucleus into the temporal lobe terminates at the amygdaloid nucleus, with which the caudate nucleus has no functional relationship, and consists of an attenuated, interrupted strand of gray matter in some human brains.

The head of the caudate nucleus bulges into the anterior horn of the lateral ventricle, while the first part of the tail lies along the lateral edge of the floor of the lateral ventricle (Figs. 11–9 through 11–11). The tail follows the contour of the lateral ventricle, as noted above, continuing into the roof of the inferior or temporal horn of the ventricle. Two structures lie along the

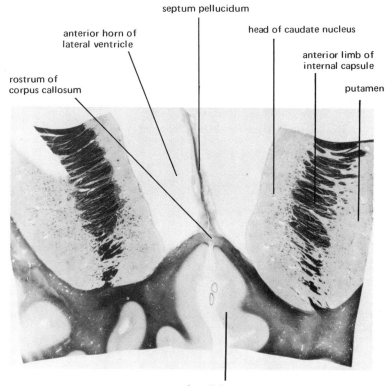

septum pellucidum

anterior horn of
lateral ventricle

head of caudate nucleus

anterior limb of
internal capsule

rostrum of
corpus callosum

putamen

cortex of medial
surface of frontal lobe

FIG. 12–5. Section through the anterior part of the corpus striatum. Weigert stain. ×2 (See Figure 11–5 for the plane of the section illustrated here.)

medial side of the tail of the caudate nucleus. These are the *stria terminalis,* a slender bundle of fibers originating in the amygdaloid nucleus, and the *terminal vein,* which drains the caudate nucleus, thalamus, internal capsule, and nearby structures (Fig. 11–11).

The anterior limb of the internal capsule intervenes between the head of the caudate nucleus and the lenticular nucleus (Figs. 12–4 and 12–5). However, the cortical afferent and efferent fibers constituting the internal capsule do not entirely separate the two components of the neostriatum. The head of the caudate nucleus and the putamen are in continuity through a bridge

of gray matter beneath the anterior limb of the internal capsule (Fig. 12–1). 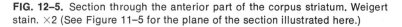The caudate nucleus and putamen are also connected by numerous gray strands extending across the internal capsule, hence the name "corpus striatum" (Fig. 12–5). In the floor of the lateral ventricle, the tail of the caudate nucleus lies next to the internal capsule as the latter merges into the medullary center of the cerebral hemisphere.

CONNECTIONS

Of the many afferent and efferent connections of the corpus striatum, only the largest and best documented are included in the following account. There are some differences with respect to the connections of the putamen and the caudate nucleus, because of the spatial separation of these two parts of the neostriatum. Similarly, the connections of the two divisions of the globus pallidus are not precisely alike. In order to avoid excessive detail, the connec-

tions of the neostriatum and paleostriatum are described without reference to their anatomic subdivisions.

NEOSTRIATUM (Fig. 12–6)

The caudate nucleus and putamen are similar histologically, as is to be expected. They consist mainly of small neurons forming

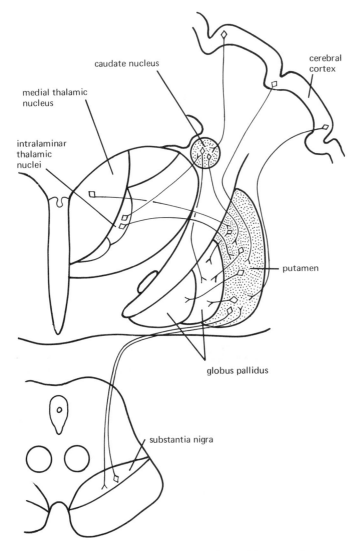

FIG. 12–6. Afferent and efferent connections of the neostriatum.

intranuclear connections or projecting to the globus pallidus. Only about 1 cell in 20 is of relatively large size; these cells send fibers to the globus pallidus and substantia nigra.

The neostriatum receives afferent fibers from the cerebral cortex, thalamus, and substantia nigra. *Corticostriate* fibers originate in widespread areas of cortex, including that of all four lobes, but especially the frontal and parietal lobes. Most of the fibers enter the neostriatum from the internal capsule, some being collateral branches of corticobulbar and corticospinal fibers, although a substantial number enter the putamen from the external capsule. *Thalamostriate* fibers from the intralaminar, medial, and ventral anterior thalamic nuclei represent a phylogenetically old afferent supply to the neostriatum, some of these connections appearing at the reptilian stage of vertebrate evolution. *Nigrostriate* fibers from the substantia nigra constitute an important afferent connection of the corpus striatum. The constituent neurons contain dopamine and the functional relationship between the substantia nigra and the striatum is prominent in current work on the pathogenesis and therapy of Parkinson's disease.

Most of the fibers leaving the neostriatum are *striopallidal,* bringing the globus pallidus under the influence and control of the neostriatum. The remaining efferents are *strionigral,* terminating in the substantia nigra.

PALEOSTRIATUM (Fig. 12–7)

The globus pallidus, which is the principal efferent part of the corpus striatum, consists of moderately large, multipolar neurons. Their axons are well myelinated, accounting for the pallor of the nucleus in fresh sections and for the name "globus pallidus." Conversely, the globus pallidus is darker than the putamen and caudate nucleus in Weigert-stained sections.

The *striopallidal* fibers noted above are the principal afferents to the globus pallidus. *Corticopallidal* and *nigropallidal* fibers have been described, but these are relatively unimportant compared with the projection from the cortex and substantia nigra to the striatum.

Fibers originating in the globus pallidus form two main efferent bundles. Some fibers penetrate the internal capsule and appear as the *lenticular fasciculus* (field H_2 of Forel) in the subthalamus, dorsal to the subthalamic nucleus; others curve around the medial border of the internal capsule further forward, forming the *ansa lenticularis.* The efferent fibers are distributed in two streams, one to the thalamus and the other to the brain stem, the former projection including the larger number of fibers in man. The *pallidothalamic* fibers enter the prerubral area (field H of Forel), where they bend in a lateral direction to enter the thalamic fasciculus (field H_1 of Forel). These fibers terminate in the ventral lateral and ventral anterior nuclei of the thalamus. The pallidothalamic fibers are joined in the prerubral area by dentatothalamic fibers proceeding to the ventral lateral nucleus. The thalamic nuclei (ventral lateral and ventral anterior) project to motor and premotor areas of the frontal lobe, bringing these cortical areas under the regulatory influence of the corpus striatum.

The remaining pallidal efferents, although including fewer fibers than the pallidothalamic projection, go to several centers and are therefore diverse in function. *Pallido-olivary* fibers contribute to the central tegmental tract and terminate in the inferior olivary complex. The latter has an extensive projection to the cerebellum, and a small olivospinal tract extends into the spinal cord. *Pallidohypothalamic* fibers

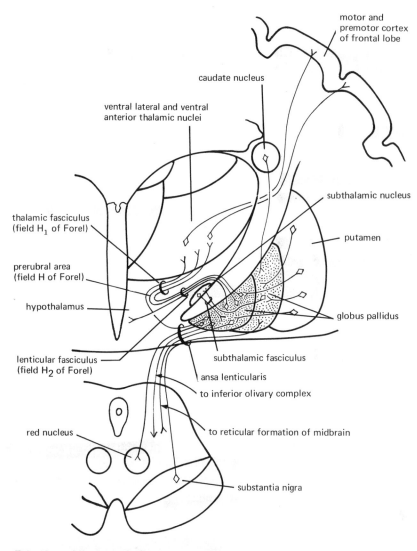

FIG. 12–7. Afferent and efferent connections of the paleostriatum.

bring the corpus striatum into relation with the autonomic nervous system (the existence of this connection has been questioned). Other pallidal efferents are the first link in a relay to lower motor neurons in nuclei of cranial nerves and the spinal cord, through which the corpus striatum influences skeletal musculature. *Pallido-rubral* fibers terminate in the large-cell portion of the red nucleus, from which im-

pulses reach lower motor neurons by way of the rubrospinal tract, and rubroreticular and reticulospinal connections. *Pallido-reticular* fibers terminate in the reticular formation of the midbrain; reticular relays, connections with motor nuclei of cranial nerves, and reticulospinal fibers establish connections with lower motor neurons at all levels. The pathway from the globus pallidus to the red nucleus and the reticular formation appears to be partially interrupted by synaptic relays involving cells situated in the prerubral area of the subthalamus (not shown in Fig. 12–7). A further connection of the globus pallidus worthy of special note is with the subthalamic nucleus. This connection consists of fibers passing in both directions across the internal capsule and making up the *subthalamic fasciculus.*

FUNCTIONS

The particular contribution of the corpus striatum to motor function is poorly understood. The connections described above provide a basis for speculation; inferences have also been drawn from the motor abnormalities which accompany degenerative changes in the corpus striatum. Unfortunately, other areas of the brain are often affected concurrently, thus detracting from the information that can be gained concerning the specific role of the corpus striatum.

The corpus striatum can be seen to participate in three main neuronal pathways. The oldest of these, already present in submammalian vertebrates, consists of fibers passing from the thalamus to the neostriatum, and from the globus pallidus to the red nucleus and reticular formation for relay to lower motor neurons. In man, this pathway may provide for motor activity of an automatic type, including responses to emotional changes.

Other pathways involve the cerebral cortex. Through corticostriate fibers and the projection from the globus pallidus to lower motor neurons via brain stem centers, cortical influences are imposed on the musculature through an extrapyramidal route. With rare exceptions, a lesion which interrupts the pyramidal pathway also interrupts fibers of extrapyramidal pathways, contributing to the signs of an "upper

motor neuron lesion." Conversely, intact extrapyramidal pathways may be in part responsible for the residual voluntary control of muscles in patients with an upper motor neuron type of disability. For example, a lesion in the internal capsule which interrupts corticospinal fibers also interrupts many extrapyramidal cortical efferents. However, some of these fibers remain intact because the external capsule includes fibers passing from the cortex to the putamen and the reticular formation of the brain stem.

The remaining pathway involving the corpus striatum is especially well developed in man. This is the circuit from the cerebral cortex, through the neostriatum, paleostriatum, and ventral thalamic nuclei to the motor and premotor areas of the frontal lobe. This circuit appears to have an important regulatory influence on cortex contributing fibers to the pyramidal system, and these cortical areas are also the source of many extrapyramidal fibers. Judging from the involuntary, hemiballistic movements which are associated with destruction of the subthalamic nucleus, the latter may have a controlling or inhibitory effect on the globus pallidus, but this is only speculation. The substantia nigra is integrated functionally with the corpus striatum and there is some evidence that the substantia nigra has an independent projection to the ventral thalamus.

DYSKINESIAS AND THE CORPUS STRIATUM

Degenerative lesions which include the corpus striatum cause motor disturbances or dyskinesia, in which involuntary movements figure prominently. The abnormal movements are regarded in part as release phenomena, i.e., a lesion in the corpus striatum or one of its parts removes a controlling influence on another center, leading to overactivity.

The involuntary movements take various forms. *Choreiform* movements are brisk, jerky, and purposeless, resembling fragments of voluntary movements. They are most pronounced in the axial and proximal limb musculature; the facial muscles and the tongue are involved at times, and there may be hypotonia of the musculature. There are two diseases in which choreiform movements are a cardinal sign. Sydenham's chorea (St. Vitus' dance) is typically a disease of childhood; it occurs more frequently in girls than in boys, and often follows an infectious disease. The pathology of Sydenham's chorea is not well understood because the disease is seldom fatal. The most common findings are scattered minute hemorrhages and capillary emboli in the corpus striatum. Huntington's chorea is a dominant hereditary disorder, onsetting in middle life, in which there is neuronal degeneration in the corpus striatum, most marked in the neostriatum. Concurrent loss of neurons in the cerebral cortex leads to progressive mental deterioration.

Athetoid movements are slow, sinuous, and aimless, involving the distal musculature of the extremities especially. The movements tend to blend together in a continuous mobile spasm and are usually associated with varying degrees of paresis and spasticity. The muscles of the face, neck, and tongue may be affected, with grimacing, protrusion and writhing of the tongue, and difficulty in speaking and swallowing.

Athetosis is often part of a congenital complex of neurologic signs (including those of cerebral palsy) resulting from maldevelopment of the brain, birth injury, or other etiologic factors. Athetoid movements are most frequently associated with pathologic changes in the neostriatum and cerebral cortex, although lesions are sometimes present as well in the globus pallidus and thalamus.

Wilson's disease (hepatolenticular degeneration) is a special condition in which the corpus striatum is involved. The disease is caused by a genetically determined error in copper metabolism, and the pathology includes cirrhosis of the liver. The signs of Wilson's disease usually appear between the ages of 10 and 25 years; they include muscular rigidity, tremor, impairment of voluntary movements (including those of speech), and loss of facial expression. There may be uncontrollable laughing or crying without apparent cause. The degenerative changes are most pronounced in the putamen and progress to cavitation of the lenticular nucleus. There may also be cellular degeneration in the cerebral cortex, thalamus, red nucleus, and cerebellum. Dystonia musculorum deformans is a particularly disabling motor disturbance in which degenerative changes involve the corpus striatum along with many other parts of the brain. The slow, writhing, involuntary movements of the axial and limb musculature are sustained, which may lead to contractures of muscles.

SUGGESTIONS FOR ADDITIONAL READING

Beck E, Bignami A: Some neuro-anatomical observations in cases with stereotaxic lesions for the relief of Parkinsonism. Brain 91:589–618, 1968

Berke JJ: The claustrum, the external capsule and the extreme capsule of Macaca mulatta. J Comp Neurol 115:297–331, 1960

Brodal A: Some data and perspectives on the anatomy of the so-called "extrapyramidal system." Acta Neurol Scand 39 (Suppl 4): 17–38, 1963

Brodal A: Neurological Anatomy in Relation to Clinical Medicine. London, Oxford University Press, 1969

Denny–Brown D: The Basal Ganglia and Their Relation to Disorders of Movement. London, Oxford University Press, 1962

Kemp JM, Powell TPS: The connections of the striatum and globus pallidus: Synthesis and speculation. Philos Trans R Soc Lond (Biol Sci) 262:441–457, 1971

Martin JP: Remarks on the functions of the basal ganglia. Lancet 1:999–1005, 1959

Martin JP: The Basal Ganglia and Posture. Philadelphia, Lippincott, 1967

Martinez A: Fiber connections of the globus pallidus in man. J Comp Neurol 117:37–41, 1961

Nauta WJH, Mehler WR: Projections of the lenti-form nucleus in the monkey. Brain Res 1:3–42, 1966

Poirier LJ, Sourkes TL: Influence of the substantia nigra on catecholamine content of the striatum. Brain 88:181–192, 1965

Smith MC: Stereotactic Operations for Parkinson's Disease: Anatomical observations. In Williams D (ed.). Modern Trends in Neurology, pp. 21–52. London, Butterworth, 1967

Szabo J: Topical distribution of the striatal efferents in the monkey. Exp Neurol 5:21–36, 1962

Szabo J: The efferent projections of the putamen in the monkey. Exp Neurol 19:463–476, 1967

Webster KE: The cortico-striatal projection in the cat. J Anat 99:329–337, 1965

13

Topography of the Cerebral Hemispheres

The complicated folding of the surface of the cerebral hemispheres substantially increases the surface area and therefore the volume of cerebral cortex. The folds are known as *convolutions* or *gyri* and the intervening grooves as *sulci*. Two grooves appear early in fetal development and are especially deep in the mature brain; they are known as the lateral and parieto-occipital *fissures*. About two-thirds of the cortex borders the sulci and fissures and is therefore hidden from surface view.

While some convolutions are constant features of the cerebral surface, others vary from one brain to another and even between the two hemispheres of the same brain. The following account of cerebral topography is of a general nature, with little reference to variations.

MAJOR FISSURES AND SULCI

The lateral and parieto-occipital fissures, and the central and calcarine sulci, are boundaries for the conventional division of the cerebral hemisphere into frontal, parietal, temporal, and occipital lobes (Figs. 13–1 and 13–2).

The *lateral fissure* or *fissure of Sylvius* begins as a deep furrow on the basal surface of the hemisphere. This is the stem of the fissure, which extends laterally between the frontal and temporal lobes, and divides into three rami on reaching the lateral surface. The *posterior ramus* is the main part of the fissure on the lateral surface of the hemisphere, while the *anterior horizontal* and *anterior vertical rami* project for only a short distance into the frontal lobe. An area of cortex called the *insula* or *island of Reil* lies at the bottom of the deep lateral fissure and is hidden from surface view. This cortex appears to have been bound to the underlying corpus striatum during fetal development, and growth of the surrounding cortex accounts in large part for the sylvian fissure.

The *central sulcus* or *sulcus of Rolando* is an important landmark for the sensori-

208

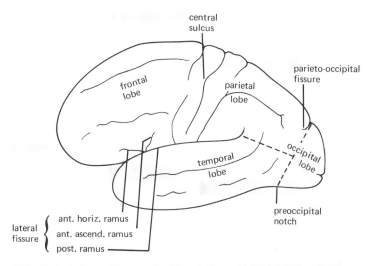

FIG. 13–1. Lobes of the cerebral hemisphere (dorsolateral surface).

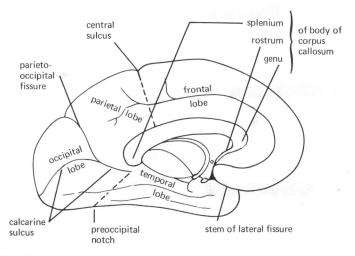

FIG. 13–2. Lobes of the cerebral hemisphere (medial and basal surfaces).

motor cortex, the general sensory strip lying behind the sulcus and the motor strip in front. The rolandic sulcus indents the superior border of the hemisphere about 1 cm behind the midpoint between the frontal and occipital poles. The sulcus slopes downward and forward at an angle of 70 degrees to the vertical, stopping just short of the lateral fissure. There are usually two bends along the course of the central sulcus. Its depth is about 2 cm and the walls of the sulcus therefore include much of the sensorimotor cortex.

The *calcarine sulcus* on the medial surface of the hemisphere begins under the posterior end of the corpus callosum and follows an arched course to the occipital pole. In some brains, the sulcus continues over the pole for a short distance on the lateral surface. The calcarine sulcus is an important landmark for the visual cortex, most of which lies in the walls of the sulcus.

The *parieto-occipital fissure,* like the lateral fissure, appears early in the development of the fetal brain. The fissure extends from the calcarine sulcus to the superior border of the hemisphere, intersects the border about 4 cm from the occipital pole, and continues for a short distance on the dorsolateral surface. This is a deep fissure with small gyri on its walls.

The longitudinal and transverse cerebral fissures are external to the hemispheres and therefore in a different category from the surface markings described above. The *longitudinal fissure* (sagittal fissure) separates the hemispheres; a dural partition called the falx cerebri extends into the fissure. The corpus callosum, which constitutes the main cerebral commissure, crosses from one hemisphere to the other at the bottom of the longitudinal fissure. The *transverse fissure* intervenes between the cerebral hemispheres above and the cerebellum, midbrain, and diencephalon below. The posterior part of the fissure is between the cerebral hemispheres and the cerebellum; it contains a dural partition known as the tentorium cerebelli. The fissure continues forward above the midbrain and then between the corpus callosum and the diencephalon. As described in Chapter 11, the anterior portion of the transverse fissure is triangular in outline, being bounded by the fornices as they converge in passing forward between the thalamus and the corpus callosum. This triangular space contains vascular connective tissue (tela choroidea) derived from the pia mater covering the brain. The tela choroidea is continuous with the connective tissue of the choroid plexuses of the lateral and third ventricles, and the plexuses are completed by choroid epithelium derived from the ependymal lining of the ventricles.

LOBES OF THE CEREBRAL HEMISPHERE

The cerebral hemisphere has dorsolateral, medial, and inferior or basal surfaces, on which the extent of the lobes of the hemisphere needs to be defined (Fig. 13–1 and 13–2).

The *frontal lobe* occupies the whole area in front of the central sulcus and above the lateral fissure on the dorsolateral surface. The medial surface of the frontal lobe envelops the anterior part of the corpus callosum and is bounded posteriorly by an arbitrary line drawn between the central sulcus and the corpus callosum. Such arbitrary lines are used elsewhere; they have no functional significance and can be ignored after serving their initial purpose. The basal surface of the frontal lobe rests on the orbital plate of the frontal bone.

The natural boundaries of the *parietal lobe* on the dorsolateral surface are the central sulcus and lateral fissure. The arbitrary boundaries consist of two lines; the first is drawn between the parieto-occipital fissure and the preoccipital notch, and the second line runs from the middle of the one just established to the lateral fissure. (The preoccipital notch is an unsatisfactory landmark, consisting of a shallow indentation of the brain caused by pressure of the petrous temporal bone.) On the medial surface, the parietal lobe is bounded by the frontal lobe, corpus callosum, calcarine sulcus, and parieto-occipital fissure.

The *temporal lobe* is outlined on the lateral surface by the sylvian fissure and the arbitrary lines noted above. The basal surface includes the area extending to the temporal pole from a line drawn between the anterior end of the calcarine sulcus and the preoccipital notch. Most of the *occipital lobe* appears on the medial surface of the hemisphere, where it is separated from the temporal lobe as described above and from the parietal lobe by the parieto-occipital fissure. On the lateral surface, the occipital lobe consists of the small area posterior to the arbitrary line joining the parieto-occipital fissure and the preoccipital notch.

The portion of the great cerebral commissure in and near the midline is known as the *body of the corpus callosum*, while the fibers of the commissure spreading out within the medullary centers of the hemispheres constitute the *radiations of the corpus callosum*. Names are assigned to certain regions of the body of the commissure (Fig. 13–2), and these regions are used as reference points further on. The enlarged posterior portion of the body is called the *splenium*. The anterior end is known as the *genu* of the corpus callosum; the genu thins out to form the *rostrum*, which is continuous with the lamina terminalis.

GYRI AND SULCI

Some surface markings of the hemisphere indicate the position of important functional areas; the central sulcus for sensorimotor cortex and the calcarine sulcus for visual cortex are good examples. For the most part, however, the sulci and gyri serve only as a rough frame of reference for cortical areas whose function may or may not be known. The markings can be identified according to lobes for the dorsolateral surface, but this is not practicable for the medial and basal surfaces. As noted above, there is considerable variation in detail from one brain to another.

DORSOLATERAL SURFACE OF THE HEMISPHERE (Fig. 13–3)

Frontal Lobe

The *precentral sulcus* (often broken into two or more parts) is parallel with the central sulcus; these sulci outline the *precentral gyrus*, which is a landmark for the primary motor area. The remainder of the surface of the frontal lobe is divided into *superior, middle,* and *inferior frontal gyri* by the *superior* and *inferior frontal sulci*. The superior frontal gyrus extends on the medial surface of the hemisphere. The anterior horizontal and anterior vertical rami of the lateral fissure divide the inferior frontal gyrus into *opercular, triangular,* and *orbital portions*. Over the frontal lobe, as in the other parts of the hemisphere, there are subsidiary gyri and sulci which contribute to the variability in the topography of different brains.

Parietal Lobe

The *postcentral sulcus* parallels the central sulcus; these sulci bound the *postcentral gyrus*, which is the topographic landmark for the general sensory cortex. Although the configuration of the remainder of the parietal lobe varies greatly, an *intraparietal sulcus* running backward from the postcentral sulcus can usually be identified. The intraparietal sulcus divides that part of the surface not occupied by the postcentral gyrus into *superior* and *inferior parietal lobules*. Those portions of the inferior lobule that surround the upturned ends of the lateral fissure and superior temporal sulcus are called the *supramarginal gyrus* and the *angular gyrus*, respectively.

Temporal Lobe

Superior and *middle temporal sulci* divide the temporal surface into *superior, middle,* and *inferior temporal gyri,* the last-named continuing on the basal surface. The surface of the temporal lobe presents many variations; in particular, the middle temporal sulcus is often discontinuous and difficult to identify. The superior temporal gyrus has a large upper surface, which

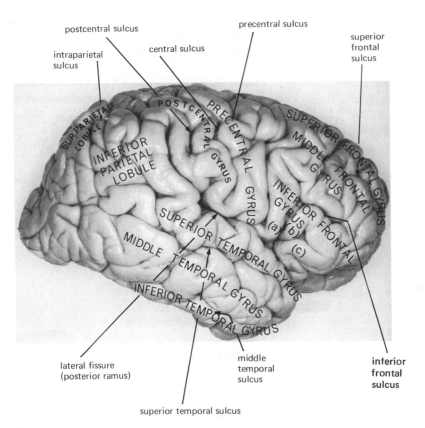

FIG. 13–3. Gyri and sulci on the dorsolateral surface of the right cerebral hemisphere. *a, b,* and *c* indicate the opercular, triangular, and orbital portions of the inferior frontal gyrus, respectively. The anterior vertical ramus of the lateral fissure separates the opercular and triangular portions, and the anterior horizontal ramus separates the triangular and orbital portions. ×⅝

forms the floor of the sylvian fissure. On this surface, *transverse temporal gyri* (also known as *Heschl's convolutions*) extend to the bottom of the lateral fissure and mark the location of the auditory area of cortex.

Occipital Lobe

In primate brains other than that of man, and in some human brains, the calcarine sulcus continues for a short distance over the occipital pole. There is then a curved *lunate sulcus* around the end of the calcarine sulcus. Except for this inconstant marking, the small area of the occipital lobe on the lateral surface has minor grooves and folds of no special significance.

INSULA

It is customary to consider the *insula* or *island of Reil* separately from the four main lobes of the hemisphere. The regions concealing the insula are known as the *frontal, parietal,* and *temporal opercula;* these must be spread apart or cut away in order to expose the insula (Fig. 13–4). The insula is outlined by a circular sulcus and divided

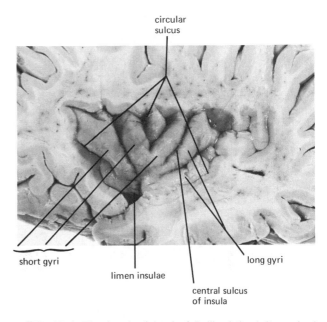

FIG. 13–4. The insula (island of Reil) of the left cerebral hemisphere. ×⅘

into two regions by a central sulcus. Several short gyri lie in front of the central sulcus and one or two long gyri behind it. The lower part of the insula in the region of the stem of the lateral fissure is known as the *limen insulae*.

MEDIAL AND BASAL SURFACES OF THE HEMISPHERE

The *cingulate gyrus* begins beneath the genu of the corpus callosum and continues above the corpus callosum as far as the splenium (Fig. 13–5). The gyrus is separated from the corpus callosum by the *callosal sulcus.* The *cingulate sulcus* intervenes between the cingulate gyrus and the extension of the superior frontal gyrus on the medial surface of the hemisphere. The cingulate sulcus gives off a *paracentral sulcus,* then divides into *marginal* and *subparietal sulci* in the parietal lobe. The

region bounded by the paracentral and marginal sulci, and surrounding the indentation made by the central sulcus on the superior border, is called the *paracentral lobule.* The anterior part of this lobule is an extension of the precentral gyrus of the dorsolateral surface, while the posterior part is continuous with the postcentral gyrus. The area above the subparietal sulcus is called the *precuneate gyrus* (quadrangular gyrus) and is continuous with the superior parietal lobule on the dorsolateral surface. The parieto-occipital fissure and calcarine sulcus bound the *cuneate gyrus* of the occipital lobe.

On the basal surface of the hemisphere (Figs. 13–5 and 13–6) a convolution extends from the occipital pole almost to the temporal pole. The posterior part of the convolution consists of the *lingual gyrus;* the anterior part forms the *parahippocampal gyrus,* which hooks sharply back-

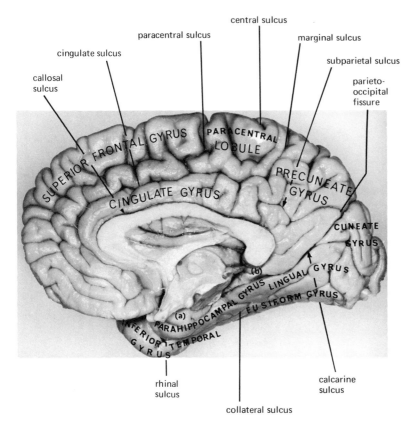

FIG. 13–5. Gyri and sulci on the medial and basal surfaces of the right cerebral hemisphere. *a*, uncus; *b*, isthmus connecting the cingulate and parahippocampal gyri. ×⅝

FIG. 13–6. Gyri and sulci on the basal surface of the right cerebral hemisphere. *a*, uncus. ×⅝

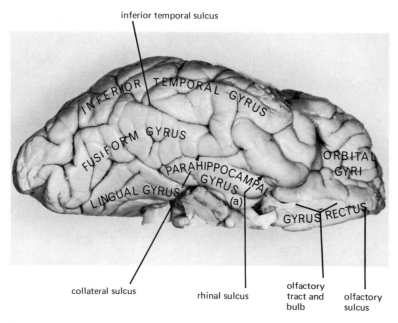

ward as the *uncus.* The *collateral sulcus* defines the lateral margin of the lingual and parahippocampal gyri, and the short *rhinal sulcus* is situated at the lateral edge of the parahippocampal gyrus anteriorly. The *fusiform gyrus,* which is inconstant in morphology and broken up by irregular sulci, lies along the lateral side of the collateral sulcus. The *inferior temporal sulcus* intervenes between the fusiform gyrus and the extension of the inferior temporal gyrus on the basal surface of the hemisphere.

On the orbital surface of the frontal lobe (Fig. 13–6), the *olfactory bulb* and *tract* lie along the *olfactory sulcus.* The *gyrus rectus* is medial to the olfactory sulcus; the large area lateral to the sulcus consists of irregular *orbital gyri.*

The cingulate and parahippocampal gyri are connected by a narrow *isthmus* beneath the splenium of the corpus callosum, forming the *limbic lobe* of the cerebral hemisphere. This is part of the limbic system of the brain, which also includes the hippocampus, dentate gyrus, and amygdaloid nucleus (all in the temporal lobe), the hypothalamus (especially the mammillary bodies), the anterior nucleus of the thalamus, and connecting fiber tracts. Because of its important specialized functions, the limbic system is discussed separately in Chapter 18.

14
Histology of the Cerebral Cortex

The cerebral hemispheres are covered by a mantle of gray matter, the cortex or pallium, lying on the medullary centers of white matter. The cerebral cortex makes up about 40 percent of the total weight of the human brain. The cortex has a characteristic histologic structure, in that the nerve cells and fibers are arranged in layers. However, there are several kinds of cortex on the basis of phylogenetic development, histology, and function.

Almost the entire cortex of submammalian vertebrates is olfactory cortex of the rhinencephalon (nosebrain). From this cortex, in which there are only three layers of cells, are derived the *paleocortex* and *archicortex* of the mammalian brain. The paleocortex retains the earlier olfactory function; the archicortex becomes incorporated in the limbic system of the brain and is present in the hippocampus, dentate gyrus, and part of the parahippocampal gyrus, all in the temporal lobe.

Neocortex, which consists of six layers of cells, is a significant feature of the brain of

mammals. Neocortex is the recipient of data for general sensation, vision, hearing, and taste; it also includes motor areas projecting to subcortical motor nuclei and lower motor neurons. The expanse of neocortex increased as higher mammals evolved, due mainly to progressively larger areas of association cortex. This trend culminated in the condition found in the human brain; 90 percent of the cerebral cortex of man is neocortex, most of which is association cortex rather than consisting of specific sensory or motor areas. Neocortex is also called *isocortex,* paleocortex and archicortex then being referred to as *allocortex*. Finally, the cortex of the cingulate gyrus is known as *mesocortex* because it is intermediate histologically between three-layered and six-layered cortices.

The present chapter deals with the histology or cytoarchitecture of the neocortex. In addition to having important sensory and motor functions, the neocortex merits special attention as the principal contributor to the intellectual capabilities of man. Human society and culture, together with the complexity and individuality of behavior, are largely the consequence of man's possessing a significantly larger volume of neocortex than any other species.

TYPES OF CORTICAL NEURONS

The number of nerve cells in the human cerebral cortex is said to be on the order of 10 billion, of which the great majority are in the neocortex. Of the morphologic varieties of neurons present, five types are especially characteristic. Pyramidal and stellate cells are the most numerous, the others being fusiform cells, cells of Martinotti, and horizontal cells of Cajal. In addition to the arrangement of cells in six layers, the principal characteristics of neocortex are the presence of pyramidal neurons and the large population of small Golgi type II neurons, the majority of the latter being stellate cells. As in gray matter elsewhere, there is a large population of neuroglial cells (protoplasmic astrocytes, oligodendrocytes, and microglial cells) and a close capillary network.

Cortical neurons fall into three categories according to the nature of their connections. *Projection* neurons transmit impulses to a subcortical center, such as the corpus striatum, thalamus, a brain stem nucleus, or the spinal cord. *Association* neurons establish connections with other cortical nerve cells in the same hemisphere. Association neurons include the vast number of Golgi type II cells whose short axons do not leave the cortex, thereby providing for complex intracortical circuits. Axons of the remaining association neurons enter the white matter and terminate in another cortical area of the same hemisphere. Axons of *commissural* neurons proceed to a cortical area in the opposite hemisphere. Most of the commissural fibers are in the corpus callosum; a relatively small number connect cortices of the temporal lobes through the anterior commissure.

The five types of cortical neurons have the following characteristics (Fig. 14–1).

Pyramidal cells derive their name from the shape of the cell body. Most of these cells fall within the range of 10–50 μ for the height of the cell body. They are classified as small, medium-sized, and large pyramidal neurons, the size increasing with the distance from the surface of the cortex. In addition, there are giant pyramidal cells, also known as *Betz cells,* with cell bodies as large as 100 μ in height; these are characteristic of the motor area of the frontal lobe.

The pyramidal cell has a branching apical dendrite directed toward the surface of the cortex and several basal dendrites. The dendritic branches bear large numbers of spines for synaptic association with axons of other neurons. The length of the axon, which arises from the base of the cell body, depends on the size of the cell. In the case of more superficially located, small pyramidal cells, the axon may terminate in a deeper cortical layer. With this exception, the axons of pyramidal neurons enter the white matter as projection, association, or commissural fibers. Collateral branches may arise from the axon while still in the cortex and establish synaptic contacts with other cortical neurons.

Stellate cells, also known as *granule cells,* are polygonal or star-shaped in outline and the cell body is about 8 μ in diameter. There are several short dendrites and the axon terminates on a neuron nearby.

Of the less numerous cell types, *fusiform cells* are located in the deepest cortical layer and the long axis of the cell body tends to be perpendicular to the surface of the cortex. Dendrites come off each pole of the perikaryon; the deep dendrite branches near the cell body, while the other one extends into more superficial layers of the cortex. The axon enters the white matter as a projection, association, or commissural

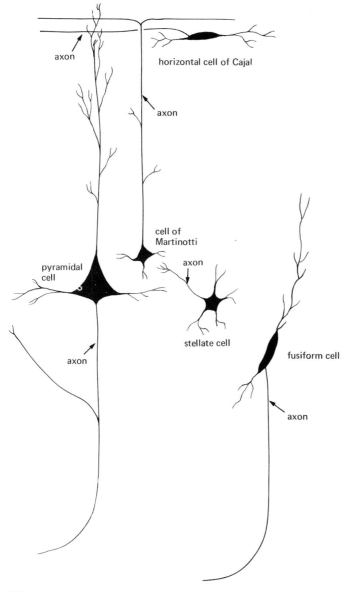

FIG. 14–1. Main types of cortical neurons.

fiber. The remaining types of cells are intracortical association neurons. *Cells of Martinotti* are present throughout the cortex, except for the most superficial layer. Short dendrites arise from the small, polygonal cell body. The identifying feature of the cell of Martinotti is that the axon is directed toward the surface, ending in any more superficial layer, but preferentially in the outermost layer. *Horizontal cells of Cajal* are restricted to the surface layer. The cell body is fusiform, with a dendrite extending from either end. The axon, which runs tangentially to the cortical surface, makes synaptic contact with dendritic branches of pyramidal neurons. These horizontal cells decrease in number during postnatal life and are therefore sparse in the outer cortical layer.

CORTICAL HISTOLOGY

The thickness of the cortex varies from 4.5 mm in the motor area of the frontal lobe to 1.5 mm in the visual area of the occipital lobe. The cortex is generally thicker over the crest of a convolution than in the depths of a sulcus. The six layers, differing in the density of cell population and the size and shape of constituent neurons, can be recognized by about the seventh month of fetal life. The details of the layers differ from one region to another, as will be discussed presently. The names and characteristics of the layers, starting at the surface and omitting regional differences, are as follows (Fig. 14–2A).

1. *Molecular layer* (plexiform layer). The superficial layer consists mainly of delicate nerve fibers, giving it a punctate or "molecular" appearance in sections stained for fibers. The dendritic branches come from pyramidal and fusiform cells. The axonal fibers originate in a cortical area

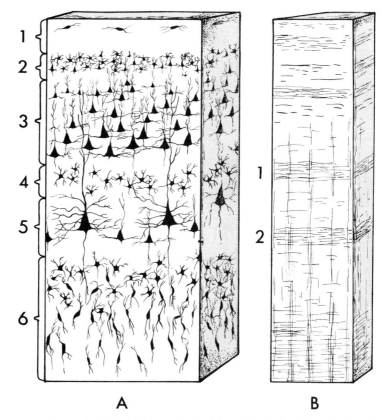

A   B

FIG. 14–2. Cortical histology. **A.** Golgi method: *1*, molecular layer; *2*, outer granular layer; *3*, pyramidal cell layer; *4*, inner granular layer; *5*, ganglionic layer; *6*, fusiform cell layer. **B.** Weigert method: *1*, outer line of Baillarger; *2*, inner line of Baillarger.

elsewhere in the same hemisphere, in the cortex of the opposite hemisphere, and in the thalamus. Cells of Martinotti in any deeper layer also contribute axons to layer 1. Sparse horizontal cells of Cajal and scattered stellate cells intervene between some axons and dendrites. The molecular layer is essentially an important synaptic field of the cortex.

2. *Outer granular layer* (layer of small pyramidal cells). This layer contains a wealth of small neurons, both small pyramidal cells and stellate cells. The dendrites of many of these cells extend into the molecular layer; most of the axons terminate in deeper layers, and the remainder enter the medullary center. The outer granular layer makes an important contribution to the complexity of intracortical circuits.

3. *Pyramidal cell layer* (layer of medium-sized and large pyramidal cells). The neurons are typical pyramidal cells, increasing in size from the outer to the inner borders of the layer. Apical dendrites extend into the synaptic field of layer 1; axons of the pyramidal cells enter the white matter and proceed to their destination as projection, association, or commissural fibers.

4. *Inner granular layer* (layer of stellate cells). The fourth layer consists of closely arranged stellate cells, many of which receive stimuli from fibers originating in the thalamus. The short axons of the stellate cells end on dendrites passing through the layer from cells in layers 5 and 6, on other stellate cells, and on cells of Martinotti. As in any nervous tissue that includes large numbers of Golgi type II neurons, the connections and circuits involving the stellate cells of layer 4 are exceedingly numerous and complex.

5. *Ganglionic layer* (inner pyramidal layer). This layer contains pyramidal cells intermingled with scattered stellate cells and cells of Martinotti. The layer owes the name "ganglionic" to giant pyramidal or Betz cells, although these are limited to the motor cortex of the precentral gyrus. Betz cells account for the 3 percent of very large fibers in the pyramidal tract.

6. *Fusiform cell layer* (layer of polymorphic cells). Although the fusiform cell is the most characteristic constituent of layer 6, there are additional cells of various shapes (hence the alternative name "polymorphic" for the layer). The deepest cortical layer is primarily efferent, giving rise to fibers proceeding to cortex elsewhere or to subcortical centers.

In the paleocortex and archicortex, there are molecular, pyramidal, and polymorphic cell layers. These correspond roughly to layers 1, 5, and 6 of neocortex. Layers 2, 3, and 4 of neocortex are therefore regarded as being a more recent acquisition phylogenetically and as having a special relation to higher cortical functions. Layers 1 through 4 of the neocortex, which include complex circuits and have an important associative function, are sometimes referred to as supragranular cortex. Layers 5 and 6, which are basically efferent in nature, are then said to compose the infragranular cortex.

The cell layers are studied in sections stained by the Nissl and Golgi techniques. When silver methods for axons and the Weigert method for myelin sheaths are used, nerve fibers within the cortex are seen to accumulate in radial bundles and tangential bands (Fig. 14–2B). The radial bundles are close together; they include axons of pyramidal and fusiform cells leaving the cortex, together with afferent fibers from the thalamus and other cortical areas. The tangential bands consist largely of collateral and terminal branches of afferent fibers. The branches leave the radial bundles and run parallel to the surface for some distance, making synaptic contact with large numbers of cortical neurons. The most prominent tangential bands are the *outer* and *inner lines of Baillarger,* located in layer 4 and the deep portion of layer 5, respectively. Thalamocortical fibers contribute heavily to the lines of Baillarger, which are therefore especially well developed in sensory areas. In the visual area in the walls of the calcarine sulcus, the outer line of Baillarger is sufficiently thick to be seen with the naked eye. In this location, the band in question is known as the *line of Gennari* (Fig. 14–3), having been first described by Francesco Gennari, an eighteenth century Italian medical student. Because of the prominent line of Gennari, the visual cortex is known alternatively as the striate area.

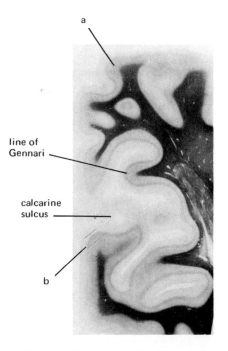

a

line of Gennari

calcarine sulcus

b

FIG. 14–3. Vertical section through the calcarine sulcus of the occipital lobe. The line of Gennari identifies the visual cortex (striate area), extending from *a* to *b* in vertical section. Weigert stain. ×2

VARIATIONS IN CYTOARCHITECTURE

The above description of cortical histology is to be regarded only as a general pattern. Six layers can be identified throughout most of the neocortex, which is said to be *homotypical* cortex. In restricted areas, known as *heterotypical* cortex, it is not possible to identify six layers. For example, in the visual area and part of the auditory and general sensory areas, the stellate cells of layer 4 overflow into adjoining layers. Layers 2 through 5 therefore merge into a single layer of small cells receiving thalamocortical fibers. This type of heterotypical cortex is called *granular cortex* or *konicortex* (*konis,* dust). The other extreme is found in the motor and premotor areas of the frontal lobe. Layers 2 through 5 again appear as a single, well developed layer, because they include large neurons of efferent type, mainly pyramidal cells (*agranular cortex*).

Students of the cerebral cortex have divided it into areas, based on differences in the thickness of individual layers, neuronal morphology in the layers, and the details of nerve fiber lamination. Such studies require infinite patience and attention to detail. The few investigators who have undertaken a meticulous analysis of cortical cytoarchitecture perhaps hoped to establish a basis for structural and functional correlations. This has been only partially fulfilled because of uncertain structural criteria and an incomplete understanding of the functional significance of many parts of the cortex. Parcelation of the cortex by different investigators varies from 20 to 200 areas, depending on the cytoarchitectural criteria used. Brodmann's map which was published in 1909 and consists of 57 areas remains the most widely used map of cortical cytoarchitectural areas.

More recent studies agree that heterotypical areas can be identified without difficulty. For example, the anterior portion of the general sensory cortex in the postcentral gyrus is granular cortex (area 3 of Brodmann); the visual cortex around the calcarine sulcus (area 17) and the central part of the auditory cortex in the superior temporal gyrus (area 41) also consist of granular cortex. The motor and premotor areas of the frontal lobe (areas 4 and 6) are agranular heterotypical cortex, as noted above, and are distinguished from one another by the easier identification of Betz cells in area 4. It is extremely doubtful that the large areas of homotypical cortex can be divided into discrete areas as shown on the Brodmann cytoarchitectural map. Nevertheless, this numbering system has been used extensively when referring to a limited area of the cortex and this practice is likely to continue for some time. The map, regardless of its validity, is useful when discussing functional areas of the cortex. It is used in this context in the following chapter, the numbers appearing in Figures 15–1 and 15–2 being derived from the cytoarchitectural map of Brodmann. It must be emphasized that the Brodmann map is referred to because the student will probably encounter the numbering system elsewhere in the neurosciences. In view of the uncertainties surrounding variations in cortical cytoarchitecture, the use of any map purporting to identify specific areas throughout the cerebral cortex is open to question.

INTRACORTICAL CIRCUITS

Studies of cortical neurons with the Golgi technique, combined with electrical recording from microelectrodes placed in the cortex, have yielded some information concerning intrinsic circuits. These are suggested in Figure 14–4; in reality, the circuits are much more complex than the figure indicates.

Afferent fibers entering the cortex are of two general kinds: fibers from the thalamus and fibers from another cortical area of the same or opposite hemisphere. Thalamocortical fibers are either specific afferents, such as those originating in sensory relay nuclei of the thalamus and terminating in sensory areas, or nonspecific afferents from other thalamic nuclei. Specific thalamocortical fibers divide into branches which synapse with cortical neurons mainly in the region of the outer line of Baillarger (line of Gennari in the visual cortex). Nonspecific thalamic afferents and fibers from other regions of cortex terminate in all cortical layers, with an emphasis on layers 1 through 3. Cortical efferent fibers are axons of the larger cells, notably pyramidal and fusiform cells. They enter the white matter for distribution as projection, association, or commissural fibers.

The histologic structure of neocortex is basically the same in all mammals, but the population of Golgi type II cells with short axons increases, the higher the mammal in the phylogenetic scale. The principal attribute of the neocortex of man is the presence of an especially large population of small neurons, notably the small pyramidal cells of layer 2 and the stellate cells of layer 4. An afferent fiber may establish synaptic contact directly with an efferent neuron, or one to many Golgi type II neurons may be inserted between afferent fibers and efferent cells. In addition, collateral branches of axons of efferent cells establish synaptic contacts with Golgi type II neurons; these, along with other intrinsic connections, provide for reverberating circuits within the cortex.

Recording from microelectrodes has shown that the cortex is functionally organized into minute vertical units which include nerve cells of all layers. This has been demonstrated best in sensory areas. All

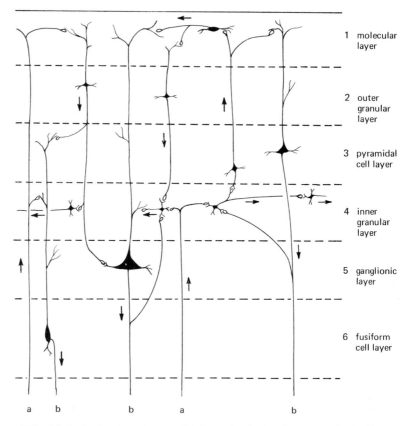

FIG. 14–4. A simple scheme of intracortical circuits. *a*, cortical afferent fiber; *b*, cortical efferent fiber.

neurons in the unit are activated by the same peripheral stimulus, whether it originates in a particular type of cutaneous receptor at a particular location or in a specific point on the retina. Adjacent functional units are integrated by means of connections established by small neurons.

SUGGESTIONS FOR ADDITIONAL READING

Bailey P, Von Bonin G: The Isocortex of Man. Illinois Monographs in the Medical Sciences, Vol. 6. Urbana, University of Illinois Press, 1951

Colonnier M: Synaptic patterns on different cell types in the different laminae of the cat visual cortex: An electron microscope study. Brain Res 9:268–287, 1968

Diamond IT, Hall WC: Evolution of neocortex. Science 164:251–262, 1969

Hubel DH, Wiesel TN: Anatomical demonstration of columns in the monkey striate cortex. Nature (London) 221:747–750, 1969

Powell TPS, Mountcastle VB: Some aspects of the functional organization of the cortex of the postcentral gyrus of the monkey: A correlation of findings obtained in a single unit analysis with cytoarchitecture. Johns Hopkins Med J 105: 133–162, 1959

Purpura DP, Carmichael MW, Housepian, EM: Physiological and anatomical studies of development of superficial axodendritic synaptic pathways in neocortex. Exp Neurol 2:324–347, 1960

Tower DB, Schadé JP: (eds.). Structure and Function of the Cerebral Cortex. Amsterdam, Elsevier, 1960

15

Functional Localization in the Cerebral Cortex

Clinicopathologic studies and animal experiments have provided evidence of functional specialization in different regions of the cerebral cortex. For example, there are three main sensory areas; they are for general sensation, vision, and hearing, to which should be added gustatory and vestibular areas. There are also motor areas from which contractions of the skeletal musculature can be elicited by electrical stimulation. The remainder of the neocortex falls under the heading of association cortex, which may be intimately related with the primary sensory areas or function at the higher level of behavior and the intellect. As noted in the preceding chapter, the trend in mammalian evolution has been toward larger areas of association cortex, and the human brain is preeminent in this respect.

DEVELOPMENT OF THE CONCEPT OF CORTICAL LOCALIZATION

The sensory and motor areas are more accessible to investigation than association cortex. In fact, our knowledge of cortical function in relation to the higher mental processes is still fragmentary, although regions of association cortex that are of special importance for language have been identified.

The first indications of functional localization came from clinical observations. Broca (1861) examined postmortem the brain of an individual who had suffered from a speech defect (motor aphasia). A lesion was found in the inferior frontal gyrus and this region is still known as Broca's motor speech area. On the basis of clinicopathologic studies, Hughlings Jackson (1864) concluded that a form of localized epilepsy (now known as jacksonian epilepsy) is caused by focal irritation of the precentral gyrus. The work of Hughlings Jackson drew attention to the probability of a motor area; experimentalists then proceeded to demonstrate such an area by electrical stimulation of the cortex in animals. An area from which motor responses were elicited on weak stimulation was demonstrated by Fritsch and Hitzig (1870) in the dog, and by Ferrier (1875), Horsley and Beevor (1894), and Sherrington and Grünbaum (1901) in the monkey and chimpanzee.

The identification of sensory areas had a somewhat parallel history. In 1870, Gudden showed that removal of the eyes from young animals interfered with full development of the occipital lobes. Ferrier (1873) found that an animal would prick up the ears if a particular region of the temporal lobe was stimulated. This region included the auditory area and stimulation produced the animal's natural response to a sound. Similarly, Dusser de Barenne (1916) showed that application of strychnine to a small area of the monkey's postcentral gyrus caused the animal to scratch the skin in one place or another, depending on the precise point at which cortical neurons were stimulated by strychnine. He was able with this technique to map the somesthetic cortex of the monkey. Head's meticulous study of patients with brain injuries received during World War I added greatly to an understanding of the sensory areas of the human cerebral cortex.

The experimental work on subhuman primates was expanded to include the human brain by neurosurgeons, notably Cushing, Foerster, and Penfield. In certain neurosurgical procedures, it is essential to identify the motor area, a sensory area, or even a particular region within these areas. Identification of sensory areas requires operating on a conscious patient under local anesthesia, a procedure made possible because the brain is insensitive to trauma or other stimuli that would be painful elsewhere in the body. Electrical stimulation of the brain surface under the above circumstances has provided information of the first importance with respect to functional localization in the cerebral cortex of man.

It is convenient to consider the neocortex as consisting of two main parts: 1) cortex of the parietal, occipital, and temporal lobes and 2) cortex of the frontal lobe. Simply stated, the former is concerned with the reception and conceptual elaboration of sensory data, while the latter is concerned with motor responses and the judgments, foresight, and moods associated with behavior. The following account of functional areas is at best a brief summary of a difficult yet important subject, and one which is in need of much further investigation.

PARIETO-OCCIPITO-TEMPORAL CORTEX

GENERAL SENSATION

The *general sensory* or *somesthetic area* occupies the postcentral gyrus on the dorsolateral surface of the hemisphere and the posterior part of the paracentral lobule on the medial surface (Figs. 15–1 and 15–2). It consists of areas 3, 1, and 2 of the Brodmann cytoarchitectural map. Area 3, most of which is in the posterior wall of the rolandic sulcus, is granular heterotypical cortex. Areas 1 and 2 are homotypical cortex, slightly thicker than area 3. It is possible to elict motor responses by stimulating the somesthetic area (which contributes fibers to the pyramidal tract), as well as sensory responses from the motor area in the precentral gyrus. The connections and functions of the two areas therefore overlap to some extent and they should be considered as a sensorimotor strip surrounding the rolandic sulcus.

The ventral posterior nucleus of the thalamus is the main source of afferent fibers for the general sensory area, the larger proportion of these fibers terminating in area 3. The fibers traverse the internal capsule and medullary center, conveying data for the various modalities of general sensation. Fibers related to cutaneous sensibility end preferentially in the anterior part of the area, and those for deep sensibility in the posterior part. The contralateral half of the body is represented as inverted. The pharyngeal region, tongue, and jaws are represented in the most ventral part of the somesthetic area, followed by the face, hand, arm, trunk, and thigh. The sensory cortex for the leg and foot is in the posterior part of the paracentral lobule on the medial surface of the hemisphere. The anal and genital regions are likewise represented on the medial surface just above the cingulate sulcus. The size of the cortical area for a particular part of the body is determined by the functional importance of the part and its need for sensitivity. Thus the area for the face, especially the lips, is disproportionately large, and a large area is assigned to the hand, particularly the thumb and index finger. There is some ipsilateral representation of the face for touch sensation, in addition to the main contralateral representation. In fact, single cell recordings from the cortex indicate that there is more ipsilateral conduction of sensory data to the sensorimotor strip than is traditionally recognized.

The contribution of the thalamus relative to the cortex, with respect to awareness of the general senses, varies form one modality of sensation to another. Pain, heat, and cold (all nociceptive sensations) are felt at the thalamic level. However, the somesthetic area is necessary for recognition of the source, severity, and quality of painful and thermal stimuli. The cortex has a larger role in appreciation of simple touch and pressure, but there is a crude awareness of these sensations in the thalamus. The sense of vibration may be included in the latter category. The neural processes inherent in the somesthetic cortex are required for any awareness of the more discriminative sensations of fine touch and position and movement of the body parts. It follows that the neurologic deficits following a destructive lesion in the postcentral gyrus include 1) a crude awareness only of pain, temperature, touch, and pressure, and 2) complete loss of discriminative touch and proprioception. The sensory deficit is contralateral to the lesion and involves the part of the body normally represented in the affected region of the postcentral gyrus. Electrical stimulation of the general sensory area in a conscious patient usually elicits modified forms of the tactile sense such as tingling or numbness.

A *secondary somatic sensory area* has been described in subhuman primates, situated in the dorsal wall of the sylvian fissure in line with the postcentral gyrus and perhaps extending on the insula. Such an area is probably present in the human brain, although damage to the area does not cause detectable sensory deficits.

The *somesthetic association cortex* occupies the superior parietal lobule on the dorsolateral surface, extending on the medial surface of the hemisphere. The region in question is said to coincide with areas 5 and 7 of the Brodmann map. There is an extensive input from the primary sensory area, as well as reciprocal connections with the dorsal tier of nuclei in the lateral mass of the thalamus. Data pertaining to the general senses are integrated in this association cortex; this permits, for example, a comprehensive assessment of the characteristics of an object held in the hand

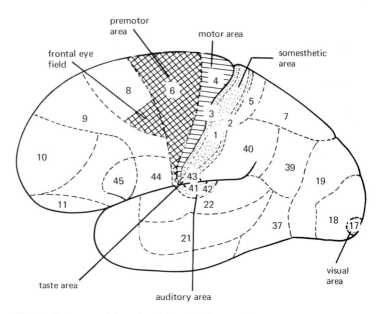

FIG. 15–1. Areas of functional localization on the dorsolateral surface of the cerebral hemisphere. The numbers are taken from the cytoarchitectural map of Brodmann.

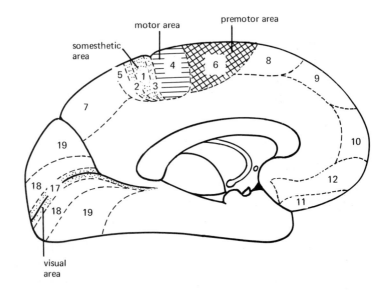

FIG. 15–2. Areas of functional localization on the medial surface of the cerebral hemisphere. The numbers are taken from the cytoarchitectural map of Brodmann.

and its identification without visual aid. When there is a lesion in the superior parietal lobule, leaving the postcentral gyrus intact, awareness of the general senses persists but the significance of the information received on the basis of previous experience is elusive. A defect in understanding the significance of sensory information is called *agnosia*, of which there are several kinds, depending on the sense that is most affected. A lesion causing destruction of a large proportion of the somesthetic association area causes tactile agnosia and astereognosis, which are closely related. They combine when a person is unable to identify a common object, such as a pair of scissors, held in the hand with the eyes closed. It is impossible to correlate the surface texture, shape, size, and weight of the object or to compare the sensations with previous experiences. Astereognosis includes a loss of awareness of the "body scheme" or "body image" (the spatial relations of body parts).

VISION

The *visual area* surrounds the calcarine sulcus on the medial surface of the occipital lobe, extending over the occipital pole in some brains (Fig. 15–2). The area is more extensive than the illustration suggests because most of it is in the walls of the deep calcarine sulcus, on which there are secondary folds. The visual cortex is thinner than cortex elsewhere, being only about 1.5 mm in thickness. It is granular heterotypical cortex, corresponding to area 17 of the Brodmann map. The visual area is also called the *striate area* because of the prominent line of Gennari.

The chief source of afferent fibers to area 17 is the lateral geniculate nucleus of the thalamus by way of the geniculocalcarine tract. It is worth noting that part of this tract passes forward in the medullary center of the temporal lobe, then swings back (Meyer's loop) to the striate area. A cerebral lesion causing visual field defects may therefore be located in the temporal lobe as well as in the occipital lobe.

Through a synaptic relay in the lateral geniculate nucleus, the visual cortex receives data from the temporal half of the ipsilateral retina and the nasal half of the contralateral retina. The dividing line or "watershed" runs vertically through the macula lutea, which is a specialized central region of the retina. The left half of the field of vision is therefore represented in the visual area of the right hemisphere and vice versa. There are spatial patterns within the striate area. The lower retinal quadrants (upper field of vision) project on the lower wall of the calcarine sulcus, while the upper retinal quadrants (lower field of vision) project on the upper wall of the sulcus. Another pattern is related to central and peripheral vision. The macula lutea is represented in the posterior part of area 17; proceeding from the macula to the ora serrata (anterior limit of the functional retina), the retina is represented progressively more anteriorly. The macula contains a concentration of cone photoreceptors, accounts for a disproportionately large number of fibers in the optic nerve and tract, and is responsible for central vision of maximal discrimination. Consistent with the foregoing, the part of area 17 receiving data for central vision accounts for one-third of the visual cortex.

A lesion that destroys visual cortex of a hemisphere causes a defect in the opposite visual field, the size and location of the area of blindness being determined by the extent and location of the lesion. However, central vision is found to be retained on field examination following a unilateral lesion in the occipital lobe, e.g., infarction caused by a thrombus in the posterior cerebral artery. This clinical observation is known as "macular sparing," for which there is no anatomic explanation on the basis of bilateral cortical representation of the macula. Macular sparing may be an artifact of testing, caused by the patient's shifting his fixation point a few degrees while the visual fields are being examined. Another possibility is that collateral circulation from the middle cerebral artery partially maintains the large part of area 17 responsible for central vision, following occlusion of the posterior cerebral artery or a branch of this artery supplying the occipital pole.

The *visual association cortex* is described as corresponding with areas 18 and 19 of Brodmann, which surround the primary visual area on the medial and lateral surfaces of the hemisphere. These areas receive afferent fibers from area 17 and have reciprocal connections with other cortical areas and the pulvinar of the thalamus. The role of the association cortex includes, among other complex aspects of vision, the relating of present to past visual experience, with recognition of what is seen and appreciation of its significance. A lesion involving a substantial proportion of areas 18 and 19 therefore results in visual agnosia, in which there is inability to recognize objects in the opposite field of vision. (Specific cortical areas can be ablated with some precision in experimental animals, such as the monkey and chimpanzee. It will be appreciated that naturally occurring lesions such as an infarction or a tumor include various functional areas and the subjacent white matter.)

Areas 18 and 19 send corticotectal fibers to the superior colliculus of the midbrain. A cortical reflex is thereby established for automatic scanning movements of the eyes in response to visual clues. This is distinct from an area for voluntary scanning eye movements, which is located in the frontal lobe.

HEARING

Most of the *auditory area* (acoustic area) is in the lower wall of the sylvian fissure and therefore concealed from surface view. The surface of the superior temporal gyrus forming the floor of the fissure is marked by transverse temporal gyri. The two most anterior of these, called *Heschl's convolutions,* are landmarks for the auditory area, which corresponds with areas 41 and 42 of Brodmann (Fig. 15–3). Area 41 is granular heterotypical cortex; area 42 is homotypical and may function in part as auditory association cortex.

The medial geniculate nucleus of the thalamus is the principal source of fibers ending in the auditory area, these fibers constituting the auditory radiation in the medullary center. There is a spatial representation in the auditory cortex with respect to pitch or tone of sounds. Impulses for low frequencies impinge on the anterolateral part of the area and impulses for high frequencies on the posteromedial part. Although the medial geniculate nucleus receives auditory information mainly from the organ of Corti of the opposite side, there is a substantial input from the ear of the same side. A unilateral lesion in the auditory area causes diminution in the acuity of hearing in both ears, the greater loss being in the opposite ear. However, the impairment is slight because of the bilateral projection to the cortex and the deficit is difficult to detect by simple clinical tests. Destruction of the auditory area of one hemisphere is said to impair one's ability to detect the direction from which a sound originates.

The *auditory association cortex* occupies

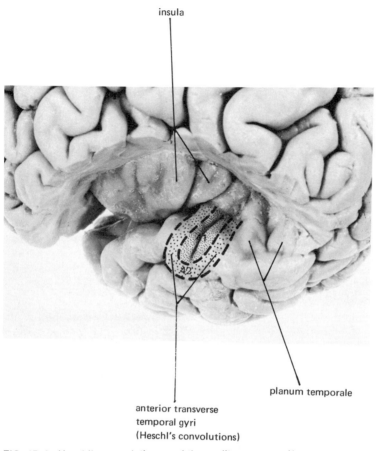

insula

anterior transverse
temporal gyri
(Heschl's convolutions)

planum temporale

FIG. 15–3. Heschl's convolutions and the auditory area. ×⅘

the floor of the sylvian fissure behind the primary auditory area (the region labeled "planum temporale" in Fig. 15–3) and the posterior part of Brodmann's area 22 on the lateral surface of the superior temporal gyrus. The region of cortex thus defined is also known as *Wernicke's area* and is of major importance in language functions.

TASTE

The *taste area* was demonstrated later than other sensory areas, but was eventually identified in the parietal operculum ventral to the somesthetic area. The gustatory area is situated mainly in the upper wall of the sylvian fissure adjacent to cortex receiving general sensory data from the tongue and pharynx, and corresponds with area 43 of the Brodmann map.

The central pathway for taste sensation is not fully known. The gustatory nucleus in the brain stem, receiving afferents from taste buds, is the rostral portion of the nucleus of the solitary tract. The available evidence suggests that fibers originating in the gustatory nucleus cross the midline and ascend near the medial lemniscus and ventral trigeminothalamic tract. These fibers terminate in the medial part of the ventral posterior nucleus of the thalamus, and the pathway is completed by thalamocortical fibers.

VESTIBULAR REPRESENTATION

The best evidence concerning the location of the *vestibular area* comes from recording of evoked potentials in the cortex during stimulation of the vestibular nerve in monkeys. On the basis of this evidence, the vestibular area is situated in the lower part of the postcentral gyrus of the parietal lobe, immediately behind the general sensory representation of the head. This cortical field presumably contributes information for higher motor regulation and conscious spatial orientation. The pathway from vestibular nuclei in the brain stem to the cortex is not known. On the basis of related pathways, the thalamic relay may be in the medial part of the ventral posterior nucleus, from where fibers for sensation from the head project to the inferior part of the postcentral gyrus.

The vestibular area was placed previously in the superior temporal gyrus in front of the auditory area. This interpretation was based on the occasional reporting of feelings of dizziness and vertigo by patients during electrical stimulation of the superior temporal gyrus, and also as auras preceding temporal lobe seizures. The presence of a vestibular area at this site gained credence from the close anatomic relationship of the vestibular and auditory systems in the membranous labyrinth of the inner ear. However, the vestibular system is essentially proprioceptive in function, and the presence of a vestibular area in the parietal lobe is entirely plausible on a physiologic basis. In view of the rather scant and conflicting evidence bearing on the cortical projection of the vestibular sys-tem, further data are needed to resolve the problem.

ASSOCIATION CORTEX

After identification of areas of the association cortex adjacent to the primary sensory areas and having a special cognitive relationship with those areas, additional association cortex remains in the inferior parietal lobule and posterior part of the temporal lobe. Data reaching the primary sensory areas and analyzed in the adjacent association cortex are correlated in the intervening region to yield a comprehensive assessment of the immediate environment.

The total expanse of association cortex in the parietal, occipital, and temporal lobes is responsible (along with association cortex of the frontal lobe) for many of the unique qualities and the potentialities of the human brain. Engrams or memory traces are laid down over the years, probably as a macromolecular phenomenon in cortical neurons having other functions. These form the basis of learning at an intellectual level. The complicated neuronal circuitry provided by the cortex permits the coalescence of memory traces in the form of ideas and conceptual, abstract thinking. The anterior part of the temporal lobe appears to have special properties related to the highest level of brain function and has been called the "psychic cortex." Electrical stimulation of this region in the conscious patient may elicit recall of objects seen, music heard, or other experiences in the recent or distant past. A patient with a temporal lobe tumor may have auditory or visual hallucinations, sometimes reproducing earlier events. The association cortex of the three "sensory" lobes has abundant connections with cortex of the frontal lobe through fasciculi in the medullary center. Complex and flexible behavioral patterns are formulated on the basis of experience; emotional tones are added; and overt expression may follow through the motor system.

FRONTAL CORTEX

The neocortex of the frontal lobe has a special role in motor activities, in the attributes of judgment and foresight, and in determining one's mood or "feeling tone."

MOTOR AREA

The *motor area* (primary motor area) has been identified on the basis of histology and the elicitation of motor responses at a low threshold of electrical stimulation. The area is located in the precentral gyrus, including the anterior wall of the central sulcus, and the anterior part of the paracentral lobule on the medial surface of the hemisphere (Figs. 15–1 and 15–2). The motor cortex is 4.5 mm in thickness, with the histologic appearance of heterotypical agranular cortex, in which the giant pyramidal cells of Betz can be most readily identified.

The main sources of input to area 4 are the premotor cortex (area 6), the somesthetic cortex, and the ventral lateral and ventral anterior thalamic nuclei. While area 4 contributes fibers to extrapyramidal pathways, the efferents that give it a special significance are those included in the pyramidal motor system (corticobulbar and corticospinal tracts). The source of all of the fibers of the pyramidal pathway has yet to be determined, the proportion originating in area 4 being about 40 percent. An additional 20 percent of fibers is said to come from the postcentral gyrus; the remainder probably emanate from frontal cortex anterior to area 4 (areas 6 and 8) and parietal cortex behind the general sensory strip, in particular areas 5 and 7. There is a good correlation between the number of Betz cells in the region of area 4 contributing fibers to the corticospinal or pyramidal tract and the number of large, thickly myelinated fibers about 10 μ in diameter in the pyramidal tract. The number is on the order of 35,000 in each instance, which accounts for about 3 percent of pyramidal tract fibers. The giant pyramidal cells of Betz therefore contribute a small population of rapidly conducting fibers to the pyramidal tract, the remainder being thin fibers with slower conduction rates.

Electrical stimulation of the motor area elicits contraction of muscles predominantly on the opposite side of the body. However, cortical influence on the musculature is not entirely contralateral; there is a significant degree of ipsilateral control, as well as control by the opposite hemisphere, over most of the muscles of the head and the axial musculature. The body is represented in the motor area as inverted— the pattern being similar to that described for the somesthetic cortex. The sequence from below upward is pharynx, larynx, tongue, and face, the region for muscles of the head constituting about a third of the whole of area 4. Continuing dorsally, there is a small region for muscles of the neck, followed by a large area for muscles of the hand, this being consistent with the importance of manual dexterity in man. Next in order are areas for the arm, shoulder, trunk, and hip, continuing into regions for the leg, foot, and anal and vesical sphincters on the medial surface of the hemisphere.

The motor area has a low threshold of excitability, compared with other regions from which contraction of voluntary muscles can be elicited by electrical stimulation. Contractions of contralateral muscles are usually elicited, as noted above, and the muscles responding depend on the particular part of area 4 that is stimulated. The response usually involves muscles that make up a functional group, although there is occasionally contraction of a single muscle. Destructive lesions of area 4 result in voluntary paresis of the affected part of the body. The paralyzed muscles are flaccid; spastic voluntary paralysis characteristically follows lesions spreading beyond area 4 into the premotor area or which interrupt motor projection fibers (including extrapyramidal fibers) in the medullary center or internal capsule. There is considerable recovery in time, the residual paralysis being most evident as impairment of movements in the distal portions of the extremities. Destruction of part of the motor area without involvement of adjacent cortex or the underlying white matter is rarely encountered clinically. Deficits resulting from ablation of area 4 are inferred from experiments on subhuman primates and on isolated instances in which a region of area 4 was ablated in man as a therapeutic procedure, usually in the treatment of epilepsy.

A *secondary* and a *supplementary motor area* have been identified by cortical stimulation in primates, including man, although they are not known to be of importance clinically. The secondary motor area is ventral to the sensorimotor strip in the dorsal wall of the sylvian fissure, overlapping the secondary somesthetic area; the supplementary motor area is on the medial surface of the hemisphere in front of the paracentral gyrus.

PREMOTOR AREA

The *premotor area,* which coincides with Brodmann's area 6, is situated in front of the motor area on the dorsolateral and medial surfaces of the hemisphere. The cytoarchitecture of area 6 is like that of area 4, except that Betz cells are less easy to identify. In addition to association and commissural connections, the premotor area receives fibers from the ventral anterior and ventral lateral thalamic nuclei.

Muscular contractions result from stimulation of area 6, although stronger stimulation is required compared with area 4. Stimulation of the posterior part of area 6 produces responses similar to those obtained from area 4, i.e., contraction of several muscles of a functional group. In the experimental animal, this type of response no longer occurs following ablation of area 4 or after an incision is made along the border between areas 6 and 4. Movements elicited by stimulation of the anterior part of area 6, or any part of the premotor area if it has been isolated from the motor area, are generalized and directional; these include turning the head, twisting the trunk, or gross movements of the limbs. These observations suggest that the functions of the premotor area are mediated in part through the motor area and in part through independent projection fibers. The latter include fibers contributed to the pyramidal tract and also extrapyramidal fibers.

By analogy with the sensory association areas, area 6 may be concerned in part with learned motor activity of a complex and sequential nature. The term *apraxia* refers to the result of a cerebral lesion, characterized by an impairment in the performance of learned movements even though there is no voluntary motor paralysis. One form of apraxia follows a lesion involving the premotor area; another is caused by a lesion in the superior parietal lobule, proprioception being a necessary background for motor proficiency. When the particular activity is that of writing, the disability is known as *agraphia.*

The *frontal eye field* in the lower part of Brodmann's area 8 on the lateral surface of the hemisphere may be included in the premotor cortex. This area controls voluntary scanning movements of the eyes, and electrical stimulation of the frontal eye field produces conjugate deviation of the eyes to the opposite side.

PREFRONTAL CORTEX

The large expanse of cortex from which motor responses are not elicited on stimulation falls under the heading of association cortex. The region enveloping the frontal pole is called *prefrontal cortex;* corresponding to areas 9, 10, 11, and 12 in Brodmann's cytoarchitectural map, the prefrontal area is well developed only in primates and especially so in man. The prefrontal cortex has extensive connections through fasciculi in the medullary center with the parietal, temporal, and occipital lobes, thus gaining access to contemporary sensory experience and the repository of data derived from previous experience. There are also abundant reciprocal connections with the dorsomedial thalamic nucleus, forming a system which determines affective reactions to situations presently encountered on a background of past experience. The prefrontal cortices appear to monitor one's behavior and contribute controls based on such higher mental faculties as judgement and foresight.

LANGUAGE AREAS

The use of language is a peculiarly human accomplishment, requiring special neural mechanisms in association areas of the cerebral cortex. Areas of cortex that have a special role with respect to language have been identified from the study of patients in whom restricted areas were damaged by occlusion of blood vessels. The most reliable information has been derived from long-term studies of patients with deficits in the use of language, and whose brains were subjected to careful postmortem ex-

amination. Two cortical areas with special importance in language functions have been demonstrated; one such area in the temporal and parietal lobes (especially the former) is concerned with sensory aspects of language, while a second area in the inferior frontal gyrus functions in relation to motor aspects of language (speech). The two areas are in communication through the superior longitudinal (arcuate) fasciculus in the medullary center. As discussed further below, the cortical areas for language are located in the left hemisphere, with few exceptions, and the left hemisphere is therefore the dominant hemisphere as a rule with respect to language.

Observations made during cortical stimulation in conscious patients led to the concept of a sensory or "ideational" language area in the temporal and parietal lobes (Fig. 15–4). This area has a considerable extent, occupying the posterior parts of the superior and middle temporal gyri and most of the inferior parietal lobule. In relation to the Brodmann map, the above sensory language area includes portions of

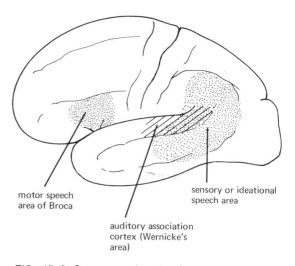

motor speech area of Broca

sensory or ideational speech area

auditory association cortex (Wernicke's area)

FIG. 15–4. Sensory and motor language areas. These areas are in communication through the superior longitudinal (arcuate) fasciculus.

areas 21, 22, and 37 in the temporal lobe, and most of areas 39 and 40 in the inferior parietal lobule (Fig. 15–1). However, clinicopathological studies of patients with speech disorders have shown quite clearly that the lesion responsible for a sensory or receptive type of language defect typically involves the auditory association cortex or Wernicke's area. A child first experiences language by hearing others talk and only later learns to read and write; it is perhaps for this reason that Wernicke's area has a special role in sensory aspects of language. In any event, association cortex in and around Wernicke's area receives data pertinent to language from the sensory areas and synthesizes these data into a comprehensive totality of the sensory aspects of language.

Broca's area or the motor speech area occupies the opercular and triangular portions of the inferior frontal gyrus, corresponding with areas 44 and 45 of Brodmann. In this area, neural processes are organized in such a way as to ensure appropriate and coordinated use of the organs of speech through the motor cortex.

A lesion involving the areas described above results in aphasia, of which there are several types, depending on the location of the lesion. Sensory aphasia (Wernicke's aphasia), in which comprehension of language, naming of objects, and repetition of phrases or sentences are all defective, is caused by a lesion in the sensory language area, more specifically in Wernicke's area. Lesions in Wernicke's area and the arcuate fasciculus may result in jargon aphasia, with fluent but unintelligible jargon. Destruction of the arcuate fasciculus connecting Wernicke's and Broca's areas may be followed by conduction aphasia, in which there is poor repetition but relatively good comprehension and spontaneous speech. Infarcts which isolate the sensory language area from surrounding parietal and tempo-

ral cortex may cause anomic aphasia, characterized by fluent but circumlocutory speech due to word-finding difficulties. Alexia refers to loss of ability to read and occurs with or without other aspects of aphasia. "Pure alexia" may result from a defect in the dominant occipital lobe and the splenium of the corpus callosum. Motor aphasia (Broca's aphasia), caused by a lesion in Broca's area of the frontal lobe, is characterized by hesitant and distorted speech with relatively good comprehension. Global aphasia is a term used for severe loss of all speech function except stereotyped utterances. Complete loss of speech or mutism is not usually an aphasic disturbance.

CEREBRAL DOMINANCE

Memory traces laid down in one hemisphere, e.g., in the cortex of the right hemisphere as a result of some particular activity involving the left hand, are in general transferred to the other hemisphere through the corpus callosum. There are therefore bilateral cortical memory patterns for one's previous experience. This does not apply to language, for which there is no fully adequate explanation. In right-handed persons and a proportion of those who are left-handed, language is a function of the left hemisphere, as pointed out above. The "talking" hemisphere is said to be dominant, relative to the "nontalking" hemisphere. A left-sided cerebral lesion is therefore more serious than one in the right hemisphere because aphasia may be added to other neurologic deficits. The reverse is true for the few individuals whose right hemisphere is the dominant one.

Factors determining cerebral dominance and handedness (these are not always related to one another) are not well known, although heredity is almost certainly involved to some extent. The planum temporale behind the primary auditory area on the upper surface of the superior temporal gyrus (Fig. 15–3) is reported as being larger in the left than the right hemisphere in 65 percent of brains, and larger on the right side in only 11 percent. This is an indication that the dominance with respect to language may be reflected in cerebral asymmetry, since the planum temporale constitutes a large part of Wernicke's area. There is evidence that the nondominant hemisphere is superior in some nonlan-

guage aspects of cortical function, notably in activities requiring three-dimensional or spatial perception. The evidence is derived from the study of patients whose corpus callosum had been sectioned as a therapeutic measure in severe epilepsy. Following commissurotomy, these persons were able to execute drawings and place blocks in a desired position better with the left hand than with the right. The right hemisphere is therefore better equipped to perform such acts, even though it is called the nondominant hemisphere.

SUGGESTIONS FOR ADDITIONAL READING

Brain WR: The physiological basis of consciousness: A critical review. Brain 81:426–455, 1958

Brain WR: Speech Disorders: Aphasia, Apraxia, and Agnosia. London, Butterworth, 1961

Crosby EC, Humphrey T, Lauer EW: Correlative Anatomy of the Nervous System. New York, Macmillan, 1962

De Reuck AVS, O'Connor M: (eds.). Disorders of Language. London, Churchill, 1964

Eccles JC: (ed.). Brain and Conscious Experience, New York, Springer, 1966

Fessard A, Gerard RW, Konorski J, Delafresnaye JF: (eds.). Brain Mechanisms and Learning. Springfield, Ill., Thomas, 1961

Frederickson JM, Figge U, Sheid P, Kornhuber HH: Vestibular nerve projection to the cerebral cortex of the Rhesus monkey. Exp Brain Res 2: 318–327, 1966

Geschwind N: The organization of language and the brain. Science 170:940–944, 1970

Geschwind N: Language and the brain. Sci Am 226/4: 76–83, 1972

Geschwind N, Levitsky W: Human brain: Left-right asymmetries in temporal speech region. Science 161:186–187, 1968

Millikan CH, Darley FL: (eds.). Brain Mechanisms Underlying Speech and Language. New York, Grune & Stratton, 1967

Mountcastle VB: (ed.). Interhemispheric Relations and Cerebral Dominance. Baltimore, Johns Hopkins Press, 1962

Penfield W, Jasper H: Epilepsy and the Functional Anatomy of the Human Brain. Boston, Little, Brown, 1954

Penfield W, Rasmussen T: The Cerebral Cortex of Man: A Clinical Study of Localization of Function. New York, Macmillan, 1950

Russell WR: Brain, Memory, Learning: A Neurologist's View. Oxford, Clarendon Press, 1959

Truex RC, Carpenter MB: Human Neuroanatomy. Baltimore, Williams & Wilkins, 1969

Zangwill OL: Cerebral Dominance and Its Relation to Psychological Function. Springfield, Ill., Thomas, 1960

16

Medullary Center, Internal Capsule, and Lateral Ventricles

Each cerebral hemisphere includes a large volume of white matter constituting the medullary center, in order to accommodate the vast number of fibers running to and from all parts of the cortex. The medullary center is bounded by the cortex, lateral ventricle, and corpus striatum. Nerve fibers that establish connections between the cortex and subcortical gray matter continue from the medullary center into the internal capsule. The paired lateral ventricles are the largest of the four ventricles of the brain and therefore have a prominent role in the dynamics of the cerebrospinal fluid system.

MEDULLARY CENTER

The nerve fibers of the medullary center are of three kinds, depending on the nature of their connections (Fig. 16–1). *Association fibers* are confined to a hemisphere, connecting one cortical area with another.

Many of these fibers accumulate in longitudinally running bundles, which can be displayed by dissection and have been assigned specific names. *Commissural fibers* connect the cortices of the two hemispheres; most of the neocortical commissural fibers constitute the corpus callosum, the remainder being included in the anterior commissure. *Projection fibers* establish connections between the cortex and such subcortical structures as the corpus striatum, thalamus, nuclei of the brain stem, and spinal cord. As noted above, these fibers of the medullary center become concentrated in the internal capsule toward the base of the hemisphere. The projection fibers are afferent (corticipetal) or efferent (corticofugal) with respect to the cortex, the former originating in the thalamus.

ASSOCIATION FASCICULI

Of the three kinds of fibers noted above, association fibers are the most numerous.

237

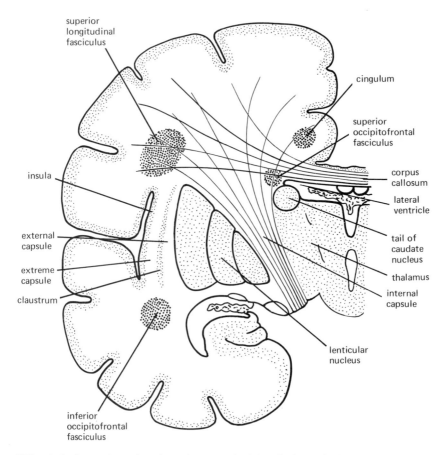

FIG. 16–1. Coronal section through a cerebral hemisphere, indicating the position of association, commissural, and projection fibers.

Operative procedures, vascular accidents, or other lesions involving the fasciculi described below may lead to dysfunction by disconnecting functionally related regions of the cerebral cortex.

The *cingulum* (Figs. 16–2 and 16–3) is an association bundle of the limbic lobe. The cingulum extends from the medial olfactory (septal) area beneath the genu of the corpus callosum, over the corpus callosum in the core of the cingulate gyrus, and through the isthmus into the parahippocampal gyrus.

The *superior longitudinal fasciculus* (Figs. 16–2 and 16–3), also known as the *arcuate fasciculus,* runs in an anteroposterior direction above the insula and many of the fibers bend downward into the temporal lobe. In common with other association bundles, this fasciculus consists of long fibers and many short fibers entering and leaving the bundle along its course. The superior longitudinal fasciculus provides an important communication between cortex of the parietal, temporal, and occipital lobes and cortex of the frontal lobe, including the sensory and motor language areas of Wernicke and Broca. An *inferior longi-*

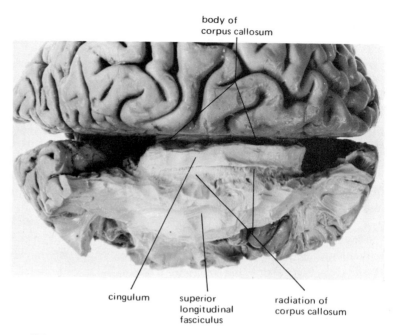

FIG. 16–2. Dissection of the right cerebral hemisphere, dorsal view. ×⅔

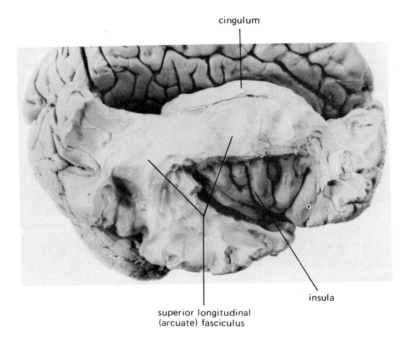

FIG. 16–3. Dissection of the right cerebral hemisphere, lateral view. ×⅔

tudinal fasciculus has been described as running superficially beneath the lateral and basal surfaces of the occipital and temporal lobes. However, this thin sheet of association fibers is difficult to demonstrate by dissection or to distinguish from other fibers at a deeper level, in particular from projection fibers of the geniculocalcarine tract.

The *inferior occipitofrontal fasciculus* and the *uncinate fasciculus* are components of a single association system (Figs. 16–4 and 16–5). The fibers are compressed into a well defined bundle between the stem of the lateral fissure below and the insula and lenticular nucleus above. The longer part of the fiber system, extending the length of the hemisphere, is the inferior occipitofrontal fasciculus. The uncinate fasciculus is that part which hooks around the lateral fissure to connect the frontal lobe, especially cortex on its orbital surface, with the region of the temporal pole.

The *superior occipitofrontal fasciculus,* also called the *subcallosal bundle,* is located deep in the hemisphere and is therefore not accessible to dissection from a lateral approach. The fasciculus is compact in the midregion of the hemisphere, where it is bounded by the corpus callosum, internal capsule, tail of the caudate nucleus, and lateral ventricle (Fig. 16–1). The fibers spread out to frontal lobe cortex and to cortex in the posterior part of the hemisphere. The fasciculus includes some projection fibers proceeding from the cortex to the caudate nucleus.

Large numbers of *arcuate fibers* connect adjacent gyri. These fibers are oriented at right angles to the gyri, bending sharply under the intervening sulci. Spread of activity along a gyrus is provided by other

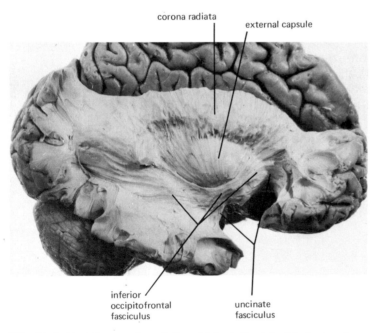

corona radiata

external capsule

inferior occipitofrontal fasciculus

uncinate fasciculus

FIG. 16–4. Medullary center of the right cerebral hemisphere, after removal of the superior longitudinal fasciculus, insula, and underlying structures down to the external capsule. ×⅔

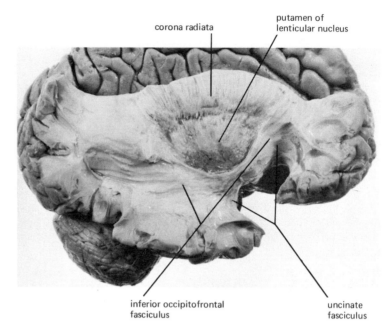

corona radiata

putamen of
lenticular nucleus

inferior occipitofrontal
fasciculus

uncinate
fasciculus

FIG. 16–5. Dissection illustrated in Figure 16–4 continued by removal of the external capsule to expose the putamen of the lenticular nucleus. ×⅔

subcortical association fibers and by the wealth of Golgi type II cells which function as intracortical association neurons.

COMMISSURES

Corpus Callosum

Most of the neocortical commissural fibers constitute the corpus callosum; the remainder are included in the anterior commissure along with fibers of other than neocortical origin. The number of fibers in the corpus callosum is on the order of 300 million; however, the commissure varies considerably in size among normal individuals.

The *body* of the corpus callosum is the compact portion of the commissure in and near the midline (Fig. 16–2). On entering the medullary center, the fibers constitute the *radiation* of the corpus callosum, which intersects association bundles and projection fibers to reach most areas of the neocortex. The interhemispheric connections are predominantly between comparable cytoarchitectural and functional areas, but there are also connections between dissimilar areas.

The body of the corpus callosum is considerably shorter than the hemispheres, accounting for enlargements of the body of the commissure at either end. These form the *splenium* behind and the *genu* in front (Fig. 13–2). The splenium and the radiations connecting the occipital lobes constitute the *forceps major* (Fig. 16–6), and the genu and radiations connecting the frontal lobes form the *forceps minor.* The genu tapers into the *rostrum* of the corpus callosum, which is continuous with the lamina terminalis. Some fibers of the radiation

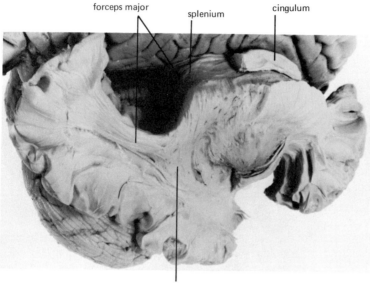

forceps major   splenium   cingulum

tapetum

FIG. 16–6. Dissection of portions of the corpus callosum. ×⅔

form a thin sheet, called the *tapetum,* over the inferior horn of the lateral ventricle (Fig. 16–6). These fibers contribute to communication between the temporal lobes, especially between cortices on the basal surfaces of these lobes.

Certain relations of the corpus callosum are of interest, even though they are anatomic rather than functional relations, resulting in part from invasion of older parts of the brain by the neocortical commissure. The dorsal surface of the body of the corpus callosum is clothed by the *indusium griseum,* a microscopically thin layer of gray matter in which are embedded two delicate strands of fibers on either side called the *medial* and *lateral longitudinal striae.* The indusium griseum is an insignificant remnant of rhinencephalic cortex; in effect, it is a vestigial gyrus whose white matter is represented by the longitudinal striae.

The corpus callosum roofs over the lateral ventricles. The fornices, originating in the hippocampi of the temporal lobes, con-verge and make contact with the undersurface of the corpus callosum in the midline. Continuing forward, the fornices turn ventrally in front of the foramina of Monro and immediately behind the anterior commissure (Fig. 11–2). The resulting interval between the fornices and the corpus callosum is bridged by the *septum pellucidum,* a thin sheet of tissue containing scattered nerve cells and covered on either side by ependyma. The septum pellucidum separates the anterior horns of the lateral ventricles; the septum is essentially a double membrane and may contain a slit-like cavity which does not communicate with the ventricles.

Anterior Commissure

The anterior commissure is a small bundle of fibers which crosses the midline in the lamina terminalis, traverses the anterior part of the corpus striatum, and provides for additional communication between the temporal lobes (Fig. 16–7). The anterior

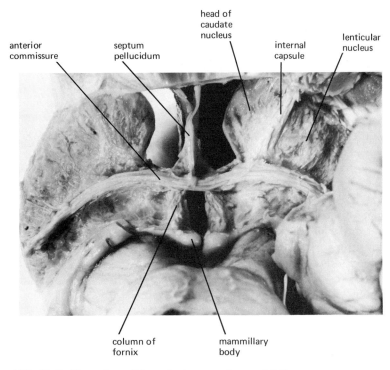

anterior commissure

septum pellucidum

head of caudate nucleus

internal capsule

lenticular nucleus

column of fornix

mammillary body

FIG. 16–7. Dissection of the anterior commissure. ×1⅔

commissure includes fibers passing between the middle and inferior temporal gyri of the two sides; this is a neocortical component similar to the corpus callosum. Other fibers run between olfactory cortex of the temporal lobes (the lateral olfactory areas), for which the uncus is a landmark. There are also commissural fibers between the olfactory bulbs, but these are a minor component of the anterior commissure in man.

Role of Cerebral Commissures

The interhemispheric connections provided by the corpus callosum and the anterior commissure contribute to the bilaterality of memory traces. The role of the neocortical commissures in interhemispheric transfer has been studied in recent years by assessing the effect of section of the corpus callosum and anterior commissure in the monkey and chimpanzee (split-brain preparation). In normal, unoperated animals, a training exercise learned with one hand is performed efficiently by the other hand because of interhemispheric transfer of the neural basis of learning. This is not so in the case of the split-brain monkey or chimpanzee. On the contrary, when a previously unfamiliar task is learned by use of the left hand, for example, that task can not be performed by the right hand unless training in the exercise is repeated with the right hand.

Similar observations, with an extension in the area of language, are available for man. There is occasionally agenesis of the corpus callosum; the developmental defect can be diagnosed by pneumoencephalography, i.e., by X-ray studies of the brain after instillation of air into the subarachnoid space and ventricular cavities. The condition is not necessarily associated with mental defect or other obvious neurologic impairment. When neurologic deficits are present, as is frequently the case, study of the patients is seldom informative with respect to the function of the corpus callosum because agenesis of the commissure is frequently accompanied by other developmental anomalies of the brain.

However, patients are available who are more informative in this respect. These are persons who suffered from severe epilepsy and in whom the corpus callosum was sectioned in order to confine the epileptic discharge to one hemisphere. There are no significant changes in intellect, behavior, or emotional responses that can be attributed to commissurotomy. Bimanual skills acquired before operation are not affected. However, an expertise learned postoperatively with one hand is not transferable to the other hand, as is to be expected from the experiments on other primates.

A particularly significant result of commissurotomy in man lies in the area of language. Let us say that the left hemisphere is dominant, as is usually the case. After section of the corpus callosum the patient is unable to describe an object held in the left hand (with the eyes closed) or seen in the left visual field, although the nature of the object is apparently understood. There is no such difficulty when the sensory data reach the left or dominant hemisphere. After commissurotomy the right hemisphere is rendered mute and agraphic because it has no access to memory for language in the left hemisphere. However, there is evidence that the subordinate hemisphere with respect to language is superior in certain activities, such as copying drawings that include perspective or arranging blocks in a predeter-

mined manner. The nondominant hemisphere therefore appears to be the more proficient side of the brain in functions requiring special competence in three-dimensional perspective.

INTERNAL CAPSULE AND PROJECTION FIBERS

The configuration of the projection system of fibers has some resemblance to that of the commissural system. In the latter, the fibers are concentrated in the body of the corpus callosum and radiate in the medullary center. Similarly, projection fibers are concentrated in the *internal capsule* and fan out as the *corona radiata* in the medullary center (Fig. 16–5).

Because of adaptation to the contours of adjacent gray masses, the internal capsule has an *anterior limb,* a *genu,* and a *posterior limb* (Fig. 16–8). The anterior limb is bounded by the lenticular nucleus and the head of the caudate, while the genu is opposite the apex of the lenticular nucleus. The posterior limb has three portions; this is based on the relation of the fibers to the lenticular nucleus, which does not extend as far posteriorly as does the thalamus. The *lenticulothalamic* portion is between the lenticular nucleus and the thalamus; the *retrolenticular* portion consists of fibers occupying the region behind the lenticular nucleus, and the *sublenticular* portion includes those fibers that pass beneath the posterior part of the lenticular nucleus.

THALAMIC RADIATIONS

Many of the projection fibers establish reciprocal connections between the thalamus and the cerebral cortex. The *anterior thalamic radiation,* which is included in the anterior limb of the internal capsule, consists mainly of fibers connecting the dorso-

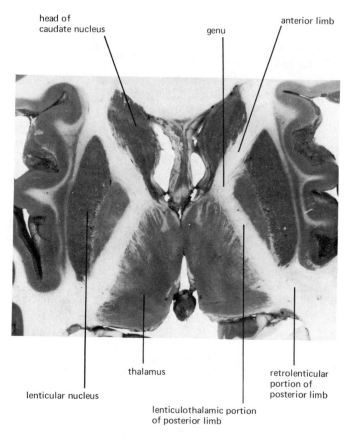

FIG. 16–8. Horizontal section of the cerebrum, stained by a method which differentiates gray matter and white matter, illustrating the regions of the internal capsule. ×1

medial thalamic nucleus with the prefrontal cortex. The *middle thalamic radiation* is included in the lenticulothalamic portion of the posterior limb. This radiation includes the projection from the ventral posterior thalamic nucleus to the somesthetic area of the parietal lobe; these fibers run in the posterior part of the lenticulothalamic region, where they are partly intermingled with pyramidal motor fibers (see below). Other fibers establish reciprocal connections between the dorsal tier of nuclei of the lateral thalamus and association cortex of the parietal lobe. Fibers from the ventral anterior and ventral lateral nuclei of the thalamus reach the motor and premotor areas of the frontal lobe by traversing the genu and adjacent region of the posterior limb of the internal capsule.

The *posterior thalamic radiation* establishes connections between the thalamus and cortex of the occipital lobe. The geniculocalcarine tract ending in the visual cortex of the occipital lobe is a particularly important component of this radiation. Originating in the lateral geniculate nucleus, the geniculocalcarine tract first traverses the retrolenticular and sublenticular regions of the internal capsule. The constituent fibers then spread out into a broad band bordering the lateral ventricle and turn backward into the occipital lobe. Some of the fibers run forward for a considerable distance into the temporal lobe above the inferior horn of the lateral ventricle before turning back into the occipital lobe; these fibers constitute Meyer's loop. The posterior thalamic radiation includes abundant reciprocal connections between the pulvinar and association cortex of the occipital lobe. The *inferior thalamic radiation* consists of fibers directed horizontally in the sublenticular portion of the posterior limb, connecting thalamic nuclei with temporal lobe cortex. Most of the fibers are included in the auditory radiation, which originates in the medial geniculate nucleus and terminates in the auditory area, for which Heschl's convolutions are a landmark. There are also scanty fibers providing reciprocal connections between the pulvinar and association cortex of the temporal lobe.

MOTOR PROJECTION FIBERS

The remaining projection fibers are corticofugal and make up tracts with motor functions. The *corticobulbar* and *corticospinal tracts,* which together constitute the pyramidal motor system, originate in the motor area, in frontal lobe cortex anterior to the motor area, and in cortex of the parietal lobe. The fibers converge as they traverse the corona radiata and enter the posterior limb of the internal capsule. From the beginning of the present century, it was believed that the corticobulbar tract occupied the genu of the internal capsule and that the corticospinal tract was situated in the posterior limb behind the genu. Evidence accumulated during the past decade, both from electrical stimulation of the internal capsule and the tracing of fiber degeneration following lesions of the capsule, shows clearly that the conventional view is incor-

rect. In the human brain, the pyramidal fibers are in fact situated in the posterior third of the lenticulothalamic portion of the posterior limb. In the region thus defined, corticobulbar fibers are most anterior, followed in sequence by corticospinal fibers related to the upper extremity, trunk, and lower extremity. However, there is considerable overlapping of fibers for the major regions of the body.

Corticopontine fibers originate from widespread areas of cortex, but in greatest numbers from the frontal and parietal lobes. Fibers of the *frontopontine tract* run through the anterior limb of the internal capsule, and probably the genu and adjacent part of the posterior limb as well. The *temporopontine tract* is inappropriately named; the majority of the constituent fibers originate in the parietal lobe and traverse the retrolenticular region of the internal capsule.,

Extrapyramidal motor fibers terminate in various subcortical centers; depending on their destination, they are called *corticostriate, corticorubral, corticonigral, corticoreticular,* and *cortico-olivary fibers.* Since these extrapyramidal fibers have their source in widespread regions of the cerebral cortex, they are distributed through various parts of the corona radiata and internal capsule. This is especially true of corticostriate and corticoreticular fibers, and fibers ending in the putamen and reticular formation are included in the external capsule as well as the internal capsule. Extrapyramidal fibers destined for the red nucleus, substantia nigra, and inferior olivary complex come mainly from the sensorimotor strip and adjoining cortex. Although their passage through the corona radiata and internal capsule has not been traced precisely, many of these fibers are probably closely related to the pyramidal fibers topographically. An infarction in the posterior part of the lenticulothalamic region of the internal capsule, spreading into the retrolenticular region, results in especially serious neurologic deficits. These include the effects of an "upper motor neuron lesion" because of interruption of pyramidal and extrapyramidal pathways, general sensory deficits through involvement of the thalamocortical projection to the somesthetic area, and visual field defects because of interruption of geniculocalcarine fibers. Stated differently, the consequences of such a lesion are voluntary motor paralysis and impairment of general sensation on the opposite side of the body, and blindness in the opposite visual field; the details vary according to the size and precise location of the lesion.

Although the composition of the *external capsule* is incompletely known, this thin layer of white matter between the putamen and the claustrum consists mainly of projection fibers. As noted above, these include corticostriate fibers ending in the putamen and corticoreticular fibers.

LATERAL VENTRICLES

The *lateral ventricles,* one in each cerebral hemisphere, are roughly C-shaped cavities lined by ependymal epithelium and filled with cerebrospinal fluid. Each lateral ventricle is described as consisting of a body in the region of the parietal lobe from which anterior, posterior, and inferior horns extend into the frontal, occipital, and temporal lobes. The principal features of the ventricular walls, now to be described, appear in Figures 16–9 and 16–10. The configuration of the entire ventricular system of the brain is illustrated in Figure 16–11.

The *body* of the lateral ventricle has a flat roof, formed by the corpus callosum. The floor includes part of the dorsal surface of the thalamus, of which the anterior

tubercle is a boundary of the foramen of Monro leading to the third ventricle. The tail of the caudate nucleus forms a ridge along the lateral border of the floor. The stria terminalis, a slender bundle of fibers originating in the amygdala of the temporal lobe, lies in the groove between the tail of the caudate nucleus and the thalamus, along with the vena terminalis. The fornix completes the floor medially, and the choroid plexus is attached to the margins of the choroid fissure separating the fornix and thalamus.

The *anterior horn* extends forward from a frontal plane through the foramen of Monro. The corpus callosum continues as the roof, and the genu of the corpus callosum limits the anterior horn in front. The septum pellucidum stretches between the fornix and the corpus callosum in the midline, separating the anterior horns of the two ventricles. The *posterior horn,* which is variable in length, is surrounded by the medullary center. There are two elevations on the medial wall of the posterior horn. The more dorsal prominence, for which the forceps major is responsible, is referred to as the *bulb of the posterior horn;* the lower prominence, formed by the calcarine sulcus, is called the *calcar avis.*

The *inferior horn* extends to within 3–4 cm of the temporal pole. There is a triangular area, called the *collateral trigone,* in the floor of the ventricle where the posterior and inferior horns diverge from the body of the ventricle. The collateral sulcus on the external surface of the hemisphere is at the site of the trigone and may produce a *collateral eminence.* The tail of the caudate nucleus, now considerably attenuated, extends forward in the roof of the inferior horn as far as the amygdaloid nucleus. This nucleus is situated above the anterior end of the inferior horn, which places it beneath the uncus on the external surface. The stria terminalis and vena terminalis run along

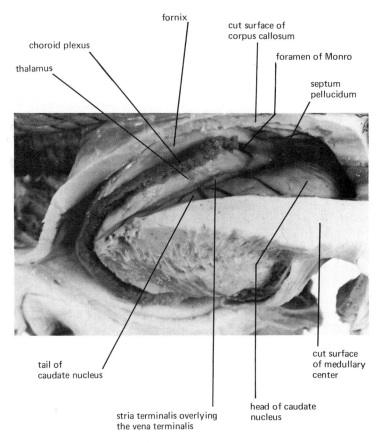

fornix

choroid plexus

cut surface of
corpus callosum

thalamus

foramen of Monro

septum
pellucidum

tail of
caudate nucleus

cut surface
of medullary
center

stria terminalis overlying
the vena terminalis

head of caudate
nucleus

FIG. 16–9. Dissection of right cerebral hemisphere, with roof of the lateral ventricle removed to show boundaries of the body and anterior horn of the ventricle. ×1¼

FIG. 16–10. Dissection of the right cerebral hemisphere to expose the inferior horn of the lateral ventricle. ×1¼

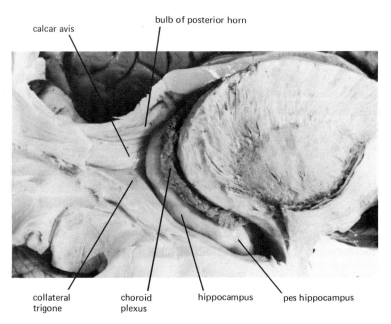

calcar avis

bulb of posterior horn

collateral
trigone

choroid
plexus

hippocampus

pes hippocampus

248

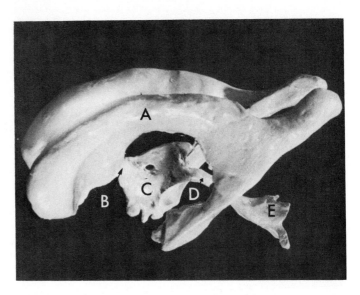

FIG. 16–11. Cast of the ventricular system of the brain. *A*, lateral ventricle, consisting of a body and anterior, inferior, and posterior horns; *B*, foramen of Monro; *C*, third ventricle; *D*, cerebral aqueduct (of Sylvius); *E*, fourth ventricle. (Prepared by Dr. D. G. Montemurro) ×⅘

the medial side of the tail of the caudate nucleus. The floor of the inferior horn includes a particularly important structure, the *hippocampus* (Fig. 16–10). The hippocampus may be visualized as an extension of the parahippocampal gyrus on the external surface, which has been "rolled into" the floor of the inferior horn. The expanded, anterior end of the hippocampus is known as the *pes hippocampus* (resembling an animal's paw). Efferent fibers from the hippocampus form a ridge or *fimbria* along its medial border. The fimbria continues as the *fornix* after the hippocampus terminates beneath the splenium of the corpus callosum. The choroid plexus of the body of the ventricle continues into the inferior horn, where it is attached to the margins of the choroid fissure above the fimbria.

The technique of pneumoencephalography permits visualization of the ventricular system of the brain and the subarachnoid cisterns in X-ray films (Figs. 16–12 and 16–13). The technique involves instillation of 20–30 ml of air into the lumbar subarachnoid space in stages; some of the air gains access to the ventricles through the apertures of the fourth ventricle. If an obstruction exists, or if there is reason to avoid a lumbar puncture, the air can be instilled directly into a lateral ventricle by means of a needle inserted through a burr hole in the skull (ventriculography). These procedures are used among other indications in the investigation of ventricular dilation (hydrocephalus) and the possible presence of a space-occupying lesion, which might produce changes in the contour or position of a part of the ventricular system. The formation, circulation, and absorption of the cerebrospinal fluid are discussed in Chapter 26.

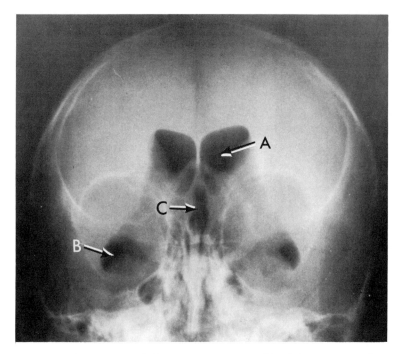

FIG. 16–12. Pneumoencephalogram of a 9-month-old child, anteroposterior view. *A*, body of lateral ventricle; *B*, inferior horn of lateral ventricle; *C*, third ventricle. (Courtesy of Dr. J. M. Allcock)

FIG. 16–13. Pneumoencephalogram of a 9-month-old child, lateral view. The head was in the brow-up position, hence the posterior horn of the lateral ventricle contains cerebrospinal fluid. *A*, anterior horn of lateral ventricle; *B*, body of lateral ventricle; *C*, inferior horn of lateral ventricle; *D*, foramen of Monro; *E*, third ventricle; *F*, cerebral aqueduct; *G*, fourth ventricle; *H*, cisterna magna. (Courtesy of Dr. J. M. Allcock)

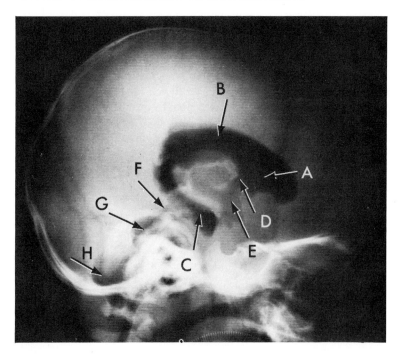

SUGGESTIONS FOR ADDITIONAL READING

Bertrand G: Stimulation during stereotactic operations for dyskinesias. J Neurosurg 24:419–423, 1966

Bertrand G, Blundell J, Musella R: Electrical exploration of the internal capsule and neighbouring structures during stereotaxic procedures. J Neurosurg 22:333–343, 1965

Ettlinger EG, De Reuck AVS, Porter R: (eds.). Functions of the Corpus Callosum. London, Churchill, 1965

Gazzaniga MS: The split brain in man. Sci Am 217/2:24–29, 1967

Gazzaniga MS: The Bisected Brain. New York, Appleton, 1970

Gazzaniga MS, Sperry RW: Language after section of the cerebral commissures. Brain 90:131–148, 1967

Smith MC: Stereotactic Operations for Parkinson's Disease: Anatomical Observations. In Williams D (ed.). Modern Trends in Neurology, pp. 21–52. London, Butterworth, 1967

Sperry RW: The great cerebral commissure. Sci Am 210/1:42–52, 1964

17

Olfactory System

The olfactory system consists of the olfactory mucosa, bulbs, and tracts, together with the cerebral cortex having olfactory functions and its projections to other centers. These structures dominate the cerebral hemispheres of lower vertebrates, in which they constitute the rhinencephalon or nosebrain. Two significant changes greatly altered the rhinencephalon during mammalian phylogeny. First, the olfactory parts of the brain regressed as non-olfactory neocortex, consisting of six layers rather than three, expanded in size and functional importance. Second, a portion of the rhinencephalic cortex remained well represented and acquired other than olfactory functions, becoming incorporated in the limbic system of the brain. These changes culminated in the situation found in the human brain. In man the olfactory system consists of the olfactory mucosa, small olfactory bulbs and tracts, and a strip of paleocortex extending from the uncus of the temporal lobe, across the anterior per-

forated substance, to the medial surface of the frontal lobe beneath the genu of the corpus callosum. The remaining rhinencephalic cortex of comparative neurology is included in the hippocampus and dentate gyrus of the temporal lobe; these are only indirectly related to the olfactory system, being included instead in the limbic system.

Lower vertebrates and many mammals rely heavily on the sense of smell for information about the environment. They are said to be "macrosmatic"; in the mammalian class, the dog is a familiar example. Man is a "microsmatic" animal, smell being much less important than other senses, especially sight and hearing. It is true that even in man olfaction is a complex sense which conjures up memories and emotions. Smell also contributes significantly to alimentary pleasures. Persons who have lost their sense of smell complain of failure of "taste," stating that everything is bland and tastes alike, and they may be unaware of their loss of ability to smell. Most of our enjoyment of "taste" is in fact an appreciation of aromas through the olfactory system. Nevertheless, loss of smell is not a serious disability. There is a technical word, anosmia, for loss of ability to appreciate odors, but there is no word in everyday use comparable to blindness and deafness.

The olfactory system has definitely fewer clinical applications than the other sensory systems; it is therefore discussed here only briefly, with omission of many details. Fiber connections and histologic details of importance in earlier stages of phylogeny are retained in the human brain; however, some of these are vestigial and not essential to a general understanding of the brain in man. The olfactory system is discussed in the context of the cerebral hemispheres rather than with other neurologic systems because it is an integral part if the telencephalon.

OLFACTORY MUCOSA AND OLFACTORY NERVES

The olfactory mucosa (Fig. 17–1) covers an area of 2.5 cm² in the roof of each nasal cavity, extending for a short distance on the lateral wall of the cavity and the nasal septum. The sensory olfactory cells are supported by pseudostratified columnar

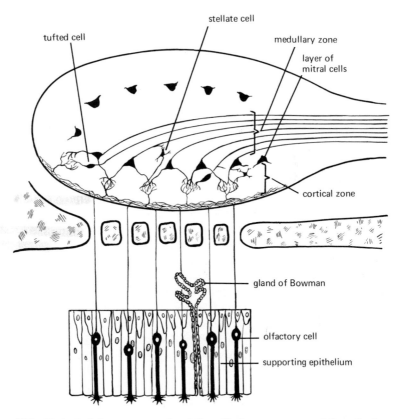

FIG. 17–1. Cellular components of the olfactory mucosa and the olfactory bulb.

epithelium, similar to that lining the respiratory passages. Glands of Bowman beneath the epithelium bathe the mucosa with a layer of serous fluid, in which odoriferous substances are dissolved. The functional cells with respect to smell, or *olfactory cells,* are bipolar neurons which are modified to serve as sensory receptors as well as conducting neurons. The major modification consists of specialization of the dendrite; this process extends to the surface of the epithelium, where it ends as an exposed bulbous enlargement bearing cilia that are exceptional in being up to 100 μ in length.

A fine unmyelinated axon with an exceptionally slow conduction velocity arises from the body of the olfactory cell. Axons from many cells converge to form the *olfactory nerves,* which pass through the foramina of the cribriform plate of the ethmoid bone and enter the olfactory bulb. The axons form a fibrous stratum beneath the surface of the olfactory bulb, then continue more deeply to terminate in specialized synaptic configurations, the *glomeruli.* The olfactory cell is a primitive type of receptor phylogenetically, being similar to the neuroepithelial cells of invertebrates. This is the only instance of an arrangement in man whereby the effective stimulus has direct access, without the intervention of non-nervous tissue, to a neuron which is specialized to serve as a receptor cell. In the semidiagrammatic representation of the olfactory mucosa and bulb (Fig. 17–1), the few olfactory cells represent some 25 million such cells in each half of the olfactory mucosa. Similarly, the axons of olfactory cells represent a corresponding number of fibers incorporated in about 20 olfactory nerve bundles on either side.

The olfactory system is exquisitively sensitive to minute traces of excitants in the air. Direct stimulation of the receptors, convergence of many sensory cells on neurons of the olfactory bulb, and facilitation by neuronal circuits in the bulb are among the factors responsible for the low threshold. Smell is a chemical sense, as is taste. In order for a substance to be detected, it must have a vapor pressure. An odoriferous substance must also be soluble in both water and lipids, in order to be taken up by the serous fluid covering the olfactory mucosa and the lipoprotein plasma membrane of the olfactory cilia. The details of excitation of olfactory cells must be very complex in view of the range of odors and aromas that are appreciated. Sensitivity to different substances appears to differ from one part of the mucosa to another and the problem of discrimination between organic odoriferous compounds must eventually be resolved at a molecular level. The olfactory system adapts rather quickly to a continuous stimulus, so that the odor becomes unnoticed. Older persons tend to have a reduced acuity of smell, caused in part by degeneration of olfactory sensory cells throughout life.

OLFACTORY BULB, TRACT, AND STRIAE

The *olfactory tract* extends forward from its point of attachment to the brain in front of the anterior perforated substance (Fig. 17–2). The *olfactory bulb* appears as a slight expansion of the tract, situated above the cribriform plate of the ethmoid bone.

The olfactory bulb has a characteristic cytoarchitecture in animals that rely heavily on the sense of smell. There are three basic layers or zones, consisting of a *cortical zone,* a *layer of mitral cells,* and a *medullary zone* (Fig. 17–1). It is sometimes difficult to demonstrate the typical mammalian histology in the olfactory bulb of adult man, although the layers are obvious in fetal stages of development.

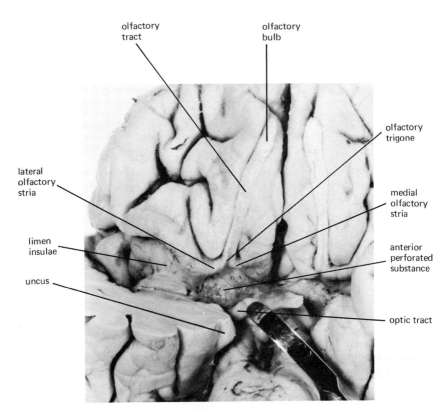

olfactory
tract

olfactory
bulb

olfactory
trigone

lateral
olfactory
stria

medial
olfactory
stria

limen
insulae

anterior
perforated
substance

uncus

optic tract

FIG. 17–2. Portions of the olfactory system. ×1

The most prominent cellular component consists of the *mitral cells* (shaped like a bishop's miter). The dendrites of these cells terminate in the complex synaptic configurations (glomeruli) of the cortical zone. (The glomeruli are of historical interest because they were among the first synapses to be studied, by Ramón y Cajal, after the introduction of silver staining methods.) There is tremendous convergence of olfactory receptors on mitral cells; several thousand olfactory cell axons enter a single glomerulus, and a mitral cell contributes dendrites to several glomeruli. There is some evidence that different glomeruli, or perhaps groups of glomeruli, function in relation to different odors. Axons arising from mitral cells enter the medullary zone,

give off collateral branches to Golgi type II neurons, and continue to olfactory areas of the brain through the olfactory tract.

There are numerous *stellate cells* (Golgi type II neurons) throughout the olfactory bulb. They are intercalated between collateral branches of mitral cell axons and dendrites of mitral cells, the latter synapse being in a glomerulus. Intrabulbar circuits are thereby established, which have a facilitating and regulatory influence on neuronal activity within the olfactory bulb. The olfactory tract contains a modest number of fibers traveling to the bulb, where they end on stellate cells; these fibers originate in the opposite bulb or in olfactory cortex. There are neurons known as *tufted cells* in the cortical zone; they are similar to mitral cells, in that dendrites participate in the glomeruli and axons pass centrally in the olfactory tract. A small group of nerve cells, making up the *anterior olfactory nucleus,* is situated at the transition between the olfactory bulb and tract. Collateral branches of axons of mitral and tufted cells terminate in this nucleus; fibers originating in the anterior olfactory nucleus reach the opposite olfactory bulb through the anterior commissure.

In lower animals, the well developed olfactory tract expands caudally into a prominent *olfactory trigone,* from which large *lateral* and *medial striae* (gyri) continue to the cortex of the olfactory system. The tract, trigone, and striae of such animals are covered with a layer of paleocortex. Although the basic pattern persists in man, the gray layer is vestigial and the fibers are greatly reduced in number. The olfactory trigone and striae are therefore poorly represented in the human brain and may not be obvious on casual inspection (Fig. 17–2). In any event, impulses from the olfactory bulb are conveyed to cortical olfactory areas for awareness of odors and aromas. These areas also establish connections with other parts of the brain for emotional and autonomic responses to olfactory stimuli. The medial olfactory stria includes the fibers which originate in the anterior olfactory nucleus of one side, cross the midline in the anterior commissure, and terminate in the contralateral olfactory bulb.

OLFACTORY CORTICAL AREAS

The anatomy of the olfactory areas and the projections from these areas to other parts of the brain are important topics in the discipline of comparative neurology. The details are many and complex, in view of the dominance of smell in the lives of lower animals. These topics are barely touched on here, because of the regression of the olfactory system in primate evolution and the infrequency with which disorders of this system are encountered in clinical neurology.

It was noted at the beginning of the chapter that the olfactory paleocortex consists of a strip extending from the uncus of the temporal lobe, across the anterior perforated substance, to the medial surface of the frontal lobe. The strip can not be considered as a unit, however, because of functional variations in different regions. Three components have therefore to be considered; these are the lateral, intermediate, and medial areas.

LATERAL OLFACTORY AREA

The *lateral olfactory area* receives afferents from the olfactory bulb through the lateral stria. The area includes the uncus in the temporal lobe and the region of the limen insulae (Fig. 17–2). Part of the amygdaloid nucleus (amygdala) is also included in the lateral area; this nucleus is situated above the tip of the inferior horn of the lateral ventricle beneath the lenticular nucleus (Fig. 18–3). The amygdala is a nuclear complex, consisting of a dorsomedial portion continuous with the cortex of the uncus and a larger ventrolateral portion. The dorsomedial part receives olfactory fibers and is included in the lateral olfactory area, while the ventromedial part is a component of the limbic system. The lateral olfactory area is the principal region for awareness of olfactory stimuli and is therefore called the *primary olfactory area.* The three-layered cortex of the uncus merges into six-layered cortex of the parahippocampal gyrus. This anterior part of the parahippocampal gyrus is called the *entorhinal area* and functions as olfactory association cortex. Through association fibers, there are connections between the entorhinal area and other areas of temporal lobe cortex. The special functions of the olfactory cortex are thereby integrated with those of the neocortex generally, including other aspects of sensation. The uncus, limen insulae, and entorhinal cortex are known as the *pyriform area* (or lobe) because they have a pear-shaped outline in animals with a well developed olfactory system.

INTERMEDIATE OLFACTORY AREA

The anterior perforated substance, situated between the olfactory trigone and the optic tract (Fig. 17–2), derives its name from the penetration of many small blood vessels into the brain in this region. The thin paleocortex at this site receives fibers from the olfactory trigone and is designated the *intermediate olfactory area*. A zone of gray matter lying between the superficial cortex and the base of the lenticular nucleus is known as the *innominate substance*. The *diagonal band of Broca* consists of a band of fibers beneath the cortex, immediately in front of the optic tract. This fasciculus includes fibers connecting the different regions of olfactory cortex.

MEDIAL OLFACTORY (Septal) AREA

The *medial olfactory area* is on the medial aspect of the frontal lobe, beneath the genu and rostrum of the corpus callosum and in front of the lamina terminalis. Groups of cells, called *septal nuclei*, lie beneath the cortex and extend as scattered neurons into the septum pellucidum. The medial olfactory area, known alternatively as the *septal area*, receives scanty olfactory fibers through the medial olfactory stria and is connected with the other olfactory areas by the diagonal band of Broca. It is doubtful, however, that the septal area makes a significant contribution to the sense of smell at a conscious level. Rather, the septal area appears to be more closely integrated with the limbic system, sharing the function of the limbic system with respect to emotions. In support of this interpretation, the septal area has been shown to be a "pleasure zone" of the brain in rats. Animals with electrodes implanted in the area self-stimulate by pressing on a lever until they are exhausted, preferring the effect to pleasurable activities such as eating.

PROJECTIONS FROM OLFACTORY AREAS

The olfactory system is notable for triggering autonomic responses, such as salivation, when there is a pleasing aroma connected with food, or reactions associated with nausea if an odor is particularly unpleasant. In view of the ancient lineage of the olfactory system, it is not surprising that the projections to autonomic centers are numerous and complicated. In brief, the main projections are through the medial forebrain bundle and the stria medullaris thalami. All olfactory areas contribute to these tracts; however, more fibers originate in the septal area than elsewhere, and these are shown in Figure 17–3.

The *medial forebrain bundle*, which is a small fasciculus in man, traverses the lateral area of the hypothalamus, giving off fibers to hypothalamic nuclei. Some fibers continue into the brain stem (olfactotegmental fibers) for distribution to autonomic nuclei, including the salivatory nuclei, the dorsal motor nucleus of the vagus nerve, and autonomic centers in the reticular formation. The *stria medullaris thalami* runs along the dorsomedial border of the thalamus and ends in the habenular nucleus. The pathway continues as the habenulo-interpeduncular fasciculus to the interpeduncular nucleus, then to the dorsal teg-

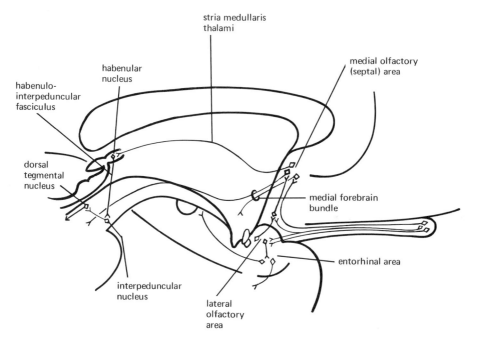

FIG. 17–3. Projections of the olfactory cortex.

mental nucleus, and finally to autonomic nuclei in the brain stem through the dorsal longitudinal fasciculus.

The sense of smell is powerful in arousing emotions, for which spread of activity into the limbic system through the following connections is apparently responsible. The olfactory association cortex (entorhinal area) projects to the hippocampal formation, and the septal area is in communication with cortex of the cingulate gyrus through the association bundle of the gyrus (the cingulum). Although the fornix is mainly an efferent tract of the hippocampus, it includes fibers proceeding from the septal area to the hippocampus.

Neurologic signs caused by dysfunction of the olfactory system are not often encountered, but they may have considerable diagnostic importance when present. A tumor, usually a meningioma, in the floor of the anterior cranial fossa may interfere with the sense of smell through pressure on the olfactory bulb and tract. Since olfactory loss is likely to be unilateral, it is important to test for smell through each nostril separately. A lesion in the temporal lobe may cause olfactory hallucinations, which are usually of disagreeable odors and may be combined with visual hallucinations. The symptom is known as an "uncinate fit," since it may be the aura preceding a seizure if the lesion is epileptogenic in nature.

SUGGESTIONS FOR ADDITIONAL READING

Amoore JE: Molecular Basis of Odor. Springfield, Ill., Thomas, 1970

Amoore JE, Johnston JW Jr, Rubin M: The stereo-

chemical theory of odor. Sci Am 210/2:42–49, 1964

Bargmann W, Schadé JP: (eds.). The rhinencephalon and related structures. Progr Brain Res 3, 1963

Moulton DG, Beidler LM: Structure and function in the peripheral olfactory system. Physiol Rev 47:1–52, 1967

Mozell MM: Olfactory discrimination: Electrophysiological spatiotemporal basis. Science 143: 1336–1337, 1964

Zotterman Y: (ed.). Olfaction and Taste. New York, Macmillan, 1963

18

Limbic System

Certain components of the cerebral hemispheres and the diencephalon are brought together under the heading of the *limbic system*. The concept of a limbic system of the brain with special functions developed from comparative neuroanatomic studies and neurophysiologic investigations. The following regions of gray matter are included within the term limbic system: the limbic lobe, consisting of the cingulate and parahippocampal gyri, the hippocampal formation, a large part of the amygdaloid nucleus, the hypothalamus (especially the mammillary bodies), and the anterior nucleus of the thalamus. The fornix, mamillothalamic tract, and stria terminalis are fiber bundles of the limbic system.

Although the essential anatomy of the limbic system can be described briefly, ultrastructural and functional aspects are exceedingly complex. They constitute an important component of current research in the neurosciences. In general terms, the limbic system is functionally associated with 1) emotional aspects of behavior related to the survival of the individual and

the species, together with visceral responses accompanying these emotions, and 2) the brain mechanisms for memory. Because of the visceral responses to activity within the limbic system, it is also known as the *visceral brain*. Research on this system is far from being of only academic value. On the contrary, there is urgency to understand the limbic system in health and disease, since pathophysiology in this part of the brain may be responsible for certain types of mental illness.

The limbic system includes intrinsic neural circuits involving its components; there is therefore no obligatory "origin" or "starting-point" for neural activity within the system, and the description begins somewhat arbitrarily with the hippocampal formation of the temporal lobe.

HIPPOCAMPAL FORMATION

The *hippocampal formation* consists of the hippocampus, dentate gyrus, and the portion of the parahippocampal gyrus that is in direct continuity with the hippocampus.

The *hippocampus* develops in the fetal brain by a process of continuing expansion of the medial edge of the temporal lobe. It does so in such a way that the gyrus comes to occupy the floor of the inferior horn of the lateral ventricle (Fig. 16–10). In the mature brain, therefore, the parahippocampal gyrus on the external surface is continuous with the hippocampus along the medial edge of the temporal lobe. The hippocampus is C-shaped in coronal section (Fig. 18–1). The outline bears some resemblance to a ram's horn, and the hippocampus is sometimes called Ammon's horn, Ammon being the name of an Egyptian diety with a ram's head. The ventricular surface of the hippocampus consists of a thin layer of white matter called the *alveus*, which consists of fibers originating

in the hippocampal cortex. The fibers course over the hippocampus to its medial border, where they collect as the *fimbria of the hippocampus*. The fimbria continues as the fornix when the hippocampus terminates beneath the splenium of the corpus callosum.

A further extension of the hippocampus in the fetal brain forms the *dentate gyrus* (Fig. 18–1). This gyrus occupies the interval between the fimbria of the hippocampus and the parahippocampal gyrus, as viewed from the medial aspect. Its surface is toothed or beaded, hence the name "dentate gyrus." The *hippocampal sulcus* is between the parahippocampal and dentate gyri. The *choroid fissure* is above the fimbria of the hippocampus.

The cortex of most of the parahippocampal gyrus consists of neocortex. In the

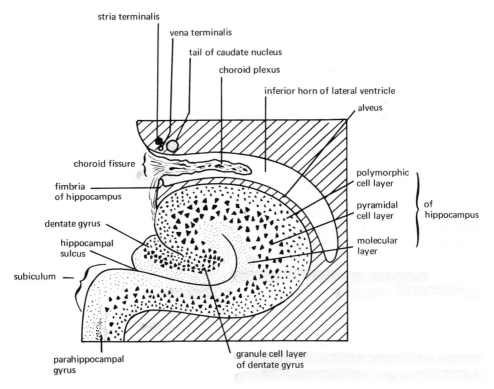

FIG. 18–1. Coronal section through the hippocampal formation.

region known as the *subiculum* (Fig. 18–1), there is a gradual transition between six-layered cortex and the archicortex of the hippocampus, in which there are the following three layers. 1) The *molecular layer,* consisting of delicate nerve fibers and scattered small neurons, is continuous with the outermost layer of neocortex. 2) The prominent *pyramidal cell layer* is composed of large neurons, many of them having a pyramidal outline. Dendrites of cells in this layer extend into the molecular layer, while axons enter the alveus and continue into the fornix. 3) The *polymorphic cell layer* is similar to the innermost layer of the neocortex. This layer includes neurons which contribute fibers to the fornix; other neurons are comparable to the cells of Martinotti of neocortex, because the axons of these cells extend into the molecular layer.

The dentate gyrus likewise has three layers. The cytoarchitecture differs from that of the hippocampus in that the pyramidal cell layer is replaced by a *granule cell layer* of small neurons. Efferent fibers from the gyrus terminate in the hippocampus; very few enter the fornix. The cytoarchitecture and connections of the dentate gyrus suggest that it is largely a reinforcing and regulating part of the hippocampal formation.

AFFERENT CONNECTIONS OF THE HIPPOCAMPAL FORMATION

Although direct connections between the lateral olfactory area and the hippocampal formation are few or lacking, the entorhinal area or olfactory association cortex is a source of afferent fibers. Fibers reaching the hippocampus from the septal area constitute the longitudinal striae embedded in the indusium griseum. In addition, the fornix, although primarily an efferent tract of the hippocampus, includes a few fibers running from the septal area to the hippocampus. While the afferent connections noted above convey olfactory information, among other data, they are presumably concerned with emotional responses to odors and aromas. There is no good evidence that the hippocampal formation contributes to conscious appreciation of smell, this being a function mainly of the lateral olfactory area.

The hippocampal formation receives many fibers from the cortex of the parahippocampal gyrus, and the latter cortex is in communication with widespread areas of the cerebral cortex through association fibers of the medullary center. These fibers include those of the cingulum, or association bundle of the limbic lobe, through which the cortex of the parahippocampal and cingulate gyri are in communication.

EFFERENT CONNECTIONS OF THE HIPPOCAMPAL FORMATION

The connections bringing data to the hippocampal formation from the cerebral cortex generally are paralleled by association fibers through which activity in the hippocampal formation spreads to other regions of the cerebral cortex. In addition, the fornix constitutes a large and discrete efferent pathway of the hippocampus.

The *fornix,* which contains in excess of a million fibers in man, consists of myelinated axons of cells in the pyramidal and polymorphic cell layers of the hippocampus. The fibers first form the *alveus* on the ventricular surface of the hippocampus, as noted above, then accumulate as the *fimbria* along the medial edge of the hippocampus (Fig. 18–1). The fimbria continues as the *crus* of the fornix, which begins at the posterior limit of the hippocampus beneath the splenium of the corpus callosum (Fig. 18–2). The crus curves over the

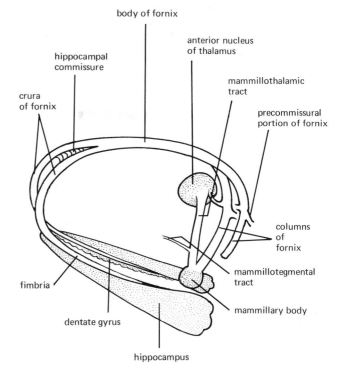

FIG. 18–2. Fornix and related connections of the limbic system.

thalamus, the two crura converging to form the *body* of the fornix, which adheres to the undersurface of the corpus callosum. A small *hippocampal commissure* at the convergence of the crura consists of decussating fibers joining the hippocampi of the two sides. The body of the fornix separates into two *columns*, each of which curves ventrally in front of the foramen of Monro. The column of the fornix continues through the hypothalamus, where it is the landmark for dividing the hypothalamus into medial and lateral areas. Most of the fibers terminate in the mammillary body, with a smaller number ending in the ventromedial hypothalamic nucleus. Fibers leave the column in considerable numbers immediately below the foramen of Monro and turn backward into the anterior nucleus of the

thalamus. Other fibers separate off from the fornix just above the anterior commissure; these constitute the *precommissural portion* of the fornix and are distributed to the septal area and the anterior region of the hypothalamus. The septal area sends fibers to various parts of the hypothalamus by way of the medial forebrain bundle.

There are reciprocal connections between the mammillary body and the anterior thalamic nucleus through the *mammillothalamic tract* (bundle of Vicq d'Azyr), which is readily demonstrable by gross dissection (Fig. 11–14). The anterior thalamic nucleus is in communication with the cortex of the cingulate gyrus by means of fibers running in both directions through the medullary center of the hemisphere. The structures composing the limbic system are therefore closely integrated, with abundant provision for feedback within the system.

AMYGDALOID NUCLEUS

The larger part of the *amygdaloid nucleus* (amygdala) is included with the limbic system. As noted in the preceding chapter, the amygdala is situated between the tip of the inferior horn of the lateral ventricle and the basal surface of the lenticular nucleus (Fig. 18–3). The dorsomedial portion of the amygdala, which blends with the cortex of the uncus, receives fibers from the olfactory bulb and is therefore included in the lateral olfactory area. The larger ventrolateral portion of the amygdaloid nucleus has no direct olfactory afferents. Although there are connections with the dorsomedial portion and the entorhinal area, the ventrolateral part of the amygdala is considered as a component of the limbic system on the

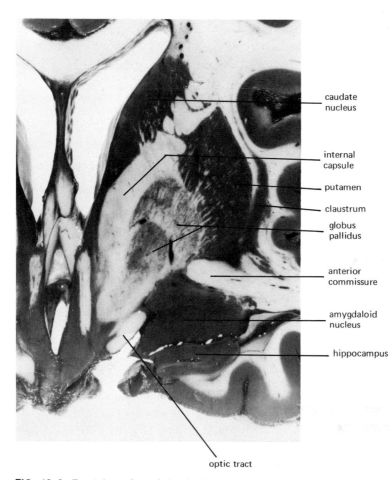

caudate nucleus

internal capsule

putamen

claustrum

globus pallidus

anterior commissure

amygdaloid nucleus

hippocampus

optic tract

FIG. 18–3. Frontal section of the brain through the region that includes the amygdaloid nucleus. Stained by a method which differentiates gray matter and white matter. ×2

basis of stimulation and ablation experiments. In addition to connections with neocortex of the temporal lobe, the amygdala gives rise to a slender efferent bundle called the *stria terminalis*. The stria follows the curvature of the tail of the caudate nucleus, continuing between the caudate nucleus and the thalamus in the floor of the lateral ventricle. The constituent fibers diverge in the region of the foramen of Monro; the majority terminate in the septal area and the anterior portion of the hypothalamus, while the remainder turn caudally to reach the habenular nucleus through the stria medullaris thalami. The projections from the amygdala through the stria terminalis are similar in some respects to those of the hippocampus through the fornix.

SOME FUNCTIONAL CONSIDERATIONS

Ablation or stimulation of portions of the limbic system in monkeys and other experimental animals gives some indication of its function. Bilateral ablation of the temporal lobes, which include the hippocampal formation and the amygdala, is followed by docility and lack of emotional responses, such as expressions of fear or anger, to situations that normally arouse those responses. The animals are not only hypersexed, but the sexual drive may be perverted, being directed toward either sex, a member of another species, or even inanimate objects. Lesions confined to the amygdala produce comparable changes in behavior, although sexual behavior is less affected. The intimate anatomic and functional relation of diencephalic and telencephalic components of the limbic system is demonstrated by the observation that penile erection and ejaculation in the monkey is readily obtained from electrical

stimulation in the preoptic area of the hypothalamus and the anterior thalamic nucleus. Further, this response to stimulation is often followed by after-discharges in the hippocampus.

In man, bilateral removal of the temporal lobes results in the Klüver-Bucy syndrome, which is characterized by a voracious appetite, increased (sometimes perverse) sexual activity, and docility. There is also loss of recognition of people and a memory defect (see below). It has been reported that electrical stimulation of the amygdala in man induces feelings of fear or anger.

Studies of the type indicated above led to the view that the limbic system represents a phylogenetically old part of the brain, and that it is responsible for emotions having a broad biologic importance with respect to preservation of the individual and the species. These include such strong affective reactions as fear and anger and emotions associated with sexual behavior. Changes in visceral function are a natural result of these emotions, and electrical stimulation of the hippocampus, amygdala, or cingulate gyrus has been shown to produce a wide variety of visceral responses in experimental animals. These include changes in respiration, changes in gastrointestinal movements and secretion, piloerection, and pupillary dilation. The visceral responses to activity within the limbic system are mediated mainly through the hypothalamus (Chapter 11).

The assignment of a role in memory to the limbic system, in particular the hippocampus, is an interesting development of recent years. Impairment of memory is most evident following bilateral temporal lobectomy, or when arterial occlusion, having caused an infarction in the hippocampal formation of one side, is followed at a later time by a similar infarction in the other hemisphere. Interruption of the major circuit within the limbic system, such as occurs when the mammillary bodies are involved in a lesion, may also result in a memory defect. Persons with such lesions forget information obtained recently and are unable to commit anything to memory. It is not implied that memory traces are stored in the hippocampus. Although there are only hypotheses at this point, one possibility is that memory is a function of neurons of the cerebral cortex generally, depending on macromolecular changes in these neurons superimposed on their other activities. It is further proposed that there is a tendency for these macromolecular changes to decay with time; there would therefore be no memory beyond a short interval in the absence of a mechanism that encourages retention of memory traces in neuronal macromolecules. It is envisaged

that the hippocampus may provide a bias against "forgetting" through its numerous and diversified connections, direct and indirect, with all parts of the cerebral cortex. When the hippocampi are no longer functional, memories of earlier events are retained, these having already been established. But there is amnesia for events occurring subsequent to the lesion, because the mechanism for retention or consolidation of memory is no longer in operation. As noted in Chapter 11, amnesia may also follow bilateral lesions in the dorsomedial nuclei of the thalamus, as in Korsakoff's syndrome. It may not be a coincidence that the hippocampus and the dorsomedial thalamic nucleus both contribute to affective aspects of brain function and to the brain mechanisms for memory.

SUGGESTIONS FOR ADDITIONAL READING

Douglas RJ: The hippocampus and behavior. Psychol Bull 67:416–442, 1967

Green JD: The hippocampus. Physiol Rev 44: 561–608, 1964

Livingston KE, Escobar A: Anatomical bias of the limbic system concept: A proposed reorientation. Arch Neurol 24:17–21, 1971

MacLean PD: The limbic system with respect to self-preservation and the preservation of the species. J Nerv Ment Dis 127:1–11, 1958

MacLean PD, Ploog DW: Cerebral representation of penile erection. J Neurophysiol 25:29–55, 1962

Penfield W, Milner B: Memory deficit produced by bilateral lesions in the hippocampal zone. Arch Neurol Psychiatry 79:475–497, 1958

Raisman J, Cowan WM, Powell TPS: The extrinsic efferent, commissural and association fibres of the hippocampus. Brain 88:963–996, 1965

Symonds C: Disorders of memory. Brain 89:625–644, 1966

Terzian H, Dalle Ore G: Syndrome of Klüver and Bucy: Reproduced in man by bilateral removal of the temporal lobes. Neurology (Minneap) 5: 373–380, 1955

Victor M: The amnesic syndrome and its anatomical basis. Can Med Assoc J 100:1115–1125, 1969

Young JZ: What can we know about memory? Br Med J 1:647–652, 1970

Review of the
Major Systems

19
General Sensory Systems

Impulses arising in receptors for general sensation are incorporated in reflex arcs involving the spinal cord, brain stem, and cerebellum. These reflexes are of the first importance in the physiology of the nervous system. Interference with reflex pathways by disease may result in clinical signs which are usually manifest as some form of motor dysfunction. However the present chapter deals with the pathways from general sensory receptors to the thalamus and cerebral cortex, where the sensations attain a conscious level. With knowledge of the anatomy of these pathways, an appraisal of sensory deficits gives valuable information concerning the location of a lesion in the central nervous system. Although the components of the general sensory pathways leading to the cerebral cortex were described in earlier chapters, it is worthwhile bringing the material together so that the systems can be reviewed in their entirety.

By way of introduction it may be noted that sensory fibers entering the spinal cord segregate in such a way that there are two main general sensory systems. The phylogenetically older system includes a relay in the dorsal gray horn to the crossed spinothalamic tracts in the lateral and ventral white columns. This sensory system is for pain and temperature (lateral spinothalamic tract) and simple touch and pressure (ventral spinothalamic tract). The spinothalamic system is partly protective in function, especially with respect to pain. Emotional responses are easily aroused at the thalamic level. In the more recent phylogenetic pathway dorsal root fibers ascend in the ipsilateral dorsal white column and end in the nuclei gracilis and cuneatus of the medulla. Fibers from the latter nuclei constitute the crossed medial lemniscus, which terminates in the thalamus. This pathway is for proprioception (position and movement of body parts), fine touch, and vibration. The sensations are discriminative and closely related to mental activity at the cortical level; emotional responses are minimal or lacking.

As a further generalization, the pathways

from receptors to cerebral cortex consist of a series of three neurons: the primary, secondary, and tertiary sensory neurons. The cell bodies of *primary sensory neurons* are in dorsal root ganglia and ganglia of cranial nerves (mainly the trigeminal nerve); dendrites traverse peripheral nerves to receptors, and axons enter the spinal cord or brain stem. The cell bodies of *secondary sensory neurons* are located in the gray matter of the cord (for spinothalamic tracts), in the gracile and cuneate nuclei of the medulla (for the medial lemniscus), and in sensory trigeminal nuclei (for the trigeminothalamic tract). *Tertiary sensory neurons* in the ventral posterior nucleus of the thalamus project to the somesthetic cortical area in the parietal lobe. However, the concept of a simple relay along a series of three neurons does not reflect the true situation because small neurons with short axons may be interposed between the major neurons of the pathways. In addition the secondary sensory neurons of a specific system (the pain and temperature pathway for example) are influenced by nerve impulses from various sources, including the cerebral cortex; therefore message transmission along the pathway is subject to changes or "editing." Further, the ventral posterior nucleus of the thalamus has connections with other thalamic nuclei; the thalamic organization is such that there is awareness of some aspects of general sensation at the thalamic level and emotional overtones are added.

PATHWAY FOR PAIN AND TEMPERATURE (Fig. 19–1)

RECEPTORS

The receptors for pain consist of unencapsulated endings of peripheral nerve fibers; these fibers are the smaller components of group A, with thin myelin sheaths, and unmyelinated group C fibers. Simple, undifferentiated endings are phylogenetically old receptors; although not concerned with pain exclusively, these simple endings appear to be the only type of receptor that responds to painful stimuli. Pain may be felt as two waves, separated by a very short interval. The first is sharp and localized, with conduction along group A fibers. The second wave, which is rather diffuse and still more disagreeable, depends on the slower conduction of group C fibers.

The identity of receptors for temperature is still not resolved. The view that specific encapsulated endings, in particular the end-bulbs of Krause and Ruffini, are sensors of cold and warmth, respectively, is no longer tenable. In the absence of reliable evidence about the nature of temperature receptors unencapsulated endings similar to those functioning for pain, together with some form of end-bulb yet to be specifically identified, are regarded as sensors of temperature differences between body surfaces and the immediate environment. The nerve fibers are of similar caliber to those conducting impulses for pain.

PATHWAY FOR THE BODY

The cell bodies in dorsal root ganglia are small and of intermediate size. Their axons traverse the dorsal roots and enter the *dorsolateral fasciculus* (zone of Lissauer) of the spinal cord, in which ascending and descending branches travel for a length corresponding to one segment or two segments at the most. These fibers, which give off many collateral branches in their short course, terminate in the *substantia gelatinosa* Rolandi of the dorsal gray horn.

The substantia gelatinosa consists of Golgi type II neurons whose axons are confined to the nucleus or run for short distances in the zone of Lissauer, connecting adjacent regions of the substantia gelatinosa. The nucleus does not include "tract cells," i.e., the cell bodies of the main secondary sensory neurons, which are situated instead in the chief nucleus of the dorsal gray horn. Dendrites of tract cells ramify extensively in the substantia gelatinosa, making synaptic contact with the Golgi type II cells of the nucleus and with dorsal root fibers. The transmission of messages from pain and temperature receptors is apparently subject to alteration in the substantia gelatinosa. The second order neurons with dendritic ramifications in the nucleus may be inhibited or facilitated by nerve impulses reaching the substantia gelatinosa along collateral branches of fibers for other modalities of general sensation in the dorsal white column. There is inhibition, for example, when one shakes the hand vigorously in an attempt to diminish the pain from a bruised or burned finger. In addition, transmission of pain and temperature data in the substantia gelatinosa appears to be altered by nerve impulses coming from the cerebral cortex. The fibers responsible for this inhibition or facilitation originate in the sensorimotor strip (especially the somesthetic area) and accompany the corticospinal tract. Inhibition of sensory transmission by cortical activity may be exemplified by the diminished awareness of pain at the time of injury in combat and in contact sports.

Axons of tract cells in the chief nucleus of the dorsal horn cross the midline in the ventral gray and white commissures. Continuing across the ventral horn of gray matter, the fibers turn upward in the *lateral spinothalamic tract*, which is situated in the ventral part of the lateral white column and separated from the surface of the cord by the ventral spinocerebellar tract. Proceeding in a cephalad direction, fibers are continually being added to the ventromedial aspect of the lateral spinothalamic tract. At upper cervical levels, therefore, fibers from

sacral segments are dorsolateral, followed by fibers from lumbar and thoracic segments, while those from cervical segments are in a ventromedial position.

The ascending tracts of the spinal cord continue into the lower medulla without appreciable change of position. In the upper part of the medulla the lateral spinothalamic tract occupies a position near the lateral surface and between the inferior olivary nucleus and the nucleus of the spinal tract of the trigeminal nerve. The lateral medullary zone thus outlined is known as Monakow's area. The lateral and ventral spinothalamic tracts and the spinotectal tract are closely associated at this level and throughout the remainder of the brain stem; together, they constitute the *spinal lemniscus*. The spinal lemniscus continues through the ventrolateral region of the dorsal pons and close to the surface of the tegmentum of the midbrain, running along the lateral edge of the medial lemniscus. Spinotectal fibers leave the spinal lemniscus in the midbrain and terminate in the superior colliculus. The spinothalamic tracts and the medial lemniscus, which together convey data for all the general senses from the body, terminate in the *ventral posterior nucleus* of the thalamus. There is a somatotopic representation of the opposite side of the body in the lateral portion of this thalamic nucleus. The somatotopic projection is such that the lower extremity is represented in the dorsolateral region of the nucleus and the upper extremity in a more ventromedial position. The most medial portion of the ventral posterior nucleus, which is often designated separately as the arcuate or semilunar nucleus, receives trigeminothalamic fibers and is therefore the region of representation of the opposite side of the head.

The ventral posterior nucleus has connections with other thalamic nuclei, especially the nuclei of the dorsal tier of the

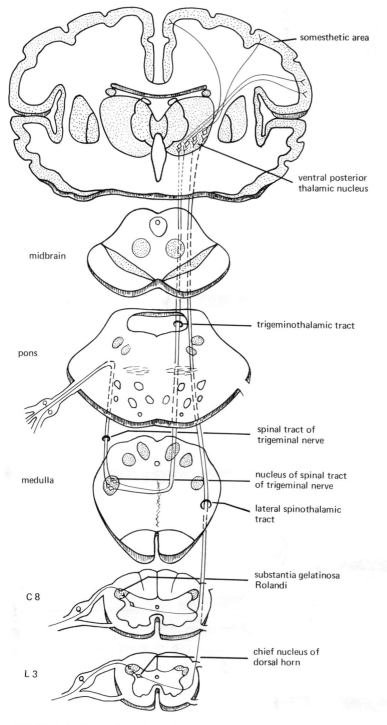

somesthetic area

ventral posterior
thalamic nucleus

midbrain

pons

trigeminothalamic tract

spinal tract of
trigeminal nerve

medulla

nucleus of spinal tract
of trigeminal nerve

lateral spinothalamic
tract

substantia gelatinosa
Rolandi

C 8

chief nucleus of
dorsal horn

L 3

FIG. 19–1. Pathways for pain and temperature.

lateral thalamus, intralaminar nuclei, and the medial nucleus. Pain, heat, and cold attain consciousness at the thalamic level and emotional reactions are elicited. Cortical analysis of sensory data is necessary for recognition of the precise source, the severity, and the quality of painful and thermal stimuli. Tertiary neurons in the ventral posterior nucleus project to the somesthetic area in the postcentral gyrus, the fibers traversing the lenticulothalamic region of the internal capsule and the corona radiata. The contralateral half of the body is represented as inverted in the dorsal two-thirds of the somesthetic area. The sequence is therefore hand, arm, and trunk, followed by representation of the leg, foot, and anogenital region on the medial surface of the hemisphere. The cortical area for the hand is disproportionately large, providing for maximal sensory discrimination. The somatotopic arrangement at various levels of the sensory pathways forms the basis for recognition of the site of stimulation.

PATHWAY FOR THE HEAD

Most of the cell bodies of primary sensory neurons of the trigeminal nerve are in the semilunar (gasserian) ganglion. The peripheral processes have a wide distribution through the ophthalmic, maxillary, and mandibular divisions of the nerve. The central processes enter the pons through the sensory root; those for pain and temperature turn caudally in the *trigeminal spinal tract*. There is a spatial arrangement of fibers in the sensory root and spinal tract corresponding to the divisions of the trigeminal nerve. In the sensory root ophthalmic fibers are dorsal, mandibular fibers ventral, and maxillary fibers in-between. Because of a rotation of fibers as they enter the pons, the mandibular fibers are dorsal and the ophthalmic fibers ventral in the trigeminal spinal tract. The fibers for pain

and temperature terminate in the pars caudalis of the *nucleus of the spinal tract,* the pars caudalis being in the lower medulla and upper three cervical segments of the spinal cord. The portion of the pars caudalis in the cervical cord receives sensory data from areas of distribution of both the trigeminal nerve and the upper cervical spinal nerves. The cellular characteristics of the pars caudalis are like those of the dorsal gray horn of the cord. A layer of small cells, identical with the substantia gelatinosa, lies external to a layer which includes larger neurons similar to those of the chief nucleus of the dorsal horn.

The dorsal part of the trigeminal spinal tract includes a small bundle of pain and temperature fibers from the facial, glossopharyngeal, and vagus nerves. The cell bodies of the primary sensory neurons are in the geniculate ganglion of the facial nerve and the superior ganglia of the glossopharyngeal and vagus nerves. Fibers in the facial and vagus nerves, and the glossopharyngeal nerve inconstantly, supply the external ear, the lining of the auditory canal, and the tympanic membrane. The glossopharyngeal and vagus nerves also supply the mucosa of the back of the tongue, pharynx, esophagus, larynx, eustachian tube, and middle ear.

The second order neurons consist of cells in the pars caudalis of the spinal trigeminal nucleus, whose axons cross over to the opposite side of the medulla and continue forward in the *trigeminothalamic tract.* This tract terminates in the medial part of the ventral posterior nucleus of the thalamus, i.e., the arcuate or semilunar nucleus, at which level painful and strong thermal stimuli are appreciated consciously. A tertiary relay from the arcuate nucleus to the lower third of the somesthetic area of the parietal lobe provides for more precise assessment of peripheral stimulation. (There are actually two trigeminothalamic tracts. The ventral tract, which is the more important one, is a crossed pathway from the whole of the spinal nucleus and the chief sensory nucleus of the trigeminal nerve. A smaller dorsal trigeminothalamic tract contains uncrossed as well as crossed fibers, the latter predominating; this tract originates in the chief sensory nuclei and also conveys data from the mesencephalic trigeminal nucleus. Since the tracts are close together in the brain stem, it is permissible in the present context to consider them as constituting a single pathway from the sensory trigeminal nuclei to the thalamus.)

SOME CLINICAL COMMENTS

The pathways described above are of considerable clinical importance, as the following comments will indicate. Inflammatory reactions in dorsal roots or peripheral nerves or pressure on spinal nerve roots by a herniated intervertebral disk stimulate pain and temperature fibers, causing painful and burning sensations in the area supplied by the affected roots or nerves. Degenerative changes in the region of the central canal of the spinal cord interrupt pain and temperature fibers as they decussate in the ventral gray and white commissures. The best example is syringomyelia, which is characterized by central cavitation of the cord. In the event that the disease process is most marked in the region of the cervical enlargement, which is frequently the case, the area of anesthesia includes the hands, arms, and shoulders (yoke-like anesthesia).

A lesion that includes the ventrolateral region of the spinal cord on one side results in loss of pain and temperature sensibility below the level of the lesion and on the opposite side of the body. If, for example, the lateral spinothalamic tract is interrupted on the right side at the level of the first thoracic segment, the anesthetic area includes the left leg and left side of the trunk. Careful testing of the upper margin of sensory impairment will show that cutaneous areas supplied by the first and second thoracic nerves are spared. Some impulses from these areas reach the opposite spinothalamic tract above its interruption because of the short ascending branches of dorsal root fibers in the dorsolateral fasciculus. Surgical section of the pain pathway (chordotomy) may be required for relief of intractable pain. The section must extend deeply in the ventral quadrant of the cord to be effective because pain and temperature fibers mingle with fibers in fasciculi adjoining the lateral spinothalamic tract as it is conventionally illustrated. Also visceral pain conduction is partly through deeply lying fibers of the white matter, including spinospinalis relays. Chordotomy is most likely to be considered in later stages of malignant disease of a pelvic viscus; interruption of the tract may be unilateral or bilateral depending on circumstances prevailing in the individual patient. Even though the chordotomy operation sections the generally accepted pathway for pain the results are occasionally disappointing. This suggests, among other possible explanations, that there are pathways in addition to those traditionally recognized for conduction of pain and other cutaneous sensations in the cord. The spinocervical tract (see below) is one such possible route.

The spinal lemniscus may be included in an area of infarction in the brain stem. An example is provided by the lateral medullary or Wallenberg's syndrome; the area of infarction usually includes both the spinal lemniscus and the spinal trigeminal tract and its nucleus. The principal sensory deficit is loss of pain and temperature sensibility on the side of the body opposite the lesion and on the ipsilateral side of the face. A lesion in or near the thalamus may result in the thalamic syndrome; the signs and symptoms include exaggerated and exceptionally disagreeable responses to cutaneous stimulation.

The standard method of testing for integrity of the pain and temperature pathway is to stimulate the skin with a pin and ask the patient whether it feels sharp or dull. Temperature perception need not be tested separately as a rule; if such testing is required, the method used is touching the skin with test tubes containing hot or cold water.

PATHWAY FOR SIMPLE (LIGHT) TOUCH AND PRESSURE (Fig. 19–2)

Central transmission for the sense of touch is not restricted to a single pathway. The quality of touch sensation conveyed in the dorsal column-medial lemniscus system is discriminative, i.e., two points touched on the skin simultaneously are both felt, even though they are close together. The alternative touch (and pressure) pathway now to be described involves ipsilateral transmission in the dorsal white column of the cord and contralateral transmission in the ventral white column. Localization of the source of a stimulus is less accurate in this pathway than in the dorsal column system, although sensitivity is high. The clinical test is to draw a wisp of cotton across the skin.

RECEPTORS

Several types of receptors respond to light contact with the skin; whether the quality of the sensation is discriminative or coarse is more dependent on the nature of the neuronal relays in the alternative pathways than on the receptors. Endings known to be sensors for touch are unencapsulated endings, including Merkel's disks and hair follicle plexuses, Meissner's corpuscles, and probably end-bulbs which have not yet been specifically identified. Pacinian corpuscles respond to the slightest deformity and these sensors in the dermis and subcutaneous tissue serve as pressure receptors.

PATHWAY FOR THE BODY

The cell bodies in dorsal root ganglia are of intermediate size; their processes are group A fibers of medium diameter with modernately thick myelin sheaths. The central processes bifurcate on entering the dorsal white column of the cord, the short descending branches giving off collaterals to the gray matter. Most of the ascending branches from which collateral branches also arise ascend in the lateral part of the dorsal column for six to eight segments, although some are longer. The fibers for simple touch and pressure are therefore spread out over many segments, effecting synaptic contact in the dorsal gray horn and intermediate zone with tract cells and with internuncial neurons for spinal reflexes. Axons of the tract cells cross the midline in the ventral gray and white commissures, continue into the ventral white column, and turn upward in the *ventral spinothalamic tract*. Because of the overlapping of fibers from several spinal nerves in the dorsal column at any particular level some tract cells receive afferents from a number of dorsal roots. This convergence and the consequent summation of excitation of second order neurons reduce the discriminative quality of touch and pressure, but they ensure a low threshold of excitation. In the upper medulla the ventral spinothalamic tract becomes part of the spinal lemniscus. The fibers continue to the ventral posterior nucleus of the thalamus as described above for the lateral spinothalamic tract. Although there may be minimal

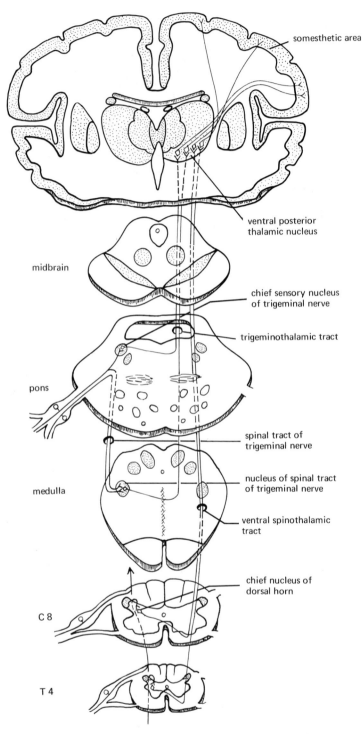

somesthetic area

ventral posterior
thalamic nucleus

midbrain

chief sensory nucleus
of trigeminal nerve

trigeminothalamic tract

pons

spinal tract of
trigeminal nerve

nucleus of spinal tract
of trigeminal nerve

medulla

ventral spinothalamic
tract

chief nucleus of
dorsal horn

C 8

T 4

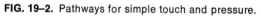

FIG. 19–2. Pathways for simple touch and pressure.

awareness of simple touch and pressure at the thalamic level, their conscious appreciation depends mainly on the cerebral cortex and is provided for by the tertiary thalamocortical relay to the somesthetic area.

PATHWAY FOR THE HEAD

As for pain and temperature, the primary sensory neurons for simple touch and pressure are located in the semilunar ganglion of the trigeminal nerve, with additional cells in the geniculate ganglion of the facial nerve and the superior ganglia of the glossopharyngeal and vagus nerves. Fibers in the sensory trigeminal root turn caudally in the spinal tract of the nerve. Most of these fibers terminate in the more rostral portions of the *nucleus of the spinal tract* (pars rostralis and pars interpolaris); only a few of these end in the pars caudalis along with fibers for pain and temperature. In addition to the afferents just described, other fibers for simple touch and pressure divide on entering the pons. One branch enters the spinal tract and the other branch terminates in the *chief* or *superior nucleus* of the trigeminal nerve, which is situated at the level of attachment of the nerve to the pons. The pathway continues as the opposite *trigeminothalamic tract* to the arcuate nucleus of the thalamus and the thalamocortical projection to the lower third of the somesthetic area. The trigeminothalamic tract includes some uncrossed fibers from the chief sensory nucleus, providing for awareness of touch in the cortices of both hemispheres.

The facial and vagus nerves (and the glossopharyngeal nerve inconstantly) include touch and pressure fibers for the external ear, the lining of the auditory canal, and the tympanic membrane. Touch fibers for the back of the tongue, pharynx, and larynx reach their destination through the glossopharyngeal and vagus

nerves. The central connections of neurons of the seventh, ninth, and tenth cranial nerves supplying the skin of the ear correspond to the connections of trigeminal neurons for touch and pressure, most of the afferent fibers joining the trigeminal spinal tract. Fibers for the sensation of touch in the mucous membranes (ninth and tenth nerves) probably terminate in the trigeminal spinal nucleus, although this is uncertain.

Compared with the other general senses, impairment of simple touch and pressure is less frequently demonstrable clinically as a result of lesions in the central nervous system. This observation is a consequence of bilateral conduction in the spinal cord and conduction for discriminative touch in the dorsal column-medial lemniscus system. Impairment or loss of touch sensation is most readily demonstrable as a contralateral sensory deficit when a lesion interrupts the spinal and medial lemnisci in the upper part of the brain stem or, more commonly, when a lesion involves the posterior limb of the internal capsule, the medullary center of the hemisphere, or the somesthetic cortex.

The *spinocervical tract* is mentioned at this point because it provides an additional pathway in the spinal cord for transmission of data concerned with pain, temperature, touch, and pressure to the brain. While most of the studies pertain to the situation in the cat, there appears to be a small spinocervical tract in man. The cells of origin are in the nucleus proprius of the dorsal gray horn and the tract ascends ipsilaterally in the dorsal part of the lateral white column. The constituent fibers terminate in the lateral cervical nucleus which consists of a short column of cells in the dorsal horn of the upper two cervical segments, extending for a short distance into the medulla. Axons from the lateral cervical nucleus cross the midline, continue through the brain stem, and terminate in the ventral posterior nucleus of the thalamus.

PATHWAY FOR PROPRIOCEPTION, FINE TOUCH, AND VIBRATION (Fig. 19–3)

RECEPTORS

Reflexes originating in proprioceptors in muscles, tendons, and joints were established at spinal cord, brain stem, and cerebellar levels early in vertebrate phylogeny for coordination of muscles in locomotion. A proprioceptive pathway to the cerebral cortex became increasingly significant in the course of mammalian phylogeny. Proprioception is especially important in man for learned or skilled motor activities. The projection from appropriate receptors to the cerebral cortex provides awareness of the precise position of body parts, the shape and size of an object held in the hand, weights of objects, and the range and direction of movements. The proprioceptors consist of neuromuscular spindles, Golgi tendon organs, unencapsulated endings in joint capsules and ligaments, and pacinian corpuscles adjacent to joints. The last two appear to be especially important with respect to the projection to the cerebral cortex, culminating in proprioception at the conscious level.

The characteristics of fine or discriminative touch are that one can recognize the location of the stimulated point with precision and is also aware that two points are touched simultaneously, even though they are close together (two-point discrimination). Of the various receptors responding to touch, Meissner's corpuscles seem to have a special significance for discriminative touch. These corpuscles have been found only in primates. They are most abundant in hairless skin, such as that of the palmar surface of the hand, and in the borders of the lips; preferential sites for

Meissner's corpuscles correspond to those areas in which two-point discrimination is best developed.

Pacinian corpuscles and unencapsulated endings are regarded as the receptors for the sense of vibration. While the dorsal columns are the main pathway for vibratory sense, clinicopathologic studies indicate that there are alternative pathways in the lateral white columns.

PATHWAY FOR THE BODY

Primary sensory neurons for the discriminative senses are represented by the largest cells of the dorsal root ganglia; their peripheral and central processes are large group A fibers with thick myelin sheaths. The central processes bifurcate on entering the *dorsal white column.* The short descending branches tend to accumulate in the fasciculus septomarginalis in the lower half of the spinal cord, and in the fasciculus interfascicularis in the upper half of the cord. These fibers, which give off collateral branches to the gray matter, form the afferent limbs of reflex circuits. The ascending branches from which collaterals also arise proceed in the ipsilateral dorsal column to the medulla oblongata. Above the midthoracic level, the dorsal column consists of a medial *fasciculus gracilis* and a lateral *fasciculus cuneatus.* The fibers of the fasciculus gracilis, which entered the cord below the midthoracic level, terminate in the *nucleus gracilis;* fibers of the fasciculus cuneatus, coming from the upper thoracic and cervical spinal nerves, end in the *nucleus cuneatus.* More precisely, there is lamination of the dorsal column according to segments. Fibers that entered the cord in lower sacral segments are most medial, and fibers from successively higher segments ascend in an orderly manner along the lateral side of those already present. (Although this is the main pathway for conduction within the cord of impulses des-

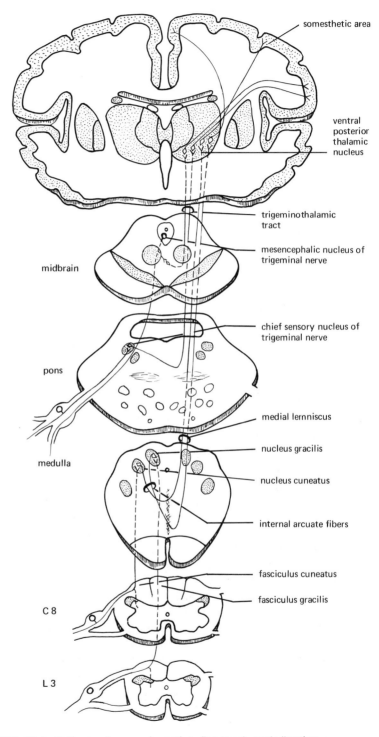

somesthetic area

ventral posterior thalamic nucleus

trigeminothalamic tract

mesencephalic nucleus of trigeminal nerve

midbrain

chief sensory nucleus of trigeminal nerve

pons

medial lernniscus

nucleus gracilis

medulla

nucleus cuneatus

internal arcuate fibers

fasciculus cuneatus

fasciculus gracilis

C 8

L 3

FIG. 19–3. Pathways for proprioception, fine touch, and vibration.

tined for the cerebral cortex, and concerned with proprioception, discriminative touch, and vibration, it is not necessarily the only such pathway. The results of animal experiments in which the dorsal white columns were sectioned, combined with the study of patients with lesions restricted to these columns, suggest that there is some conduction of these sensory modalities in other ascending or sensory pathways of the cord.)

Axons of second order neurons in the gracile and cuneate nuclei curve ventrally as *internal arcuate fibers,* cross the midline of the medulla in the decussation of the medial lemniscus, and continue to the thalamus as the *medial lemniscus.* This tract is situated between the midline and the inferior olivary nucleus in the medulla, at the junction of the dorsal and basal portions of the pons, and in the tegmentum of the midbrain just lateral to the red nucleus. The medial lemniscus and spinothalamic tracts intermingle in the dorsal region of the subthalamus, just before entering the ventral posterior nucleus of the thalamus.

An orderly arrangement of fibers according to the region from which stimuli originate is maintained throughout the medial lemniscus. In the medulla the larger dimension of the lemniscus is vertical as seen in cross-section; fibers for the lower part of the body are most ventral (adjacent to the pyramid) and fibers for the upper part of the body are most dorsal. On entering the pons, the medial lemniscus rotates through 90 degrees; from here to the thalamus fibers for the opposite foot are in the lateral part of the lemniscus, while those for the upper part of the body are included in the medial part of the tract. This conforms with the representation of the body in the ventral posterior nucleus of the thalamus, in which the body image is roughly horizontal.

There is no conscious awareness of the discriminative senses at the thalamic level,

other than a possible crude awareness of vibration. A tertiary projection to the upper two-thirds of the somesthetic area provides for one's sense of position and movement of body parts and the finer qualities of touch.

There is considerable convergence from one order of neuron to the next in the pathways for pain, temperature, simple touch, and pressure, establishing limits on the discriminative properties of these sensations. In the dorsal column–medial lemniscus system the number of primary, secondary, and tertiary neurons approaches a 1:1:1 ratio. This makes possible a detailed transmittal of information with respect to somatotopic localization and the type of receptor involved. Transmission through the nuclei gracilis and cuneatus may be facilitated or inhibited by cortical activity. The neurons responsible are in the sensorimotor cortex (especially the sensory strip) and their fibers accompany the corticospinal tract as far as the medulla.

PATHWAY FOR THE HEAD

The central connections for fine touch and proprioception differ from one another with respect to innervation of the head. For discriminative touch, which is well developed on the face, axons of large primary neurons in the semilunar ganglion terminate in the *chief sensory nucleus* of the trigeminal nerve. Information is then relayed to the somesthetic cortex through fibers of the trigeminothalamic tract (mostly crossed but some uncrossed) and thalamocortical fibers.

The primary sensory neurons for proprioception in the head area are unique in that many of them are in the brain stem rather than a sensory ganglion. These cells compose the *mesencephalic nucleus* of the trigeminal nerve, which consists of unipolar cells like most primary sensory neurons elsewhere. Peripheral process of these cells supply proprioceptors related to the tempormandibular joint and the muscles of mastication. The central processes make synaptic contact with cells in the reticular formation, and axons of the latter cells join the trigeminothalamic tract. The sensory supply of proprioceptive endings in other muscles that are innervated by cranial nerves was discussed in Chapter 8.

SOME CLINICAL COMMENTS

Since awareness of position, movement, fine touch, and vibration depends on cortical function, there is impairment or loss of these sensations if a lesion interrupts the pathway anywhere along its course. There is bilateral degeneration of the dorsal columns in tabes dorsalis; the dorsal and lateral white columns are sites of symmetrical demyelination in subacute combined degeneration of the cord. Among lesions interrupting the pathway in the spinal cord or the brain, including the sensory cortex, are trauma, infarction, and the plaques of disseminated sclerosis. When interpreting deficits in relation to the location of a lesion, it is essential to bear in mind that conduction is ipsilateral as far as the medulla, then contralateral. Joint movement and the direction of movement, which are important aspects of proprioception, are tested by the examiner's moving a finger or toe of the patient, who is asked to report when the movement begins and the direction of movement. The Romberg test in which un-steadiness is noted when the patient stands with the feet together and the eyes closed, evaluates proprioception in the lower extremities. Another useful test is to ask the patient to identify an object held in the hand with the eyes closed. Proprioception is especially helpful in recognizing the object on the basis of shape and size (stereognosis) as well as its weight. This is a sensitive test which the patient may perform unsuccessfully when there is a lesion in the parietal association cortex, even though the pathway to the somesthetic area is intact.

Another test of the integrity of the dorsal column–medial lemniscus system is to ask the patient if he feels vibration as well as touch or pressure when a tuning fork, preferably with a frequency of 128 cps, is placed against a bony prominence such as the internal malleolus at the ankle or a finger joint. The sense of vibration is often reduced in elderly persons, but minimal vibration should be felt in the young. Routine testing for fine touch is not necessary because the other tests are sufficient to detect an interruption of the pathway. If a test of two-point touch discrimination is desired, two pointed objects are applied lightly to the skin simultaneously. A suitable test object can be devised from a paper clip. A normal person is able to appreciate stimuli applied simultaneously to the finger tips when they are 3–4 mm apart, or even less.

SUGGESTIONS FOR ADDITIONAL READING

Calne DB, Pallis CA: Vibratory sense: A critical review. Brain 89:723–746, 1966

Gordon G, Jukes MGM: Descending influences on the exteroceptive organizations of the cat's gracile nucleus. J Physiol 173:291–319, 1964

Kuypers HGJM: Some projections from the pericentral cortex to the pons and lower brain stem in monkey and chimpanzee. J Comp Neurol 110:221–255, 1958

Rasmussen AT: The Principal Nervous Pathways. New York, Macmillan, 1957

Sinclair D: Cutaneous Sensation. London, Oxford University Press, 1967

Walberg F: Corticofugal fibers to the nuclei of the dorsal columns: An experimental study in the cat. Brain 80:273–287, 1957

Wall PD: The sensory and motor role of impulses travelling in the dorsal columns towards cerebral cortex. Brain 93:505–524, 1970

20

Visual System

The visual pathway begins with photoreceptors in the retina from which impulses reach the visual cortex in the occipital lobe through a series of three neurons. There are two classes of photoreceptor cells; rod cells have a special role in peripheral vision and vision under conditions of low illumination, while cone cells are responsible for central, discriminative vision and the detection of color. Action potentials generated in the photoreceptors are transmitted by bipolar cells to ganglion cells within the retina, and axons of the latter neurons reach the lateral geniculate nucleus of the thalamus through the optic nerve and tract. The final relay is from the lateral geniculate nucleus to the visual cortex by way of the geniculocalcarine tract. Some fibers from the retina terminate in the brain stem and constitute the afferent limbs of visual reflex arcs.

The following account of the visual system is restricted to nervous elements and presupposes a general understanding of the structure of the eye.

RETINA

Optic vesicles evaginate from the prosencephalon of the neural tube at an early stage of embryonic development. The anterior part of the optic vesicle caves in to form the optic cup, which therefore consists of two layers; the vesicle is connected with the neural tube by the optic stalk (future optic nerve). The outer layer of the optic cup becomes the pigment epithelium of the retina and the inner layer differentiates into the complex neural layer of the retina. In addition to the photoreceptors, bipolar cells, and ganglion cells, the neural layer includes association neurons and neuroglial cells. The complex neuronal pattern of the retina resembles the gray matter of the brain. Similarly, the histology of the optic nerve corresponds to that of white matter rather than to that of a peripheral nerve. The retina and optic nerve may therefore be viewed as outgrowths of the brain which are specialized for sensitivity to light, some modifications of the sensory data, and transmission of the resulting information to the thalamus and cerebral cortex.

SOME RETINAL LANDMARKS

Certain specialized regions or landmarks need to be identified before the cellular components of the retina are described.

The basic layers of the retina, listed from the choroid membrane to the vitreous body, are the pigment epithelium, rod and cone cells, bipolar cells, and ganglion cells (Fig. 20-1). Axons of ganglion cells run toward the posterior pole of the eye and enter the optic nerve at the *optic papilla* or *optic disk.* The papilla is slightly medial to the posterior pole, about 1.5 mm in diameter, and pale pink in color. The nerve fibers are heaped up as they converge at the margin of the papilla, then pass through the fibrous tunic (sclera) of the eyeball into the optic nerve. The optic papilla is a blind spot because it contains only nerve fibers.

The *macula lutea,* or central area in line with the visual axis, is a specialized region of the retina 6 mm in diameter and abutting on the lateral edge of the optic papilla. The name macula lutea or "yellow spot" is derived from the presence of a diffuse yellow pigment (xanthophyll) among the neural elements in this location. However, the yellow color is apparent only when the retina is examined with red-free light, and the macula is therefore not ordinarily seen when the ocular fundus is inspected with an ophthalmoscope. The macula is specialized for acuity of vision; the function of the yellow pigment is probably to screen out much of the blue part of the visible spectrum, thus protecting the photoreceptors from the dazzling effect of strong light.

The *fovea* (or fovea centralis) is a depression in the center of the macula; the fovea is about 1.5 mm in diameter and separated from the edge of the optic disk by a distance of about 2 mm. Visual acuity is greatest at the fovea, the center of which contains only cone receptors. The capillary network present elsewhere in the retina is absent from the center of the fovea, although the adjacent choroid capillaries are still present. When the retina is viewed with an ophthalmoscope, the fovea appears distinctly darker than the reddish hue of the retina generally, because the black melanin pigment of the choroid and pigment epithelium is not screened by capillary blood. The visible fovea centralis is frequently referred to as the "macula" in an ophthalmoscopic examination of the retina.

The functional retina terminates anteriorly along an irregular border, the *ora serrata.* Forward of this line the ciliary portion of the retina consists of a double layer of columnar epithelium, the outer layer being pigmented.

PIGMENT EPITHELIUM

Consisting of a single layer of cells, the *pigment epithelium* reinforces the light-absorbing properties of the choroid membrane to reduce scattering of light within the eye. Each cell has a flat hexagonal base which is adherent to Bruch's membrane of the choroid. The basal portion of the cell contains the nucleus and a few pigment granules. Processes extending from the free surface of the cell interdigitate with the outer, photosensitive regions of rod and cone cells. The processes, which are filled with granules of melanin pigment, isolate individual photoreceptors and enhance visual acuity. In lower vertebrates there is a flow of pigment granules further into the processes in response to high light intensity; such a response has not been described in mammals, including man.

While the pigment epithelium is fixed to

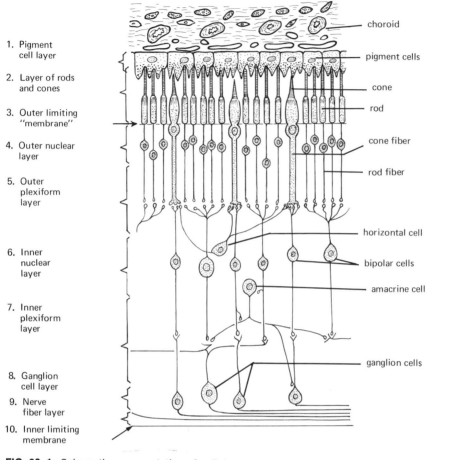

1. Pigment cell layer
2. Layer of rods and cones
3. Outer limiting "membrane"
4. Outer nuclear layer
5. Outer plexiform layer
6. Inner nuclear layer
7. Inner plexiform layer
8. Ganglion cell layer
9. Nerve fiber layer
10. Inner limiting membrane

choroid — pigment cells — cone — rod — cone fiber — rod fiber — horizontal cell — bipolar cells — amacrine cell — ganglion cells

FIG. 20–1. Schematic representation of cellular components of the retina.

the choroid, it is not so firmly attached to the neural part of the retina. Detachment of the retina, such as may follow a blow to the eye, consists of separation of the neural layers from the pigment epithelium, i.e., at the junction of the two layers of the optic cup.

PHOTORECEPTORS

The light-sensitive part of the photoreceptor cell is the outer portion adjacent to the pigment epithelium. The "inverted" retina is characteristic of vertebrates, while in

some invertebrates the layers are reversed and light impinges on the receptors without first traversing the retina. The inverted retina does not introduce a significant barrier to light because the retina is transparent and at no point more than 0.4 mm in thickness.

Rod Cells

The number of rod cells in the human retina is on the order of 130 million, outnumbering cone cells by nearly 20:1. Rod cells are lacking in the central part of the fovea and become progressively more numerous from that point to the ora serrata. The distribution is such that rod cells are important for peripheral vision. Each rod cell consists of an outer portion, the *rod* (or rod proper), and an inner portion, the *rod fiber*. Rods are about 2 μ in thickness and vary in length from 60 μ near the fovea centralis to 40 μ at the periphery of the retina. The unspecialized rod fiber consists of a slender filament which includes the nucleus in an expanded region and terminates as an end-bulb in synaptic contact with bipolar and association neurons.

The rod consists of outer and inner segments, of which the former is light-sensitive. In electron micrographs most of the *outer segment* is occupied by about 700 double-layered, membranous disks or flatened saccules (Figs. 20–2 and 20–3). The surfaces of the rods (and cones), which are grooved longitudinally, are shown in Figure 20–4. The membranous disks include the pigment *rhodopsin* (*visual purple*), which gives the retina a purplish-red color when removed from the eye and viewed under dim light. Rhodopsin consists of retinine (an aldehyde form of vitamin A) combined with a protein named opsin. The compound is broken down into its major constituents by light, causing the retina to bleach, and is restored in the dark. Studies of the photochemical reactions show that there are primary and secondary steps in the transduction of light energy to produce a nerve impulse. The primary step is absorption of a quantum of light by rhodopsin and a change in configuration of the pigment molecule. The secondary step consists of a series of reactions, still poorly understood, which produce an action potential that travels along the surface membrane of the rod cell as a nerve impulse.

The photochemical properties of rhodopsin together with summation of excitation

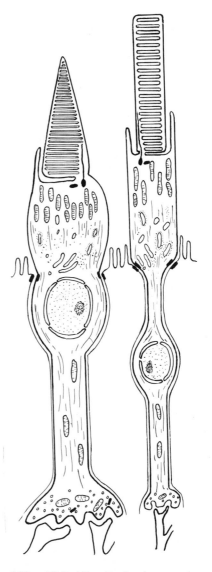

FIG. 20–2. Ultrastructural components of rod and cone cells. (Slightly modified from Figure 7 in Missotten, L: The Ultrastructure of the Human Retina, 1965. Copyright by Editions ARSCIA, Brussels, Belgium)

in the visual pathway through the retina are responsible for the sensitivity of the rod system to low illumination (twilight or night vision). The rod-free area of the

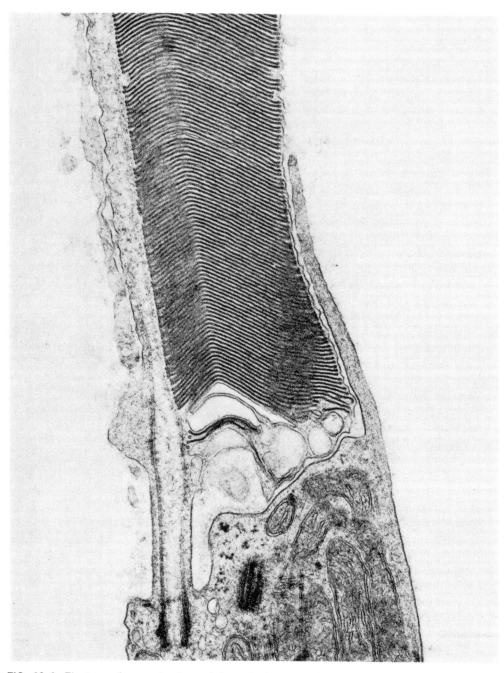

FIG. 20–3. Electron micrograph of a rod from the human retina showing a portion of the outer segment and the adjoining region of the inner segment. (Courtesy of Dr. M. J. Hogan) ×36,000

fovea is night-blind and a faint point of light such as a star of low magnitude is best detected by looking slightly away from it.

The *inner segment* of a rod is less differentiated than the outer segment and includes organelles found in cells generally. A region adjacent to the outer segment, known as the *ellipsoid*, contains large numbers of elongated mitochondria. A cilium extends into the outer segment from one of two centrioles situated at the junction of the outer and inner segments. The re-

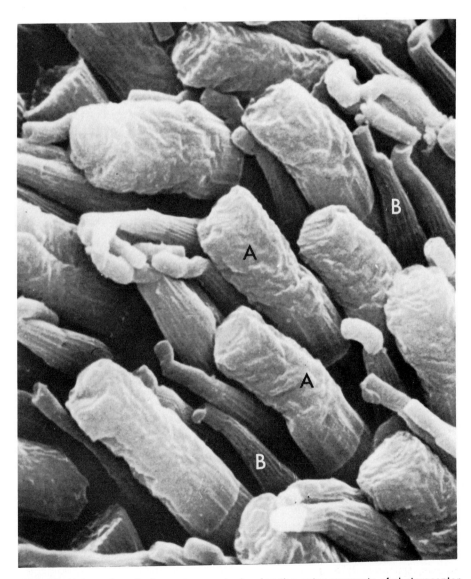

FIG. 20–4. Scanning electron micrograph showing the outer segments of photoreceptor cells of the newt after removal of the pigment epithelium. *A.* rods; *B.* cones. (Courtesy of Dr. D. H. Dickson and Dr. M. J. Hollenberg) ×4,500

mainder of the inner segment contains neurofibrils and vesicles with round or oval profiles, some of which are covered with ribosomes (granular endoplasmic reticulum). The latter region is known as the *myoid* because it is contractile in lower vertebrates and responds to changes in light intensity. A contractile property has not been established for this region in higher vertebrates, including man.

Cone Cells

The cone photoreceptors, although less numerous than rod photoreceptors, are especially important because of their role in visual acuity and color vision. Like the rod cell the cone cell consists of an outer portion, the *cone* (or cone proper), and an inner portion, the *cone fiber;* the cone likewise has outer and inner segments, the former being light-sensitive.

The tapering *outer segment* of a cone consists principally of double-layered disks, varying in number from 1000 in cones at the fovea to several hundred at the periphery of the retina (Fig. 20–2). There are differences in detail between the disks of cones and rods, including somewhat closer stacking of the disks in cones. Since cones are responsible for color vision, the chemistry of the membranous disks is of special interest. A substance called *iodopsin,* chemically related to rhodopsin, has been described. However, the photochemistry of the cone outer segment is still under investigation. The presence in separate cones of minute amounts of three photosensitive pigments has been suggested, providing differential stimulation by red, green, and blue light. The *inner segment* of a cone, compared with that of a rod, is thicker; the ellipsoid is larger, and there is more granular endoplasmic reticulum.

The *cone fiber* is thicker than a rod fiber, and the nucleus is in an enlargment of the fiber adjacent to the cone. The fiber expands terminally and establishes synaptic contact with bipolar and association neurons.

The human retina contains about 7 million cone cells. The central part of the fovea, or the foveola, contains about 35,000 cone cells and no rod cells; there are some 100,000 cone cells in the whole of the fovea. The proportion of cone cells to rod cells remains high through the macular area for central vision, but steadily decreases from the macula to the periphery of the retina. The fovea is specialized in other ways for visual acuity. In this region the cones are longer and more slender than elsewhere (75 by 1.0–1.5 μ at the fovea and 40 by 6 μ at the periphery). The cone fibers and bipolar cells diverge from the center of the fovea producing the slight concavity at this point and eliminating any slight impediment to light passing through the retina. Such diffusion of light as may be caused by capillary blood flow is eliminated by absence of a retinal capillary network in the center of the fovea. In brief, central vision with maximal acuity is provided by the concentration of cones in the macula lutea, especially the fovea centralis. Photochemical properties of the outer cone segments permit detection of colors.

BIPOLAR CELLS

Bipolar cells (Fig. 20–1) are true neurons interposed between photoreceptor cells and ganglion cells. One bipolar cell receives stimuli from numerous rod cells (10 near the macula to 100 at the periphery); the summation of excitation is an important factor in producing the low threshold of the rod system. The ratio between cone cells and bipolar cells is 1:1 at the fovea, as required for maximal visual acuity. Elsewhere, variable numbers of cone cells converge on a bipolar cell, and some of the latter receive stimuli from both rods and cones.

GANGLION CELLS

Ganglion cells (Fig. 20–1) are rather large neurons with clumps of Nissl material, forming the last retinal link in the visual pathway. Impulses are received from bipolar cells through axodendritic and axosomatic synapses. A ganglion cell receives impulses from one bipolar cell in the foveal region in order to maintain the discrete relay from cone photoreceptors that is required for maximal acuity of vision. Outside the fovea the number of bipolar cells converging on a ganglion cell increases toward the periphery of the retina. Ganglion cell axons form a layer of nerve fibers adjacent to the vitreous body. The fibers converge on the optic papilla from all directions, those from the lateral part of retina curving above and below the macula. On reaching the papilla, bundles of fibers pass through foramina in the sclera and then constitute the optic nerve. The axons acquire myelin sheaths only after traversing the sclera.

ASSOCIATION NEURONS

Impulse transmission in the retina is subject to modification by association neurons (Fig. 20–1). *Horizontal cells* are in the outer part of the zone occupied by the cell bodies of bipolar cells. The processes of these cells, which are essentially dendrites, establish synaptic contact with either cone cells or rod cells, so that in this respect there are two classes of horizontal cells. The horizontal cell had no axon in the usual sense; instead, small protuberances from the cell processes make synaptic contact with the dendrites of bipolar cells. *Amacrine cells* are located in the inner part of the layer occupied by bipolar cells. Each

cell has a single process, whose branches end in the synaptic complexes between bipolar and ganglion cells or on the cell bodies of ganglion cells. Axon collaterals of bipolar cells are in synaptic contact with the cell body of an amacrine cell or with branches of its single process.

The impulses received by association neurons and the influence of these neurons on other cells may be excitatory or inhibitory. The effect is to modify visual data picked up by photoreceptors in transit through the retina. An example of such modification is the enhancement of information passed to the brain about borders and contours, with an increase in contrast. A further example is found in the central discharge from ganglion cells. Some cells discharge when photoreceptors are first stimulated; some discharge when stimulation ceases, and others discharge throughout photic stimulation—the number of impulses per second being determined by the intensity of stimulation.

NEUROGLIAL CELLS

The retina, in particular the inner layers, contains neuroglial cells similar to those present in the gray matter of the brain. There are also large numbers of modified neuroglial cells called the *cells of Müller*. These extend from the interface between the innermost fiber layer of the retina and the vitreous body to the junction of the rod and rod fiber, and the cone and cone fiber. Microvilli project from the outer end of a Müller's cell, and the cell is connected to photoreceptor cells by desmosomes (Fig. 20–2). Müller's cells therefore extend through most of the retina; lateral processes are given off which intervene between the neuronal elements of the retina and give these modified neuroglial cells a supporting role among other possible functions.

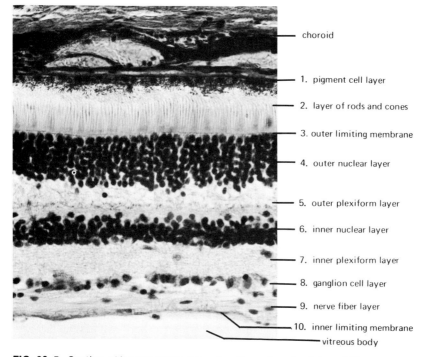

choroid

1. pigment cell layer

2. layer of rods and cones

3. outer limiting membrane

4. outer nuclear layer

5. outer plexiform layer

6. inner nuclear layer

7. inner plexiform layer

8. ganglion cell layer

9. nerve fiber layer

10. inner limiting membrane

vitreous body

FIG. 20–5. Section of human retina. Hematoxylin and eosin stain. ×350

HISTOLOGIC LAYERS OF THE RETINA

When studied in sections stained with hematoxylin and eosin rather than by the Golgi method, the retina is described as consisting of 10 layers (Fig. 20–5). These layers can now be defined in relation to the cells which constitute the retina (Fig. 20–1). Layer 1 is the *pigment epithelium* and layer 2 consists of *rods* and *cones*. Layer 3 is called the *outer limiting membrane* because it appears as a delicate line in histologic sections. In fact, it is not a membrane but rather the row of desmosomes where the outer ends of Müller's cells make contact with photoreceptor cells. Layer 4, the *outer nuclear layer*, consists of nuclei of rod and cone cells. Layer 5, or the *outer plexiform layer*, includes principally rod and cone fibers and bipolar cell dendrites. Layer 6 is called the inner nuclear *layer;* it is made up of nuclei of bipolar neurons together with nuclei of horizontal cells, amacrine cells, and cells of Müller. Layer 7, or the *inner plexiform layer*, consists mainly of bipolar cell axons and ganglion cell dendrites. The cell bodies of *ganglion cells* are in layer 8, and the axons of these cells constitute layer 9 or the *nerve fiber layer*. Layer 10 is an *inner limiting membrane* formed by the inner ends of Müller's cells.

BLOOD SUPPLY OF THE RETINA

The retina receives nourishment from two sources. The central artery of the retina enters through the optic disk and its branches spread out over the inner surface of the retina. Fine branches penetrate the retina and form a capillary network extending to the outer border of the inner nuclear layer. The capillary bed drains into retinal veins which converge on the papilla to form the central vein of the retina. The other source of nourishment is from the capillary layer of the choroid which is separated from the retina by the semipermeable Bruch's membrane. The outer part of the retina, extending from the pigment epithelium to the outer border of the inner nuclear layer, is devoid of capillaries.

PATHWAY TO VISUAL CORTEX

There is a point-to-point projection from the retina to the lateral geniculate nucleus and from the latter to the visual cortex of the occipital lobe. The cortex therefore receives a spatial pattern of excitation which corresponds with the retinal image of the visual field. Prior to a discussion of the components of the pathway, certain general rules concerning the central projection of the retina may usefully be established.

For the purpose of describing the retinal projection, each retina is divided into nasal and temporal halves by a vertical line passing through the fovea centralis. A horizontal line, also passing through the fovea, divides each half of the retina into upper and lower quadrants. The macular area for most acute vision is represented separately from the peripheral part of the retina. Figure 20–6 illustrates the following rules with respect to the central projection of retinal areas. 1) Fibers from the right halves of the two retinae terminate exclusively in the right lateral geniculate nucleus, and the visual information is then relayed to the visual cortex of the right hemisphere. The converse holds true, of course, for the contralateral projection. 2) Fibers from the upper quadrants peripheral to the macula end in the medial part of the lateral geniculate nucleus, and impulses are relayed to the anterior two-thirds of the visual cortex

above the calcarine sulcus. 3) Fibers from the lower quadrants peripheral to the macula end in the lateral portion of the geniculate nucleus, with a relay to the anterior two-thirds of the visual cortex below the calcarine sulcus. 4) The macula projects to a relatively large posterior region of the lateral geniculate nucleus, which in turn sends fibers to the posterior third of the visual cortex in the region of the occipital pole. The portions of the lateral geniculate nucleus and visual cortex receiving fibers from the macula (which is only 6 mm in diameter) are disproportionately large because of the role of the macula in central vision with maximal discrimination.

Visual defects result from interruption of the pathway at any point from the retina itself to the visual cortex. Such defects are described in terms of the visual field rather than the retina. The retinal image of an object in the visual field is inverted and reversed from right to left, just as an image on the film in a camera is inverted and reversed. The following rules therefore apply to the nuclear and cortical representation of regions of the visual field. 1) The left visual field is represented in the right geniculate nucleus and the visual cortex of the right hemisphere. 2) The upper half of the visual field is represented in the lateral portion of the geniculate nucleus and the visual cortex below the calcarine sulcus. 3) The lower half of the visual field is projected on the medial portion of the geniculate nucleus and the visual cortex above the calcarine sulcus.

OPTIC NERVE, CHIASMA, AND TRACT

Each *optic nerve* in man contains about 1 million fibers, all of them myelinated; the large number of optic fibers is indicative of the importance of human vision. The nerve is surrounded by extensions of the meninges; the pia mater adheres to the nerve and

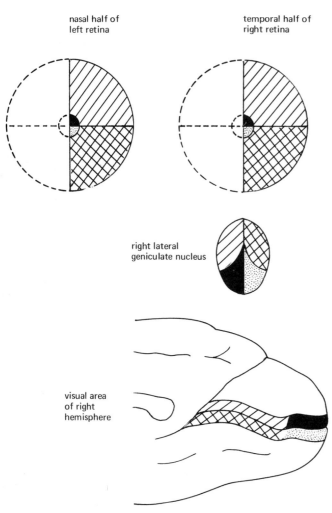

FIG. 20–6. Projection of the retina on the lateral geniculate nucleus and the visual cortex.

is separated from the arachnoid by an extension of the subarachnoid space. The dura mater forms an outer sheath, and the meningeal extensions around the nerve fuse with the fibrous scleral coat of the eyeball. The nerve fibers are arranged in groups or fasciculi which are separated by connective tissue septa continuous with the pial sheath. Each group of fibers is further divided into small bundles by neuroglial cells, whose processes penetrate between individual fibers. The myelin sheaths are formed by oligodendrocytes rather than neurilemma cells of Schwann because the optic nerve is comparable to a tract within the central nervous system.

The central artery and vein of the retina traverse the meningeal sheaths and are included in the anterior part of the optic nerve. An increase in pressure of cerebrospinal fluid around the nerve impedes the return of venous blood. Edema or swelling of the optic disk (papilledema) results; this is a valuable indication of an increase in intracranial pressure.

The partial crossing of optic nerve fibers in the *optic chiasma* is the basis of binocular vision. Fibers from the nasal or medial half of each retina decussate in the chiasma and join uncrossed fibers from the temporal or lateral half of the retina to form the *optic tract*. Impulses conducted to the right hemisphere by the right optic tract therefore represent the left half of the field of vision, while the right visual field is represented in the left hemisphere. Immediately after crossing in the chiasma fibers from the nasal half of the retina loop forward for a short distance in the optic nerve. A lesion affecting the optic nerve just in front of the chiasma may therefore cause a temporal field defect with respect to the opposite eye, in addition to blindness in the eye whose optic nerve has been interrupted. The optic tract winds around the rostral end of the cerebral peduncle and ends in the lateral geniculate nucleus of the thalamus.

LATERAL GENICULATE NUCLEUS, GENICULOCALCARINE TRACT, AND VISUAL CORTEX

The *lateral geniculate nucleus* produces a small swelling, the lateral geniculate body, under the posterior projection of the pulvinar of the thalamus. The nucleus is the site of termination of all optic tract fibers except the few which serve as afferent limbs of reflex arcs. The lateral geniculate nucleus consists of six layers of cells, numbered consecutively from its ventral surface. Within the general pattern shown in Figure 20–6 and described above, crossed fibers of the optic tract terminate in layers 1, 4, and 6, while uncrossed fibers end in layers 2, 3, and 5. Although the lateral geniculate nucleus contains small

intercalating neurons, axons of most of its constituent cells extend to occipital cortex adjacent to the calcarine sulcus.

Fibers of the *geniculocalcarine tract* first traverse the retrolenticular and sublenticular portions of the internal capsule; the fibers then pass around the lateral ventricle, curving posteriorly toward their termination in the visual cortex (Fig. 20–7). Some of the geniculocalcarine fibers travel far forward over the temporal horn of the lateral ventricle. These fibers, which constitute the temporal or Meyer's loop of the geniculocalcarine tract, terminate in the cortex below the calcarine sulcus. It will be apparent from the retinal projection shown in Figure 20–6 that a temporal lobe lesion involving Meyer's loop will cause a defect in the upper visual field on the side opposite the lesion. A lesion in the parietal lobe, on the other hand, may involve geniculocalcarine fibers proceeding to the cortex above the calcarine sulcus; the result is then a defect in the lower visual field on the side opposite the lesion.

The *visual cortex* occupies the upper and lower lips of the calcarine sulcus on the medial surface of the hemisphere. The area is much larger than suggested by the usual cortical maps because of the depth of the calcarine sulcus. The visual cortex is thin, heterotypical cortex of the granular type (area 17 of Brodmann); it is marked by the line of Gennari and known alternatively as the striate area. There is a detailed point-to-point projection of the retina on the lateral geniculate nucleus and the visual cortex. The size of the retinal point is reduced to the diameter of a single cone for most acute vision in the central part of the fovea. Precise coordination of movements of the two eyes ensures that the retinal patterns of excitation in the two eyes correspond with one another, as required for binocular vision. The visual association cortex, corresponding roughly to areas 18 and 19 of

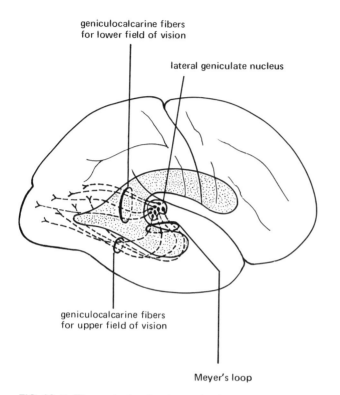

geniculocalcarine fibers
for lower field of vision

lateral geniculate nucleus

geniculocalcarine fibers
for upper field of vision

Meyer's loop

FIG. 20–7. The geniculocalcarine projection.

Brodmann, is responsible for recognition of objects, perception of color and depth, and other complex aspects of vision.

VISUAL DEFECTS CAUSED BY INTERRUPTION OF THE PATHWAY

Certain general rules governing defects in the visual field as a result of a lesion involving the visual pathway are indicated in Figure 20–8. The first example is an obvious one; severe degenerative disease or trauma involving an optic nerve results in blindness in the corresponding eye. Example 2 refers to interruption of decussating fibers in the optic chiasma which causes bitemporal hemianopsia if the full thickness of the chiasma is interrupted. The most common lesion affecting the optic chiasma is a pituitary tumor pressing on the chiasma from below, which first interrupts fibers from the inferior nasal quadrants of both retinae. The visual defect begins as a scotoma in each superior temporal quadrant of the visual field, and spreads throughout the temporal fields as the chiasma is increasingly affected. Pressure on the lateral edge of the chiasma (example 3) happens infrequently, but may occur when there is an aneurysm of the internal carotid artery in this location. The field defect, in the case of pressure on the right edge of the chiasma, is nasal hemianopsia for the right eye. Interruption of the right optic tract (example 4) causes left homonymous hemianopsia.

Example 5 refers to lesions involving the geniculocalcarine tract or the visual cortex.

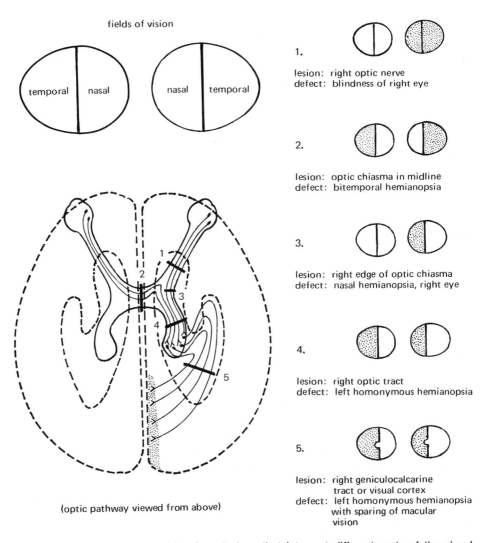

FIG. 20-8. Visual defects resulting from lesions that interrupt different parts of the visual pathway.

An extensive right-sided lesion causes left homonymous hemianopsia like that caused by interruption of the optic tract, except that central vision is usually spared. There is no fully satisfactory explanation for "macular sparing" and searches for decussating fibers that would provide bilateral cortical representation of the macula have been unsuccessful. The phenomenon may be an artifact, caused by the patient's shifting his fixation point slightly during field examination. Another possibility is that the large region of visual cortex and subjacent white matter concerned with central vision may be partially maintained by a collateral circulation from the middle cerebral artery following occlusion of the posterior cerebral artery or one of its branches. Smaller lesions involving the geniculocalcarine fibers or visual cortex cause less extensive visual field defects than one approaching hemianopsia. An example is provided by the upper quadrantic defect in the opposite visual field following interruption of fibers in Meyer's loop.

VISUAL REFLEXES

A small bundle of fibers from the optic tract enters the superior brachium. These fibers, which constitute the afferent limb of reflex arcs, terminate in the pretectal nucleus and the superior colliculus.

The *pupillary light reflex* is tested in the routine neurologic examination; the response consists of constriction of the pupil when light, as from a pen flashlight, is directed into the eye. Impulses from the retina impinge on the pretectal nucleus, which is a small group of cells immediately rostral to the superior colliculus. Impulses are relayed to the Edinger–Westphal nucleus of the oculomotor complex, then to the ciliary ganglion in the orbit, and finally to the constrictor pupillae muscle of the iris. Both pupils constrict in response to light entering one eye, because the pretectal nucleus sends fibers to parasympathetic neurons supplying the constrictor pupillae muscles of both eyes.

Visual impulses reaching the superior colliculus are concerned with reflex responses through tectobulbar and tectospinal connections. These responses include directing the gaze toward the source of a visual stimulus, together with closing the eyes and perhaps raising the arms for protection against a rapidly approaching object. However, the number of afferent fibers to the superior colliculus from the retina is small in man, the largest single component of the superior brachium being corticocollicular fibers. The latter originate

in visual association cortex and end in the superior colliculus, from which impulses are relayed to the oculomotor, trochlear, and abducens nuclei. The connections thus established provide for automatic scanning movements of the eyes, such as occur when reading. Corticocollicular fibers probably function as well in the accommodation reflex, next to be discussed.

The *accommodation reflex* (or accommodation-convergence reaction) consists of ocular convergence, pupillary constriction, and thickening of the lens when attention is directed to a near object. The reflex is tested in the routine neurologic examination by asking the patient to focus on an object held about a foot from the eyes after gazing into the distance, and noting whether there is pupillary constriction. When attention is directed to a near object the medial recti muscles contract for convergence of the eyes. At the same time, contraction of the ciliary muscle allows the lens to thicken, increasing its refractive power, and pupillary constriction sharpens the image on the retina.

The pathway for the accommodation reflex is not fully understood, although it is thought to include the cerebral cortex. Impulses from the visual association cortex may reach the midbrain through fibers in the superior brachium, probably being relayed to the oculomotor nucleus through the superior colliculus. Alternatively, although less likely, impulses may pass from the visual association cortex to the motor cortex of the frontal lobe through association fibers of the hemisphere, then reach the oculomotor nucleus by way of corticobulbar fibers. The pathways for the light and accommodation reflexes are assumed to be different because they may be dissociated by disease. This occurs, for example, in central nervous system syphilis, in which there is loss of pupillary constriction in response to light but not to accommodation

(Argyll Robertson pupil). The lesion may involve the pretectal nucleus or its immediate connection, but this is at present uncertain.

Pupillary dilation occurs in response to severe pain or strong emotional states. The pathway begins with fibers from the thalamus and hippocampal formation going to the hypothalamus, from which impulses reach the intermediolateral cell column of the upper thoracic cord through a relay in the reticular formation. The pathway continues through a synaptic relay in the superior cervical sympathetic ganglion and postganglionic fibers in the carotid plexus to the dilator pupillae muscle.

SUGGESTIONS FOR ADDITIONAL READING

Dowling JE: Foveal receptors of the monkey retina: Fine structure. Science 147:57–59, 1965

Hollenberg MJ, Bernstein MH: Fine structure of the photoreceptor cells of the ground squirrel (Citellus tridecemlineatus tridecemlineatus.) Am J Anat 118:359–373, 1966

Michael CR: Retinal processing of visual images. Sci Am 220/5:105–114, 1969

Missotten L: The Ultrastructure of the Human Retina. Brussels, Editons ARSCIA, 1965

Moses RA: Adler's Physiology of the Eye, 5th ed. St. Louis, Mosby, 1970

Polyak SL: The Vertebrate Visual System. Chicago, University of Chicago Press, 1957

Straatsma BR, Hall MO, Allen RA, Crescitelli F (eds.): The Retina: Morphology, Function and Clinical Characteristics. Los Angeles, University of California Press, 1969

Tokuyasu K, Yamada E: The fine structure of the retina studied with the electron microscope. IV. Morphogenesis of outer segments of retinal rods. J Biophys Biochem Cytol 6:225–230, 1959

21
Auditory System

Hearing is the second in importance among the special senses of man, yielding first place only to sight. Language accounts to a large extent for the paramount place of vision and hearing in humans.

The auditory system consists of the outer and middle ears, the cochlea of the inner ear, the cochlear nerve, and pathways in the central nervous system. The outer (external) ear includes the pinna or auricle, external auditory meatus, and tympanic membrane; its function is to collect sound waves, which cause resonant vibration of the tympanic membrane. The vibrations are transmitted across the middle ear cavity by a succession of three ossicles. The malleus is attached to the tympanic membrane and articulates with the incus, which in turn articulates with the stirrup-shaped stapes. The foot-plate of the stapes occupies the oval window (fenestra vestibuli) in the medial wall of the middle ear and is attached to the margin of the window by a ring of connective tissue called the annular

ligament. The ossicles function as a lever with the longer of the two arms attached to the tympanic membrane, and the foot-plate of the stapes is considerably smaller than the tympanic membrane. Because of these factors, the vibratory force of the stapes is about 10 times that of the tympanic membrane.

The inner ear, which has a dual function, consists of a membranous labyrinth encased in a bony labyrinth. Certain parts of the inner ear include sensory areas for the vestibular system, which will be discussed in the following chapter. The cochlear portion of the bony labyrinth contains the organ of Corti, from which nerve impulses arise in response to pressure waves induced in the fluid within the cochlea by vibrations of the stapes. The impulses are conducted to the brain stem by the cochlear division of the vestibulocochlear nerve, reaching the auditory cortex through several synaptic relays or causing reflex responses to auditory stimuli. The present chapter is concerned primarily with the organ of Corti and the auditory pathways. However, the main features of the bony and membranous labyrinths are reviewed as an aid in understanding how vibrations of the stapes result in stimulation of sensory cells of the organ of Corti and initiation of nerve impulses to the brain.

BONY AND MEMBRANOUS LABYRINTHS

The *bony* or *osseous labyrinth* (Fig. 21–1) is firmly embedded in the petrous temporal bone, which forms a prominent ridge between the middle and posterior fossae of the skull. The middle part of the bony labyrinth consists of the *vestibule,* whose lateral wall is shared by the medial wall of the middle ear cavity. This wall has an aperture, the *oval window* or *fenestra*

vestibuli, into which the stapes fits as mentioned above. Below the oval window at the junction of the vestibule and the basal turn of the cochlea there is a *round window* or *fenestra cochleae.* The round window is closed by a thin membrane which makes pressure waves possible in the fluid of the inner ear. The fluid would otherwise be enclosed in a completely rigid "box," except for the source of pressure waves at the oval window. Three *semicircular canals* extend posteriorly from the vestibule, while the *cochlea* makes up the anterior portion of the bony labyrinth. The cochlea has the shape of a snail shell; the base faces medially and abuts against the bottom of the internal auditory meatus, which opens to the posterior cranial fossa on the posterior surface of the petrous bone. Cochlear nerve fibers emerge from the base of the cochlea where they are joined by fibers of the vestibular nerve. The two divisions of the

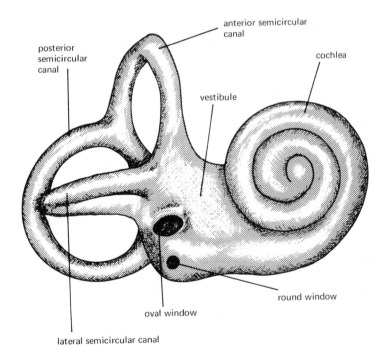

anterior semicircular canal

posterior semicircular canal

cochlea

vestibule

round window

oval window

lateral semicircular canal

FIG. 21–1. Lateral view of the right bony labyrinth.

vestibulocochlear (auditory) nerve leave the internal auditory meatus and are attached to the brain stem at the junction of the medulla and pons.

The delicate *membranous labyrinth* conforms, for the most part, to the contours of the bony labyrinth (Fig. 21–2). However, there are two dilations, the *utricle* and the *saccule*, in the vestibule of the bony labyrinth. Three *semicircular ducts* arise from the utricle. There is a patch of sensory epithelium supplied by the vestibular nerve on the inner surface of the utricle, the saccule, and each semicircular duct. The saccule is continuous with the *cochlear duct* through a narrow communication known as the ductus reuniens. The wall of the cochlear duct contains a highly specialized strip of sensory epithelium along its entire length; this is the organ of Corti,

which is the specific end-organ for hearing.

The lumen of the membranous labyrinth is continuous throughout and filled with endolymph, while the interval between the membranous and bony labyrinths is filled with *perilymph.* The vestibular portion of the membranous labyrinth is suspended within the bony labyrinth by trabeculae of connective tissue. However, the cochlear duct is firmly attached along two sides to the wall of the cochlear canal.

COCHLEA

The cochlea makes two and a half turns around a bony pillar or core, the *modiolus*, in which there are channels for nerve fibers and blood vessels. The cochlea is most conveniently described as resting on its base

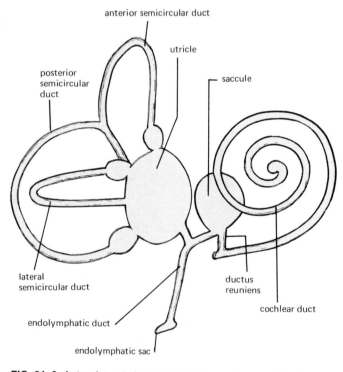

FIG. 21–2. Anterolateral view of the right membranous labyrinth.

(Fig. 21–3), although the latter in fact faces medially.

The cochlear canal is divided by two partitions into three spiral spaces. The middle of these (scala media) is the cochlear duct or that portion of the membranous labyrinth which is within the cochlea. The cochlear duct is firmly fixed to the inner and outer walls of the cochlear canal. The floor of the duct consists in part of the basilar membrane on which rests the organ of Corti; the cochlear duct is completed above by the thin vestibular or Reissner's membrane. The remaining spaces are the scala vestibuli above and the scala tympani below; they represent the lumen of the bony labyrinth and contain perilymph.

The basilar membrane is of special importance in the physiology of hearing because it responds to vibrations of the stapes in the following manner. As shown in Figure 21–4, vibrations of the foot-plate of the stapes produce resonant pressure or compression waves in the perilymph, beginning with that of the vestibule. The vestibule opens into the scala vestibuli and the latter communicates with the scala tympani through a small aperture, the helicotrema, at the apex of the cochlea. The pressure waves in the fluid produce vibrations in the membrane closing the round window, this

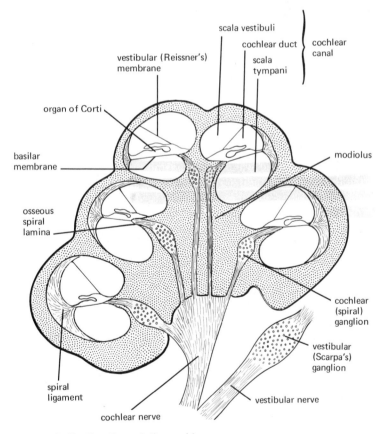

FIG. 21–3. Section through the cochlea.

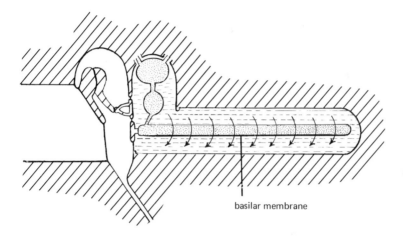

basilar membrane

FIG. 21–4. Schematic representation of the manner in which pressure waves in the perilymph and endolymph cause vibration of the basilar membrane.

being essential to eliminate the dampening effect of bone-encased fluid that would otherwise occur. The compression waves could be thought of as passing along the scala vestibuli and into the scala tympani through the helicotrema, causing vibration of the basilar membrane in transit through the scale tympani. However, the helicotrema is a minute orifice and it is more likely that the waves are transmitted from the scala vestibuli, across the cochlear duct and basilar membrane, to the scala tympani.

The scala vestibuli and scala tympani are lined by endosteal connective tissue where bounded by the bony labyrinth. All internal surfaces of the scalae are lined by a single layer of squamous cells of connective tissue origin. The perilymph filling the scalae is a watery fluid, similar in composition to cerebrospinal fluid. In fact, there is a narrow connection between the perilymph-filled spaces of the bony labyrinth and the subarachnoid space. The connection consists of a canal in the petrous bone, reaching from the scala tympani in the basal turn of the cochlea to an extension of the sub-

arachnoid space around the ninth, tenth, and eleventh cranial nerves as they traverse the jugular foramen.

The *cochlear* or *spiral ganglion* consists of cells grouped in a spiral arrangement at the periphery of the modiolus (Fig. 21–3). These primary sensory neurons are bipolar as are those of the vestibular ganglion, resembling immature sensory neurons in this respect. Bundles of dendrites enter the organ of Corti through small apertures in the osseous spiral lamina (see below), at which point myelin sheaths terminate. The myelinated axons traverse channels in the modiolus and enter the internal auditory meatus from the base of the cochlea to form the cochlear division of the eighth cranial nerve.

COCHLEAR DUCT

Certain specialized regions in the wall of the cochlear duct need to be described at this point (Fig. 21–5). The organ of Corti will be given separate consideration because of its complex structure and importance as the receptor of auditory stimuli.

Vibration of the *basilar membrane* is inherent in most theories that have been proposed to explain the transduction of a mechanical stimulus to the action potential of a nerve impulse in the organ of Corti. The inner edge of the basilar membrane is attached to the *osseous spiral lamina,* which projects from the modiolus like the thread on a screw. The outer edge of the membrane is attached to the *spiral ligament,* consisting of a thickening of the endosteum along the outer wall of the cochlear canal. The basilar membrane is made up of collagen fibers and sparse elastic fibers embedded in a ground substance, most of the fibers being directed across the membrane. The surface presenting to the scala tympani consists of a thin layer of connective tissue covered by squamous cells of mesenchymal origin. Contrary to what one might expect the basilar membrane is narrowest in the basal turn of the cochlea and widest at the apex. The width of the basilar membrane at any point determines the particular pitch to which the membrane at this point responds maximally. High tones therefore cause maximal vibration in the basal turn of the cochlea and low tones at the apex. The range of audible frequencies in the human ear is from 20 to 20,000 cps. (With advancing age there is a gradual decrease in perception of high frequencies.) The range extends over 11 octaves, of which 7 are used in musical instruments such as the piano. Ordinary conversation falls within the range of 300–3000 cps.

The *vestibular* or *Reissner's membrane* consists of two layers of simple squamous epithelium separated by a trace of connective tissue. The outer wall of the cochlear duct is specialized as the *stria vascularis* for production of endolymph. The epithelium here consists principally of cuboidal cells containing numerous mitochondria; capillaries extend into the epithelium from the underlying, vascular connective tissue. Endolymph is a rather viscous fluid; it is similar in composition to intracellular fluid in that there is a high concentration of potassium ions and a low concentration of sodium ions. Endolymph produced in the stria vascularis fills the membranous labyrinth; absorption takes place into venules surrounding the endolymphatic sac in the dura mater on the posterior surface of the petrous bone. This sac is an expansion of the endolymphatic duct arising from the communication between the saccule and the utricle (Fig. 21–2).

The epithelial lining of the membranous labyrinth, including the specialized sensory areas for the auditory and vestibular systems, is ectodermal in origin. The epithelium differentiates from the cells lining the otic vesicle, the latter being formed by an invagination of ectoderm at the level of the hindbrain of the early embryo.

ORGAN OF CORTI

The *organ of Corti* (Fig. 21–5) consists of cells specialized for a supporting role and sensory cells for conversion of a mechanical stimulus into the ionic and electrical events which constitute a nerve impulse.

Supporting cells containing bundles of tonofibrils are of two types, pillar cells and phalangeal cells. There are two rows of *pillar cells,* inner and outer, on either side of the *tunnel of Corti.* The number in each row is on the order of 5000, although the inner pillar cells are rather more numerous than the outer cells. Each cell consists mainly of a compact bundle of tonofibrils (the pillar), extending from the basilar membrane to the free surface of the organ of Corti. The tonofibrils appear in electron micrographs as compact arrays of microtubules. The inner and outer pillars converge and each ends in a flange directed outward, the flange of the inner pillar being

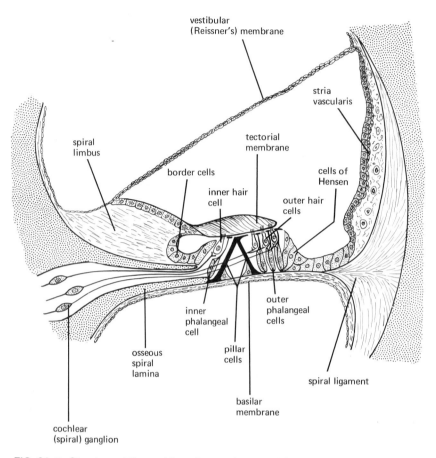

FIG. 21–5. Structure of the cochlear duct and organ of Corti.

above that of the outer pillar. The nucleus of the pillar cell is in a cytoplasmic region in the acute angle between the pillar and the basilar membrane.

The *phalangeal cells* afford intimate support for the sensory cells; they are arranged as a single row of inner phalangeal cells and three to five rows of outer phalangeal cells, the number of rows increasing from the base to the apex of the cochlea. The base of the slender, flask-shaped phalangeal cell rests on the basilar membrane, and a bundle of tonofibrils (microtubules) extends the length of the cell. Some of the

tonofibrils form a supporting shelf for the base of the shorter sensory cells, while the remainder continue alongside the sensory cell to the free surface of the organ of Corti. At this surface, the tonofibrils of phalangeal and pillar cells form a thin plate in which holes accommodate the ends of sensory cells. The organ of Corti is completed on the inner side by *border cells* and on the outer side by *cells of Hensen.*

The sensory cells are called *hair cells* because of peculiar hair-like projections from their free ends. There is a single row of inner hair cells, numbering about 7000;

the outer hair cells, of which there are some 25,000, are arranged in three rows in the basal turn of the cochlea, increasing to five rows at the apex. The hairs project from the cell along a V- or W-shaped line, their tips being embedded in the tectorial membrane. The number of hairs per cell varies from 50 to 150, the largest number being on hair cells at the base of the cochlea and the smallest number on cells at the apex. The hairs are microvilli of an unusual type; there is also a single cilium extending from a basal body, but the cilium disappears in the adult. The inner and outer hair cells differ not only in their position but also in certain details of ultrastructure and innervation. The roles of the inner and outer hair cells are probably different in some respects, although their separate contributions to auditory input to the brain have yet to be fully determined.

Dendritic terminals of primary sensory neurons are in synaptic contact with the hair cells. For the most part, a sensory neuron receives stimuli from a small group of hair cells, which is therefore the smallest sensory unit in the organ of Corti. However, the dendritic fields overlap so that a single hair cell is innervated by more than one neuron. The cochlear nerve includes efferent fibers originating in the superior olivary nucleus in the pons (see below). These fibers also terminate on the hair cells, on which they have a suppressor effect. The axonal terminals of the efferent fibers can be distinguished from dendritic terminals of cochlear ganglion cells in electron micrographs because the former contain synaptic vesicles. Probably because of minute holes in the basilar membrane, the fluid in the tunnel of Corti and the interstitial fluid in much of the organ of Corti has a chemical composition similar to that of perilymph rather than endolymph. The high concentration of potassium ions in endolymph would prevent impulse conduction along

the unmyelinated fibers crossing the tunnel of Corti to reach the outer hair cells.

The *tectorial membrane* is a ribbon-like structure consisting of a gelatinous type of connective tissue and attached to the *spiral limbus* or endosteal thickening on the osseous spiral lamina. The tectorial membrane extends over the organ of Corti and, as stated above, the tips of the hairs of the sensory cells are embedded in the membrane.

It is basic to the physiology of the cochlea that a particular region of the basilar membrane, depending on the tone or pitch of sound, responds by maximal vibration. Through a complex mechanism of transduction, bending of the hairs produces a change in the ionic polarization of the surface membrane of the hair cells and stimulation of dendritic terminals. Regardless of the pitch of sound, vibration of the basilar membrane begins at the base of the cochlea and travels along the membrane with increasing magnitude to a point determined by the pitch or tone. At this point the vibration suddenly dies away and impulses reaching the brain from the place of maximum stimulation of the organ of Corti are interpreted as a particular pitch or tone of sound. Tonotopic localization is sharpened by the suppressor effect of efferent fibers in the cochlear nerve and by feedback circuits in the central pathway to the auditory cortex. Increase in intensity of sound causes maximal vibration in a larger region of the basilar membrane, thereby activating more hair cells and neurons. Persistent exposure to excessively loud sounds is known to cause degenerative changes in the organ of Corti at the base of the cochlea. This results in high tone deafness, which is prone to occur in workers who are exposed to the sound of compression engines or jet engines, and in those who work for long hours on farm tractors. High tone deafness was formerly encountered most frequently among workmen in boiler factories and is still sometimes known as "boiler-makers' disease."

AUDITORY PATHWAYS

The cochlear nerve occupies the internal auditory meatus in company with the vestibular nerve (forming the auditory, vestibulocochlear, or eighth cranial nerve), the facial nerve, and the internal auditory artery. On emerging from the meatus, the cochlear nerve continues to the junction of the medulla and pons. The constituent fibers then bifurcate, one branch ending in the *dorsal cochlear nucleus* and the other branch in the *ventral cochlear nucleus*. The cochlear nuclei lie on the surface of the upper end of the medulla adjacent to the root of the inferior cerebellar peduncle (Fig. 21–6). A tonotopic pattern of axonal endings (from base to apex of the cochlea) has been demonstrated in both nuclei in experimental animals. Although such a pattern undoubtedly exists in man, the details have yet to be established. The dorsal and ventral cochlear nuclei differ in their cellular organization, and the pattern of axon endings in the ventral nucleus is more precise than in the dorsal nucleus. It is therefore probable that the two nuclei also differ in their contribution to the central pathways and to the overall functioning of the auditory system.

PATHWAY TO AUDITORY CORTEX

The pathway to the cortex is characterized by one or more synaptic relays between the cochlear nuclei and the specific thalamic nucleus for hearing, the medial geniculate nucleus (Fig. 21–6). There is an obligatory relay in the inferior colliculus, and additional synaptic interruptions may occur in the superior olivary nucleus or in the nucleus of the lateral lemniscus. The path-

way is also characterized by a significant ipsilateral projection to the cortex. In view of the complicated nature of the pathway the transmission of auditory data to the cortex can best be described after certain components of the pathway in the brain stem have been identified.

The small *superior olivary nucleus* is situated in the ventrolateral corner of the dorsal pons at the level of the motor nucleus of the facial nerve. Auditory fibers crossing the pons in the ventral part of the tegmentum constitute the *trapezoid body;* these auditory fibers pass ventral to the ascending fibers of the medial lemniscus or intersect these fibers. Cells scattered among the trapezoid fibers constitute the *nucleus of the trapezoid body,* whose connections are similar to those described below for the superior olivary nucleus. The *lateral lemniscus,* which is the principal ascending auditory tract, extends from the region of the superior olivary nucleus, through the lateral part of the pontine tegmentum, and close to the surface of the brain stem in the isthmus region between the pons and the midbrain. The *nucleus of the lateral lemniscus* consists of cells situated among the fibers of the tract in the pons.

The projection from the cochlear nuclei to the inferior colliculus and then to the medial geniculate nucleus, through the components of the pathway identified above, is as follows. Fibers from the *ventral cochlear nucleus* proceed to the region of the ipsilateral superior olivery nucleus, in which some of the fibers terminate. The majority continue across the pons, with a slight forward slope; these fibers, together with others contributed by the superior olivary nucleus constitute the trapezoid body. On reaching the region of the superior olivary nucleus on the other side of the brain stem the fibers either turn abruptly upward in the lateral lemniscus or terminate in the superior olivary nucleus, from which fibers are added to the lateral lem-

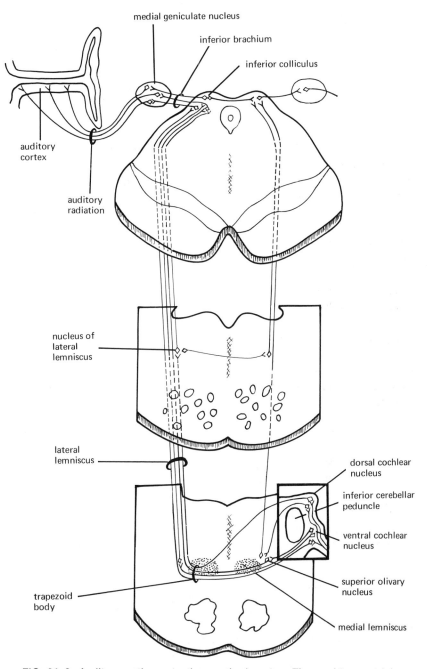

FIG. 21–6. Auditory pathway to the cerebral cortex. The cochlear nuclei are situated at a slightly lower level than that shown in the bottom-most section in this figure.

niscus. Fibers from the *dorsal cochlear nucleus* pass over the root of the inferior cerebellar peduncle and continue obliquely to the region of the contralateral superior olivary nucleus. Most of the fibers join the lateral lemniscus; the remainder end in the superior olivary nucleus, from which axons are contributed to the lateral lemniscus.

Impulses carried by the lateral lemniscus reach the *inferior colliculus* with or without a synaptic relay in the *nucleus of the lateral lemniscus*. Fibers from the inferior colliculus traverse the inferior brachium and end in the *medial geniculate nucleus*. (A few auditory fibers of the lateral lemniscus have been described as by-passing the inferior colliculus and proceeding directly through the inferior brachium to the medial geniculate nucleus. However, the existence of fibers thus identified is in question.) The termination of axons in the medial geniculate nucleus of experimental animals is such as to produce a spiral pattern for tones corresponding to the spiral of the cochlea, and a similar pattern is probably present in man. Some awareness of sounds is known to occur at the thalamic level in subprimates. However, any conscious appreciation of sounds at subcortical levels is minimal at best in man.

The last link in the auditory pathway consists of the *auditory radiation* in the sublenticular portion of the internal capsule, through which the medial geniculate nucleus projects on the *auditory cortex* of the temporal lobe. The auditory area, which consists of areas 41 and 42 of Brodmann, is in the floor of the lateral fissure, extending only slightly on the lateral surface of the hemisphere. A landmark is provided by the two most anterior of the transverse temporal gyri (Heschl's convolutions) on the upper surface of the superior temporal gyrus. The tonotopic pattern in the auditory area is such that fibers for sounds of low frequency end in the anterolateral part of the area while those for high frequency sounds terminate in the posteromedial part of the auditory cortex. Analysis of auditory stimuli at a higher neural level, notably the recognition and interpretation of sounds on the basis of past experience, occurs in the auditory association cortex of the temporal lobe, also known as Wernicke's area. This area makes an important contribution to sensory aspects of language.

The auditory pathway is described above as an entirely crossed pathway, yet it is well known that deafness in the opposite ear does not ensue from unilateral destruction of the auditory cortex. There is, instead, slight diminution in acuity of hearing in both ears, most noticeably in the opposite ear, together with some difficulty in judging the direction and distance of the source of sounds. The impairment may not be detected unless special audiometric tests are used. These observations are explained in part by a contribution to the lateral lemniscus from the ipsilateral cochlear nuclei, probably with a synapse in the superior olivary nucleus. A bilateral cortical projection from each organ of Corti is also provided by interneurons establishing cross-connections between the nuclei of the lateral lemniscus and between the inferior colliculi (Fig. 21–6).

DESCENDING FIBERS IN THE AUDITORY PATHWAY

Parallel with the neurons conducting information from the organ of Corti to the auditory cortex, there are descending and efferent neurons conducting impulses in the opposite direction thereby providing for feedback circuits. These consist of a complement of nerve fibers connecting the auditory and adjacent cortex with the medial geniculate nucleus and the inferior colliculus; others run from the geniculate nucleus to the inferior colliculus. Finally, fibers from the inferior colliculus proceed to the cochlear nuclei and the superior olivary nucleus. The *olivocochlear bundle of Rasmussen* is a predominantly crossed bundle originating in the superior olivary nucleus. The fibers leave the brain stem with the vestibular nerve, join the cochlear nerve in the internal auditory meatus, and terminate as synaptic end-bulbs on hair cells of the organ of Corti. The central transmission of data from the sensory hair cells is therefore far more than just a relay to the cortex. In the various cell stations of the pathway, there is a complex processing of auditory data, providing for refinement of such qualities as pitch, timbre, and volume of sound perception. In particular, feedback inhibition sharpens tone perception, especially through the efferent bundle of Rasmussen. This is accomplished by suppression of impulses from regions of the organ of Corti other than the particular region in which the basilar membrane is responding by maximal vibration to a particular tone (auditory sharpening).

AUDITORY REFLEXES

Connections provide for reflex turning of the head and eyes toward the source of sounds, one such pathway being through the tectum of the midbrain. Impulses are relayed from the inferior to the superior colliculus, where they reach nuclei controlling extraocular muscles and motor neurons of the cervical cord through tectobulbar connections and the tectospinal tract. There is an additional reflex pathway for ocular responses to auditory stimuli, which begins as fibers from the superior olivary nucleus in a small bundle known as the *peduncle of the superior olive*. Some of these fibers terminate in the abducens nucleus while others join the medial longitudinal fasciculus and end in the trochlear and oculomotor nuclei. Fibers from the superior olivary nucleus, and probably the nucleus of the lateral lemniscus, terminate in the motor nuclei of the trigeminal and facial nerves for reflex contraction of the tensor tympani and stapedius muscles, respectively. Contraction of these muscles in response to loud sounds dampens the vibration of the tympanic membrane and the stapes. As noted earlier in the appropriate chapters, both auditory and visual data reach the cerebellum and the reticular formation of the brain stem.

SUGGESTIONS FOR ADDITIONAL READING

Dallos P, Billone MC, Durrant JD, Wong C-y, Raynor S: Cochlear inner and outer hair cells: Functional differences. Science 177:356–358, 1972

Engström H, Wersäll J: Structure and innervation of the inner ear sensory epithelia. Int Rev Cytol 7:535–585, 1958

Friedmann I: The cytology of the ear. Br Med Bull 18:209–213, 1962

Galambos R: Neural mechanisms of audition. Physiol Rev 34:497–528, 1954

Goldberg JM, Moore RY: Ascending projections of the lateral lemniscus in the cat and monkey. J Comp Neurol 129:143–155, 1967

Hawkins JE Jr, Johnsson L-G: Light microscopic observations in the inner ear in man and monkey. Ann Otol Rhinol Laryngol 77:608–628, 1968

Kimura RS, Schuknecht HF, Sando I: Fine morphology of the sensory cells in the organ of Corti of man. Acta Otolaryngol (Stockh) 58:390–408, 1965

Rasmussen GL, Windle WF (eds.): Neural Mechanisms of the Auditory and Vestibular Systems. Springfield, Ill., Thomas, 1960

Smith CA: Electron microscopy of the inner ear. Ann Otol Rhinol Laryngol 77:629–643, 1968

Smith CA, Rasmussen GL: Recent observations on the olivocochlear bundle. Ann Otol Rhinol Laryngol 72:489–506, 1963

Whitfield IC: The Auditory Pathway. Monographs of the Physiological Society, No. 17. London, Arnold, 1967

22

Vestibular System

Three principal sources of sensory information are used by the nervous system for the purpose of maintaining equilibrium. These are the eyes, proprioceptive endings throughout the body, and the vestibular portion of the inner ear. The role of the vestibular system, vis-à-vis visual information especially, is illustrated by the individual with congenital atresia of the vestibular apparatus, usually accompanied by cochlear atresia and deaf-mutism. A person so afflicted is able to orient himself satisfactorily by visual guidance, but becomes disoriented in the dark or if submerged while swimming. In addition, vestibular impulses signaling movements of the head cause appropriate movements of the eyes to maintain visual fixation on an object. In order to serve the above functions with respect to equilibrium and coordination of head and eye movements, impulses from the vestibular labyrinth are distributed to motor neurons through reflex pathways in the spinal cord, brain stem, and cerebellum. There is also a cortical projection, the details of which are not fully known.

The peripheral vestibular apparatus consists of two parts which differ in certain structural and functional aspects. The *static labyrinth* represented by the utricle and saccule signals the position of the head in space and influences chiefly the distribution of muscle tone throughout the body. The *kinetic labyrinth* consists of the three semicircular ducts; it signals movements of the head and has a special relationship to ocular movements in order to maintain visual fixation.

STATIC LABYRINTH

The *utricle* and *saccule* are endolymph-containing dilations of the membranous labyrinth, enclosed by the vestibule of the bony labyrinth (Figs. 21–1 and 21–2). Except at the maculae or specialized sensory areas, the utricle and saccule are lined by

310

simple cuboidal epithelium which is derived from the otic vesicle of the embryo and supported by a thin lamina propria of connective tissue. The utricle and saccule are suspended from the wall of the vestibule by connective tissue trabeculae, and they are surrounded by a perilymphatic space lined by a single layer of squamous cells (mesenchymal epithelium).

Each dilation includes a specialized area of sensory epithelium, the macula, about 2 by 3 mm in size. The *macula utriculi* is in the floor of the utricle and parallel with the base of the skull, while the *macula sacculi* is vertically disposed on the medial wall of the saccule. The two maculae are identical in histologic structure, that of the utricle being illustrated in Figure 22–1.

The columnar *supporting cells* of the maculae are continuous with the low cuboidal epithelium lining the utricle and saccule elsewhere. The sensory *hair cells*, of which two types have been identified in electron micrographs, are basically similar to hair cells of the organ of Corti. Type 1 hair cells are flask-shaped with a round base and a constricted neck region; type 2 cells have a more slender and uniform shape. From 40 to 80 straight hairs project from each cell together with a single cilium arising from a basal body (Fig. 22–2A). The hairs are microvilli of an unusual type, like those of hair cells of the organ of Corti except for their greater length (up to 100 μ). The hairs are embedded in the *otolithic membrane,* which consists of gelatinous, noncellular material and contains crystals of calcium carbonate and protein (otoliths).

The bipolar cell bodies of the primary sensory neurons are in the *vestibular ganglion,* also known as Scarpa's ganglion, at the bottom of the internal auditory meatus. The dendrites enter the maculae, with loss

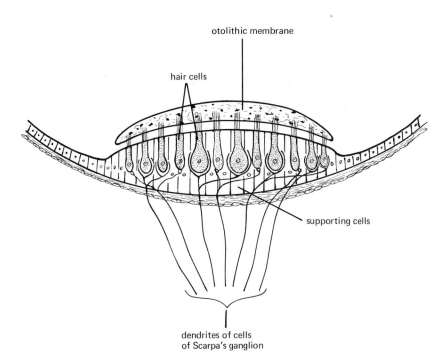

otolithic membrane

hair cells

supporting cells

dendrites of cells
of Scarpa's ganglion

FIG. 22–1. Structure of the sensory area of the utricle.

of myelin sheaths while traversing the lamina propria, and end on the hair cells. The dendritic terminals on type 1 hair cells take the form of chalice-like expansions surrounding the cells, while minute terminal swellings of dendrites make contact with type 2 hair cells. In addition, efferent fibers in the vestibular nerve terminate as synaptic end-bulbs on the hair cells.

The otoliths give the otolithic membrane a higher specific gravity than the endolymph, thereby causing bending of the hairs in one or another direction except when the macula is in a strictly horizontal

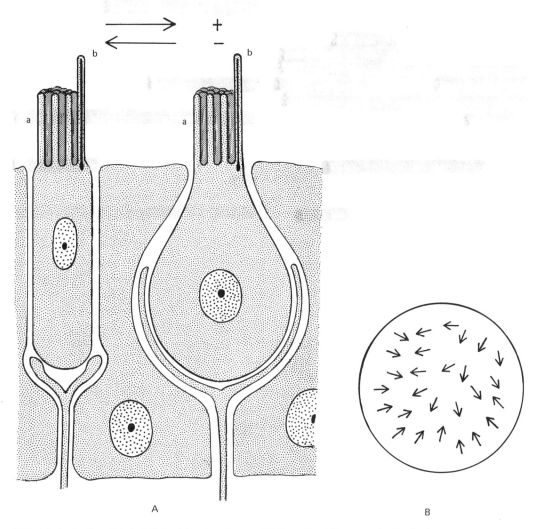

FIG. 22–2. *A.* Simplified sketch of the two types of hair cells of the macula. Excitation occurs when the hairs or microvilli (a) are bent in the direction of the cilium (b), while inhibition of the hair cells occurs when the bending of the hairs is in the opposite direction. *B.* Surface of the macula, showing that hair cells in different regions are stimulated and different nerve fibers activated according to the direction of gravitational pull on the otolithic membrane. This pattern results from variations in the position of the cilium relative to the tuft of hairs from one region of the macula to another.

plane. The detailed sensory output of the macula is, however, quite complicated. In each hair cell the cilium lies to one side of the tuft of hairs, and the position of the cilium around the periphery of the hairs differs from one region of the macula to another. The hair cells are excited when the hairs are bent in the direction of the cilium and they are inhibited when there is bending of the hairs in the opposite direction (Fig. 22–2A). The pattern of afferent impulses conducted by the constituent fibers of the vestibular nerve to the vestibular nuclei and cerebellum differs, therefore, according to the orientation of the macula to the direction of gravitational pull (Fig. 22–2B). Appropriate changes in muscle tonus follow, depending on the particular position of the head.

Although primarily static organs, signaling the position of the head in space, the maculae also respond to quick tilting movements and to linear acceleration and deceleration. Motion sickness is caused predominantly by prolonged, fluctuating stimulation of the maculae. The utricle and saccule are not as efficient sensors of orientation in man as they are in lower animals. This is illustrated by the pilot of a small aircraft flying through clouds without instruments, who may emerge from a cloud bank upside down without having been aware of changing orientation.

KINETIC LABYRINTH

The three semicircular ducts are attached to the utricle and enclosed in the semicircular canals of the bony labyrinth (Figs. 21–1 and 21–2). The *anterior* and *posterior semicircular ducts* lie in vertical planes, the former being transverse to and the latter parallel with, the long axis of the petrous temporal bone. The *lateral semicircular duct* slopes downward and backward at an angle of 30 degrees with the horizontal. The ducts of the two sides form spatial pairs; the horizontal ducts are in the same plane while the anterior duct of one side and the opposite posterior duct are in corresponding planes. The sensory areas of the semicircular ducts respond only to movement, the response being maximal when movement is in the plane of the duct.

Each duct has an expansion or *ampulla* at one end, in which a *crista* of sensory epithelium covers a transverse septum formed by a thickening of the lamina propria (Fig. 22–3). Among the columnar supporting cells are situated the sensory *hair cells*, whose structural details conform to those described above for hair cells of the static labyrinth. The hairs are embedded in gelatinous material forming the *cupula*, in which otoliths are lacking.

The cristae are sensors of movement, as has been indicated. More specifically, they

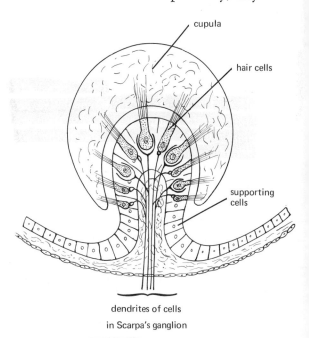

cupula

hair cells

supporting cells

dendrites of cells

in Scarpa's ganglion

FIG. 22–3. Structure of the sensory area of a semicircular duct.

respond to changes in the direction of movement often called angular movement or angular rotation, especially when accompanied by acceleration or deceleration. Rotation as slow as 2 degrees a second can be detected and the direction interpreted. During such movement in or near the plane of a semicircular duct, the endolymph lags because of inertia and the cupula swings like a door in a direction opposite to that of head movement. The momentum of the endolymph causes the cupula to swing momentarily in the opposite direction when the head stops. The hairs of the sensory cells bend accordingly, initiating a process of transduction which alters the electrical polarization of the surface membrane of the hair cells.

The cilium is consistently on the side of the tuft of hairs nearest the opening of the ampulla into the utricle. Excitation of the hair cells therefore occurs when the flow of endolymph is from the ampulla into the adjacent utricle, while there is inhibition of the hair cells when the flow is in the opposite direction. (There is a slight tonic discharge from the hair cells of both the maculae and the cristae even in the absence of bending of the hairs.) The hair cells of the cristae like those of the maculae are supplied by primary sensory neurons whose bipolar cell bodies are in the *vestibular ganglion.* The pattern of nerve fiber conduction, i.e., the particular fibers of the vestibular nerve that are conducting impulses to the vestibular nuclei and cerebellum at any given moment, varies according to the direction of head movement.

VESTIBULAR PATHWAYS

On entering the brain stem at the junction of the medulla and pons, most of the vestibular nerve fibers bifurcate in the usual manner of afferent fibers and end in the vestibular nuclear complex. The remaining fibers enter the cerebellum through the juxtarestiform body of the inferior cerebellar peduncle.

VESTIBULAR NUCLEI

The *vestibular nuclei* are situated beneath the area vestibuli, which makes up the lateral part of the floor of the fourth ventricle (Fig. 22–4). Four vestibular nuclei are recognized on the basis of cytoarchitecture and the details of afferent and efferent connections. The *lateral vestibular nucleus,* also known as *Deiters' nucleus,* consists mainly of large multipolar neurons; they have widely branching dendrites, long axons, and prominent Nissl bodies, resembling typical motor neurons. The *superior, medial,* and *inferior vestibular nuclei* consist of small and medium-sized cells. In transverse sections stained by the Weigert method the inferior nucleus can be identified by the presence of fine fasciculi consisting of the descending branches of vestibular nerve fibers.

CONNECTIONS WITH THE CEREBELLUM

The vestibular portion of the cerebellum or *archicerebellum* consists of the flocculonodular lobe, the adjacent region (uvula) of the inferior vermis, and the fastigial nuclei. The archicerebellum receives fibers from the superior, medial, and inferior vestibular nuclei in addition to a modest number of fibers directly from the vestibular nerve. In the reverse direction fibers from the archicerebellum terminate throughout the vestibular nuclear complex. The role of the archicerebellum in maintaining equilibrium is exerted through pathways from vestibular nuclei to lower motor neurons, and through cerebelloreticular and reticulospinal connections. The cortex of the *paleocerebellum,* which influences muscle tonus in the context of posture and locomotion, projects to the fastigial, globose, and emboliform nuclei of the cerebellum. The paleocerebellum therefore influences the musculature through both the vestibular nuclear complex and the red nucleus. The afferent input to, and the efferent output from, the archicerebellum are mediated through nerve fibers in the juxtarestiform body or medial portion of the inferior cerebellar peduncle.

CONNECTIONS WITH THE SPINAL CORD

The principal connections between the vestibular nuclei and the spinal cord are descending fibers in the vestibulospinal tract and the medial longitudinal fasciculus. However, clinical findings suggest that the vestibular nuclei receive *spinovestibular fibers.* These apparently ascend in the ventral white column of the cord in the region assigned to the vestibulospinal tract and probably convey impulses from touch, pressure, and proprioceptive endings. It has been known for a long time that syringomyelia or a lesion pressing on the ventral cord, when involving the second to fourth cervical segments, may produce nystagmus in addition to the anticipated neurologic signs. (Nystagmus is an oscillatory movement of the eyes and is discussed further below.) It is probable that the nystagmus is caused by irritation of spinovestibular fibers and disturbance of the normal flow of impulses from the vestibular nuclei to nuclei controlling extraocular muscles.

Of the two tracts projecting from the vestibular nuclei to the spinal cord, the vestibulospinal tract (also known as the lateral vestibulospinal tract) extends the length of the cord; the descending portion of the medial longitudinal fasciculus (also known as the medial vestibulospinal tract) is limited to the cervical region of the cord.

The *vestibulospinal tract,* which is uncrossed, originates in the lateral vestibular or Deiters' nucleus exclusively. The fibers traverse the medulla dorsal to the inferior olivary nucleus and continue into the ventral white column of the cord. Vestibulospinal fibers terminate on alpha and gamma motor neurons at all levels of the spinal cord, but most abundantly in the regions of the cervical and lumbosacral enlargements. This tract is of prime importance in regulating muscle tone throughout the body in such a manner that balance is maintained.

Fibers from the medial vestibular nucleus, perhaps with some contribution from the inferior nucleus, project toward the midline and turn caudally in the *medial longitudinal fasciculi* of both sides. This fasciculus is adjacent to the midline, close to the floor of the fourth ventricle, and just ventral to the central canal of the medulla more caudally. The fibers continue into the sulcomarginal fasciculus of the ventral white column of the cord, terminating on ventral horn cells throughout the cervical region. The white matter referred to topographically as the medial longitudinal fasciculus in the medulla and the sulcomarginal fasciculus in the cord includes, in addition to vestibulospinal fibers, reticulospinal fibers and other descending axons from small nuclei in the midbrain. The medial bundle of vestibulospinal fibers just described provides for changes in the tonus of neck muscles as required to support the head in various positions and during head movements. The pathway may also function in reflex arm movements as appropriate to maintain balance.

CONNECTIONS WITHIN THE BRAIN STEM

The ascending portion of the *medial longitudinal fasciculus* is situated adjacent to

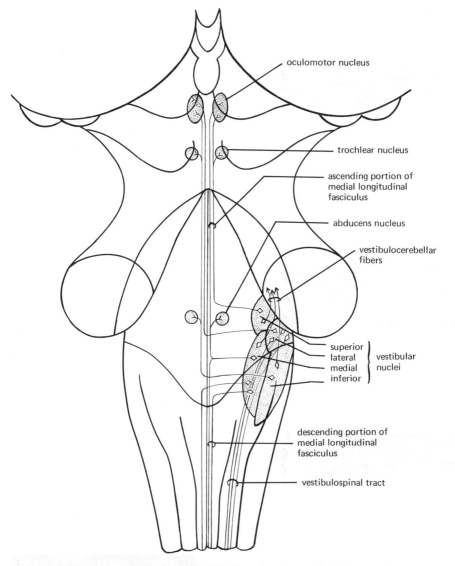

oculomotor nucleus

trochlear nucleus

ascending portion of
medial longitudinal
fasciculus

abducens nucleus

vestibulocerebellar
fibers

superior ⎫
lateral ⎬ vestibular
medial   ⎬ nuclei
inferior ⎭

descending portion of
medial longitudinal
fasciculus

vestibulospinal tract

FIG. 22–4. Vestibular pathways to the spinal cord and nuclei of the abducens, trochlear, and oculomotor nerves.

the midline in the pons and midbrain, just
ventral to the floor of the fourth ventricle
and the periaqueductal gray matter further
forward. The constituent fibers connect the
vestibular nuclei with the nuclei of
the abducens, trochlear, and oculomotor
nerves. More specifically, fibers from the
superior vestibular nucleus are uncrossed;
those from the lateral and inferior nuclei
are crossed, and the medial vestibular
nucleus contributes fibers to both fasciculi
(Fig. 22–4). This portion of the medial
longitudinal fasciculus provides for synchronized or conjugate movements of the
eyes, coordinated with movements of the
head, in order to maintain visual fixation.

Such coordination relies heavily on information received by the vestibular nuclei from the semicircular ducts or kinetic labyrinth.

The vestibular control of eye movements needs to be considered in the larger context of multiple neural mechanisms that bear on movements of the eyes. These include the frontal eye field for volitional scanning movements and visual association cortex for automatic scanning movements. There are also connections for reflex turning of the eyes toward the source of visual and auditory stimuli, and the vestibular coordination of eye and head movements described above. It should be noted that the precise synchronization of ocular movements and position as required for binocular vision is controlled in the brain stem, notably through fibers in the medial longitudinal fasciculus. In addition to the vestibular fibers just described, the fasciculus includes axons of internuncial neurons connecting the three cranial nerve nuclei supplying the extraocular muscles. A "center for lateral gaze" is postulated in the pons for specific coordination of the lateral rectus muscle of one eye with the medial rectus muscle of the other eye. The center may consist of a group of neurons in the reticular formation adjacent to the abducens nucleus, and it is therefore called the *parabducens nucleus.* This nucleus is thought to send fibers to the adjacent abducens nucleus while other fibers run in the medial longitudinal fasciculus to cells of the contralateral oculomotor nucleus supplying the medial rectus muscle. Lesions involving the parabducens nucleus or the medial longitudinal fasciculus rostral to this nucleus result in paralysis of lateral gaze.

Excessive or prolonged stimulation of the vestibular system may result in nausea and vomiting. The connections responsible for these effects appear to be collateral branches of efferent fibers from vestibular nuclei; the branches end mainly in the autonomic centers in the reticular formation of the brain stem. Excessive input from the labyrinth to the vestibular nuclei is probably reduced to some extent by a feedback through efferent fibers of the vestibular nerve. These fibers, which are of small caliber and few in number compared with afferent fibers, originate in the vestibular nuclei and possibly the fastigial nucleus. They terminate on hair cells of the maculae and cristae, on which they have an inhibitory effect.

CORTICAL REPRESENTATION

Although the vestibular system functions mainly at brain stem, cerebellar, and spinal cord levels, there is a poorly understood projection from the vestibular nuclei to the cerebral cortex. Evoked potentials have been recorded in the parietal lobe of the monkey during electrical stimulation of the vestibular nerve. The vestibular area thus identified is situated in the lower part of the postcentral gyrus, immediately behind the general sensory area for the head. There are reports of sensations of rotation or bodily displacement being elicited in man by stimulation of the parietal lobe. The vestibular cortical field probably contributes information for higher motor regulation and conscious spatial orientation. The pathway from the vestibular nuclei to the parietal cortex has not been established. There is presumably a relay in the thalamus, possibly in the medial part of the ventral posterior nucleus along with other sensory data from the head, although this is only conjecture.

It is frequently stated that the vestibular area is located in the superior temporal gyrus in front of the auditory area. This statement is based on the occasional occurrence of vertigo or of a feeling of dizziness on electrical stimulation of the superior temporal gyrus in conscious patients. The close anatomic relationship between the vestibular and auditory systems in the membranous labyrinth seemed to support the concept of adjoining cortical areas. However, the vestibular system is essentially proprioceptive in function and the presence of a cortical area in the parietal lobe is entirely plausible on physiologic grounds. The cortical projection of vestibular data is obviously in need of further investigation.

SOME CLINICAL CONSIDERATIONS

The vestibular projections to the spinal cord and brain stem nuclei can be demonstrated by strong stimulation of the labyrinth. This may be done by rotating a person around a vertical axis about 10 times in 20 seconds, then stopping the rotation abruptly. The responses are most pronounced if the head is bent forward 30 degrees to bring the lateral semicircular ducts in a horizontal plane. On stopping rotation, the endolymph flows past the cupulae because of inertia. Displacement of the cupulae bends the hairs of the sensory hair cells and there is a sudden increase in the rate of firing of nerve fibers supplying the crista of the right or left horizontal semicircular duct, depending on the direction of rotation.

The following signs appear on stopping rotation. Impulses carried by the ascending fibers of the medial longitudinal fasciculus cause nystagmus, i.e., a conjugate movement of the eyes consisting of alternating fast and slow components. The direction of nystagmus, right or left, is designated by that of the fast component which is opposite to the direction of rotation. The fast component is generally considered to be a compensatory reaction mediated by corticobulbar connections. However, both components persist in experimental animals following transection at the rostral end of the midbrain, indicating that the fast component is triggered by a center in the brain stem. The individual serving as a subject deviates in the direction of rotation if asked to walk on a straight line, and the finger deviates in the same direction on pointing to an object. These responses are caused by the effect of vestibulospinal projections on muscle tonus. There is a subjective feeling of turning in a direction opposite to that of rotation, for which the cortical projection is presumably responsible. The spread of impulses to visceral centers may produce sweating and pallor, and even nausea in more susceptible persons.

It is necessary at times to test for the integrity of the vestibular system. The need arises, for example, when there are reasons to suspect a tumor of the eighth cranial nerve or brain stem damage of traumatic or other origin. The caloric test is used. This test involves in principle the setting up of convection currents in the endolymph of the semicircular ducts by irrigating the external auditory canal with warm or cold water. Each side is tested separately, the examiner noting whether the normal vestibular responses to strong stimulation, notably nystagmus, are present. Tests of vestibular function are directed to the kinetic labyrinth; no test of the static labyrinth has been designed for standard clinical use. Labyrinthine irritation or disease causes vertigo, sometimes accompanied by nausea and vomiting. There may also be pallor, a cold sweat, and nystagmus. Paroxysms of labyrinthine irritation constitute Ménière's syndrome, the cause of which is usually obscure.

SUGGESTIONS FOR ADDITIONAL READING

Brodal A, Pompeiano O, Walberg F: The Vestibular Nuclei and Their Connections, Anatomy and Functional Anatomy. Edinburgh, Oliver & Boyd, 1962

Christoff N, Anderson PJ, Nathanson M, Bender MB: Problems in anatomic analysis of lesions of the medial longitudinal fasciculus. Arch Neurol 2:293–304, 1960

Engström H, Wersäll H: The ultrastructural organization of the organ of Corti and of the vestibular sensory epithelia. Exp Cell Res (suppl) 5:460–492, 1958

Flock Å: Structure of the macula utriculi with special reference to directional interplay of sensory responses as revealed by morphological polarization. J Cell Biol 22:413–431, 1964

Fredrickson JM, Figge U, Schied P, Kornhuber HH: Vestibular nerve projection to the cerebral cortex of the rhesus monkey. Exp Brain Res 2:318–327, 1966

Mickle WA, Ades HW: Rostral projection pathway of the vestibular system. Am J Physiol 176:243–246, 1954

Penfield W: Vestibular sensation and the cerebral cortex. Ann Otol Rhinol Laryngol 66:691–698, 1957

Rasmussen GL, Windle WF (eds.): Neural Mechanisms of the Auditory and Vestibular Systems. Springfield, Ill., Thomas, 1960

23

Motor Systems

Overt expression of activity within the central nervous system depends on the motor or efferent neurons supplying somatic muscles and viscera. The control of motor neurons for the skeletal musculature, although discussed in a fragmentary way in earlier chapters, is summarized in this chapter because of the importance of the motor systems in clinical neurology. The efferent supply of viscera through the autonomic nervous system is discussed in the following chapter.

Neurons supplying the somatic muscles are situated in motor nuclei of cranial nerves and the ventral gray horns of the spinal cord. Known as "lower motor neurons," they are also said to constitute a "final common pathway" (Sherrington) through which the pyramidal and extrapyramidal systems exert their final control over motor activity. The presence of a pyramidal system is essentially restricted to the mammalian class because the cells of origin are confined to the neocortex. The

extrapyramidal system is much more complex; it includes several regions of gray matter and their connections, most of which antedate the pyramidal system in phylogeny.

PYRAMIDAL SYSTEM

The *pyramidal system* is responsible for certain aspects of voluntary movement (the contributions of the pyramidal and extrapyramidal systems to voluntary motor activity are discussed at the conclusion of the chapter). The term "pyramidal tract" refers specifically to the corticospinal tract which occupies the pyramid of the medulla. However, the corticobulbar tract has the same relationship to motor nuclei of cranial nerves as does the corticospinal tract with respect to ventral horn cells of the cord. Both tracts are therefore included under the heading "pyramidal system."

CORTICAL AREAS FOR PYRAMIDAL PATHWAYS

All the pyramidal fibers originate in the neocortex, but their source is not restricted to a single cytoarchitectural or functional area. The main area, however, is the primary motor cortex in the precentral gyrus of the frontal lobe, and extending on the paracentral lobule of the medial surface of the hemisphere (Figs. 15–1 and 15–2). A large proportion of this area occupies the anterior wall of the central or rolandic sulcus. The primary motor cortex contributes about 40 percent of the fibers of the pyramidal system.

The lowest cortical threshold of electrical stimulation for eliciting motor responses is found in the primary motor area, i.e., area 4 of Brodmann. This cortex is thicker (4.5 mm) than elsewhere and contains a wealth of pyramidal cells which obscure the six-layered pattern of much of the neocortex. Area 4 is therefore included in heterotypical agranular cortex. Giant pyramidal cells of Betz are present in the fifth or ganglionic layer of this primary motor cortex. Excitation of area 4 is reflected in the contralateral musculature primarily. This is especially true of muscles of the extremities and most of the facial muscles; there is clinically significant ipsilateral control (in addition to contralateral) of many of the muscles of the head, neck, and trunk. A somatotopic representation within the area has been demonstrated by electrical stimulation of the human brain during neurosurgical procedures. The head is represented in the lower third of area 4, a large portion being assigned to muscles used in speech. Proceeding dorsally there is a large region for muscles of the hand, followed by representation of the arm, shoulder, trunk, and thigh. The remainder of the lower extremity together with anal and vesical sphincters is represented in the paracentral lobule on the medial aspect of the hemisphere. The relatively large portions of area 4 assigned to those parts of the body with the capacity for finer and highly controlled movements reflect the increased number of underlying cortical cells that are associated with such movements.

The somesthetic cortex of the postcentral gyrus and paracentral lobule (areas 3, 1, 2 of Brodmann) contributes about 20 percent of the fibers of the pyramidal system. Also, since sensory responses can be elicited by stimulation of the precentral gyrus a strict dichotomy between the motor and general sensory areas is lacking. They should be considered instead as a sensorimotor strip with overlapping functions, surrounding the central sulcus. Of the remaining pyramidal fibers, the main source is premotor cortex of the frontal lobe (areas 6 and 8). Additional fibers originate in areas 5 and 7 of the parietal lobe; there may be still others from cortical areas not yet identified.

CORTICOBULBAR TRACT (Fig. 23–1)

Medullated axons from the lower third of area 4, together with contributions from adjacent areas as noted above, traverse the corona radiata of the medullary center and the internal capsule. Formerly thought to traverse the genu of the internal capsule, the corticobulbar fibers are now known to pass through the posterior limb where they are situated at about the junction of the anterior two-thirds and the posterior third of the lenticulothalamic region of the internal capsule. The fibers continue into the basis pedunculi of the midbrain where small bundles separate off immediately for the oculomotor and trochlear nuclei. The middle three-fifths of the basis pedunculi consists of corticospinal fibers. Corticobulbar fibers for nuclei of cranial nerves in the pons and medulla run along the medial side of the corticospinal tract, i.e., between the corticospinal and frontopontine tracts. The corticospinal tract continues through the basilar pons and medullary pyramid, but bundles of corticobulbar fibers diverge at intervals to supply motor nuclei of cranial nerves in the pons and medulla. These consist of the motor nucleus of the trigeminal nerve, the abducens nucleus, the motor nucleus of the facial nerve, the nucleus ambiguus for the glossopharyngeal, vagus, and accessory nerves, and the hypoglossal nucleus. With few exceptions, intercalated neurons in the reticular formation intervene between the corticobulbar fibers and lower motor neurons in the cranial nerve nuclei.

The majority of corticobulbar fibers cross to the opposite side of the brain stem; cortical control of the musculature of the head through this system is therefore predominantly contralateral. However, significant ipsilateral connections exist, and voluntary paralysis of most of the muscles following a unilateral lesion involving the corticobulbar system is thereby usually prevented. In fact, there is exclusive contralateral control only for the motor nucleus of the facial nerve, and even there the cells supplying the frontalis and orbicularis oculi muscles come under bilateral cortical control. A unilateral corticobulbar lesion such as may occur in the cortex, corona radiata, or internal capsule, results in paralysis of the opposite side of the face, except that the patient is able to raise the eyebrow and close the eyelids.

The motor nucleus of the trigeminal nerve and the hypoglossal nucleus receive a moderate number of ipsilateral cortical afferents. There is nearly always weakness (paresis) rather than paralysis of voluntary contraction of the muscles of mastication and tongue muscles on the side opposite the lesion; detection of the deficit may be difficult. The oculomotor, trochlear, and abducens nuclei come under still more sub-

stantial bilateral cortical control, and voluntary eye movements are therefore preserved in the presence of a unilateral corticobulbar lesion. However, fibers from the frontal eye field (lower part of area 8) may be interrupted in such a lesion, resulting in paralysis of contralateral gaze and even transient deviation of the eyes to the side of an acute lesion. Muscles of the soft palate, larynx, and pharynx function satisfactorily following a one-sided corticobulbar lesion because the nucleus ambiguus receives a substantial number of afferents from the ipsilateral cortex in addition to a larger number from the opposite side. As noted later in the chapter, extrapyramidal projections to lower motor neurons must also be taken into consideration when dealing with the physiologic basis of voluntary motor action and voluntary motor paralysis.

CORTICOSPINAL TRACT (Fig. 23–1)

Emanating from the upper two-thirds of area 4, from the premotor area, and from cortex of the parietal lobe, myelinated corticospinal fibers traverse the corona radiata and the posterior third of the lenticulothalamic portion of the internal capsule. (These fibers were previously thought to be further forward in the internal capsule.) The tract continues through the middle three-fifths of the basis pedunculi of the midbrain and is broken up into many fasciculi on traversing the basilar pons. At the latter site the bundles are separated by accumulations of cells of the pontine nuclei and by transverse strands of pontocerebellar fibers. The fasciculi coalesce in the lower pons, caudal to which they constitute the corticospinal tract in the pyramid of the medulla. There is considerable intermingling of the corticospinal fibers that influence the musculature of different parts of the body. Nevertheless, in the internal capsule fibers for the neck and upper extremity

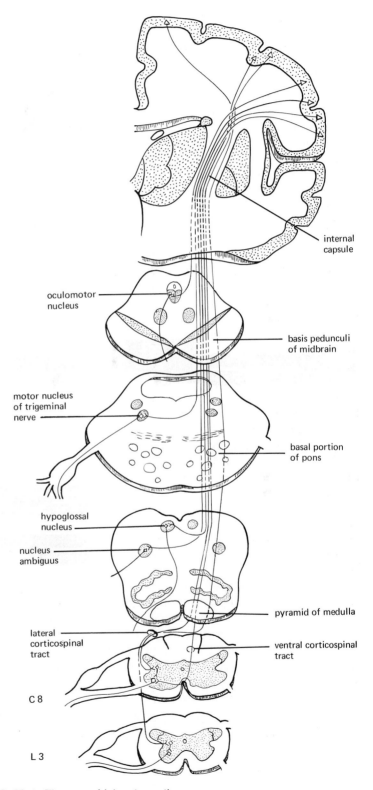

FIG. 23–1. The pyramidal motor pathway.

are concentrated in the anterior part of the region containing corticospinal fibers, followed by fibers for the trunk and then the lower extremity. Throughout the brain stem fibers for the upper part of the body tend to be medial and those for the lower part of the body lateral, although the topographical arrangement again lacks precision because of intermingling of fibers concerned with different parts of the body.

A study of the corticospinal tract based on counts in the pyramid of the medulla has shown that there are approximately 1 million fibers of various sizes. About 35,000 of these (3 percent) are distinctly larger than the remainder, measuring about 10 μ in diameter. The giant pyramidal cells of Betz are best developed in the superior two-thirds of area 4, in which the number of Betz cells corresponds closely with the number of large corticospinal fibers. It is assumed, therefore, that the Betz cells are responsible for these large, rapidly conducting fibers in the corticospinal tract. Fibers constituting the bulk of the tract are for the most part axons of pyramidal and fusiform cells in the regions of cortex from which the corticospinal tract originates.

At the caudal end of the medulla, with some variation in the exact level among different individuals, most of the corticospinal fibers cross the midline in the *decussation of the pyramids*. The proportion of crossing fibers also varies from one individual to another, the average being about 85 percent. The decussation consists of coarse bundles, the bundles from one pyramid alternating with those from the opposite pyramid. Fibers concerned with the upper extremities cross before those for the lower extremities. Having traversed the decussation, the fibers constitute the *lateral corticospinal tract* in the dorsolateral white column of the cord. The constituent fibers have a segmental topography, those ending in the highest segments being most medial

and the longest fibers most lateral. The proportions of fibers terminating in the major regions of the cord are: cervical, 55 percent; thoracic, 20 percent; and lumbosacral; 25 percent. With few exceptions, corticospinal fibers synapse with intercalating neurons, which synapse in turn with alpha motor neurons and some gamma motor neurons; only about 5 percent of the fibers synapse directly with motor cells.

About 15 percent of the fibers in a pyramid do not cross over in the pyramidal decussation. Of these, the majority continue into the ventral white column of the cord as the *ventral corticospinal tract*, the fibers terminating in the ventral gray horns of cervical and upper thoracic segments. A few fibers of the pyramid continue into the lateral corticospinal tract of the same side. These, together with those fibers of the ventral tract that terminate in the ipsilateral gray matter, account in part for bilateral cortical control of muscles of the neck and trunk. Cortical projections to extrapyramidal centers (described below) also contribute to the bilaterality of voluntary control of the musculature.

The pyramidal tracts contain a small proportion of fibers other than the motor fibers described above. These are descending fibers from the sensorimotor strip of cortex surrounding the central sulcus, proceeding with the pyramidal tract to the spinal trigeminal nucleus, the nuclei gracilis and cuneatus, and the dorsal gray horn of the cord. Through this descending pathway, cortical activity facilitates or inhibits transmission of data by second order sensory neurons to the thalamus and somesthetic cortex.

It should be added that fibers of the pyramidal system give off collateral branches, many of these being intracortical axon collaterals. Other collateral branches are given off as the pyramidal fibers traverse the internal capsule and brain stem; these terminate in such cell groups as the corpus striatum, red nucleus, pontine nuclei, inferior olivary nucleus, and the reticular formation. Through excitation or inhibition the collateral branches provide connections through which the pyramidal system influences components of the extrapyramidal motor system.

EXTRAPYRAMIDAL SYSTEM

An attempt to define the extrapyramidal system presents difficulties; agreement is lacking on components of the central nervous system that should be included under this heading. Broadly defined, the extrapyramidal system consists of all the centers and tracts, exclusive of the pyramidal system, that have a significant influence on the motor cortex or on lower motor neurons. Under this definition, the cerebellum is included together with such pathways as the tectospinal and vestibulospinal, which influence lower motor neurons. In clinical neurology attention is focused on the corpus striatum, subthalamic nucleus, and substantia nigra, because degenerative changes in these nuclei are responsible for motor disturbances of special clinical importance. Even when viewed from the latter vantage point, the ventral lateral and ventral anterior thalamic nuclei have to be considered because they are included in the pathway from the cerebellum, corpus striatum, and perhaps the substantia nigra, to motor areas of cortex. Similarly, the red nucleus and reticular formation are included peripherally because they are incorporated in pathways that lead to lower motor neurons.

The more general definition is followed in the present summary, which consists of a brief review of the centers and pathways that bear on motor performance. For convenience, the structures included in circuits from cerebral cortex to motor cortex (via thalamic nuclei) are summarized first, followed by a concise account of the nuclei and tracts that convey impulses to cells of the ventral gray horns of the cord and motor nuclei of cranial nerves.

EXTRAPYRAMIDAL COMPONENTS INVOLVED IN PROJECTIONS TO MOTOR CORTEX

The principal nuclei under this heading are the corpus striatum, substantia nigra, ventral thalamic nuclei (anterior and lateral), and the subthalamic nucleus, together with the neocerebellum (Fig. 23–2). The major connections of these nuclei are as follows.

Corpus Striatum

The corpus striatum comes under the influence of the cerebral cortex, thalamus, and substantia nigra; the afferent fibers end mainly in the neostriatum (caudate nucleus and putamen). Corticostriate fibers originate in widespread areas of cortex, but especially in that of the frontal and parietal lobes including areas from which pyramidal fibers also arise. Cortical afferents of the corpus striatum consist in part of collateral branches of corticobulbar and corticospinal fibers. Most of the fibers enter the neostriatum from the internal capsule, although a substantial number reach the putamen by way of the external capsule. Thalamostriate fibers have their origin in the intralaminar, medial, and ventral anterior nuclei of the thalamus. Most of the fibers leaving the neostriatum end in the paleostriatum (globus pallidus); a few striatal efferents terminate in the substantia nigra.

Efferent fibers of the globus pallidus make up two fasciculi, the lenticular fasciculus and the ansa lenticularis. The majority of the constituent fibers traverse the subthalamus to reach the ventral anterior and

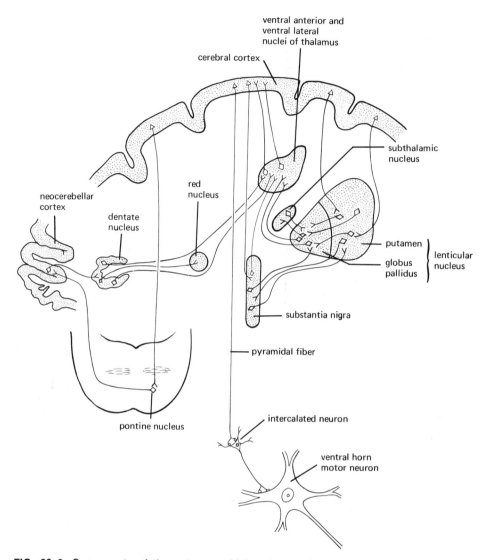

FIG. 23–2. Components of the extrapyramidal system projecting to motor and premotor cortex of the frontal lobe.

ventral lateral thalamic nuclei from which fibers project to the motor and premotor cortex of the frontal lobe.

Substantia Nigra

The connections of the substantia nigra are not fully known. However, in addition to afferent and efferent connections with the corpus striatum, red nucleus, and reticular formation, there are numerous corticonigral afferents from the frontal, parietal, and occipital lobes. Although confirmatory data are needed, fibers from the substantia nigra have been described as traversing the subthalamus and terminating in the anterior and lateral nuclei of the ventral thalamus. Through thalamocortical connections the substantia nigra would influence neural activity in the motor and premotor cortex of the frontal lobe. Along with the neocortex the substantia nigra makes its first definitive appearance in mammals and is especially well developed in the human brain.

Certainly from the clinical point of view the most important connection of the substantia nigra is the projection to the striatum. Degeneration of these neurons, in which dopamine is the neurotransmitter substance, results in paralysis agitans or Parkinson's disease.

Subthalamic Nucleus

In common with other motor nuclei the connections of the subthalamic nucleus are complex and incompletely understood. The principal connection, however, is with the globus pallidus; fibers passing in both directions constitute the subthalamic fasciculus which passes between the two nuclei across the intervening internal capsule.

In summary, the corpus striatum, substantia nigra, and ventral anterior and ventral lateral thalamic nuclei form a closely integrated group of subcortical nuclei to which the subthalamic nucleus must be added. Receiving data from the cerebral cortex and other sources, the corpus striatum and perhaps the substantia nigra project to the ventral anterior and ventral lateral nuclei of the thalamus, which in turn send fibers to the motor and premotor cortex. At the latter site, the subcortical nuclei may be expected to influence the pyramidal system since a large proportion of pyramidal fibers originate from frontal lobe cortex. Large numbers of extrapyramidal fibers arise as well from the motor and premotor areas of the frontal lobes. Thus motor activity may also be influenced by feedback circuits involving the basal ganglia and through extrapyramidal pathways to lower motor neurons discussed below.

Neocerebellum

The neocerebellum, consisting of the lateral portions of the cerebellar hemispheres and the dentate nuclei, participates in a circuit which ensures smoothly coordinated muscle action in voluntary movements. Corticopontine fibers from all cerebral lobes, but chiefly the frontal and parietal lobes, terminate in the pontine nuclei of the same side. Pontocerebellar fibers then project to the contralateral cerebellar cortex, from where fibers pass to the dentate nucleus. The efferent outflow from the dentate nucleus constitutes most of the brachium conjunctivum; the fibers cross to the opposite side of the midbrain in the decussation of the brachium conjunctivum, whereupon most of them continue rostrally through the midbrain and subthalamus to their termination in the ventral lateral nucleus of the thalamus. The circuit is completed by a thalamocortical projection to the primary motor area and a smaller projection to the premotor cortex. Neocerebellar activity therefore influences the source of many of the fibers making up the pyramidal pathway together with part of the extrapyramidal output from the cortex.

EXTRAPYRAMIDAL PATHWAYS TO LOWER MOTOR NEURONS

Several extrapyramidal pathways converge on lower motor neurons (Fig. 23–3). The red nucleus and the reticular formation receive afferents from the cerebral cortex, corpus striatum, cerebellum, and other sources; they must be included with the extrapyramidal system, however it is defined. Lower motor neurons also come under the influence of the tectum of the midbrain, the vestibular nuclei, and possibly the inferior olivary complex. Fibers from the various sources noted above end on both alpha and gamma motor neurons (an intercalated neuron often intervenes). Control of muscle tonus through the gamma reflex loop involving neuromuscular spindles is important in coordination of muscles and adjustment of muscle tonus in postural changes, locomotion, and other forms of motor activity.

Red Nucleus and Reticular Formation

The red nucleus of the midbrain (magnocellular portion) and the reticular formation of the brain stem have some connections in common; the red nucleus is sometimes considered as a specialized nucleus of the reticular formation. Corticorubral fibers originate mainly from the motor and premotor areas of the frontal lobe; they traverse the internal capsule in company with fibers of the pyramidal system. The cells of origin of corticoreticular fibers are in various parts of the cortex, including a major contribution from the sensorimotor strip. Corticoreticular fibers reach the brain stem through the internal and external capsules, terminating throughout the reticular formation but preferentially in the magnocellular nuclei of the medial area. Pallidorubral and pallidoreticular fibers leave the globus pallidus in the lenticular fasciculus and ansa lenticularis. The corpus striatum comes under the influence of the cerebral cortex, thalamus, and substantia nigra. Fibers from the paleocerebellar cortex project mainly on the emboliform and globose nuclei; efferents from the latter nuclei terminate in the red nucleus and reticular formation. Some efferent fibers of the archicerebellum also end in the reticular formation. The substantia nigra has

reciprocal connections with the corpus striatum, red nucleus, and the reticular formation; it also receives cortical afferents.

Descending fibers from the red nucleus constitute the *rubrospinal tract;* the fibers terminate above the midthoracic level although conduction may continue caudally by means of spinospinalis relays. *Reticulospinal fibers* originate in the medial part of the reticular formation, especially the magnocellular region in the medulla and caudal pons. The fibers do not form a definite fasciculus, but are scattered in the ventral and lateral white columns of the cord. In addition to reticulospinal conduction by long fibers there is polysynaptic transmission through spino-spinalis association fibers. In man, rubroreticular and reticulospinal connections probably constitute a more important descending pathway from the red nucleus than the rubrospinal tract. Comparable fibers from the red nucleus and reticular formation terminate in motor nuclei of cranial nerves innervating striated muscles.

In summary, the rubrospinal and reticulospinal tracts are pathways through which the cerebral cortex, corpus striatum, cerebellum, and substantia nigra bring their influence to bear on lower motor neurons.

Other Descending Pathways

Cells of origin of the vestibulospinal tract and the medial longitudinal fasciculus are located in the vestibular nuclear complex. This group of nuclei receives afferents from the vestibular nerve and the archicerebellum. The fibers from the cerebellum originate in the archicerebellar cortex (mainly in the flocculonodular lobe) and the fastigial nucleus. The fastigial nucleus also receives afferents from paleocerebellar cortex. The *vestibulospinal tract* originates in the lateral vestibular (Deiters') nucleus; located in the ventral white column, the

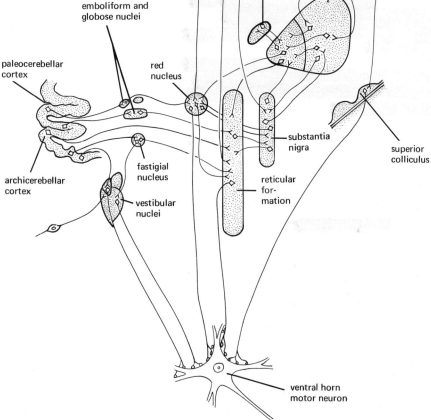

FIG. 23–3. Components of the extrapyramidal system projecting to lower motor neurons.

tract gives off fibers to the ventral gray horn throughout the spinal cord. Descending fibers of the *medial longitudinal fasciculus* arise mainly from the medial vestibular nucleus, and ascending fibers from all vestibular nuclei. The descending fibers run in the sulcomarginal fasciculus of the ventral white column of the cord and end in the ventral gray horn throughout the cervical region. The ascending fibers proceed to the abducens, trochlear, and oculomotor nuclei. The projection from the vestibular complex to motor neurons is concerned with maintenance of balance and coordination of head and eye movements.

The *tectospinal tract,* which is limited to the cervical cord (ventral white column), consists of fibers from the superior colliculus of the midbrain. The superior colliculus receives visual data from the retina, auditory data from the inferior colliculus, and general sensory data by way of the spinotectal tract. The tectospinal pathway functions in connection with reflex turning of the head and perhaps movements of the arms in response to visual, auditory, and cutaneous stimuli. Corticotectal fibers from the occipital lobe are numerous. Together with tectobulbar and tectospinal connections, they provide a pathway for automatic scanning movements of the eyes and head. The inferior olivary complex has been said to send fibers to the cervical cord through a small *olivospinal tract* adjacent to the ventrolateral sulcus. The inferior olivary complex receives afferents from the cerebral cortex, corpus striatum, red nucleus, and through the spino–olivary tract. However, the olivospinal tract is at best a minor efferent bundle of the inferior olivary complex and some even doubt its existence. Olivocerebellar fibers constitute the main outflow from the inferior olivary nucleus and the accessory olivary nuclei.

Finally, it should be pointed out that dorsal root afferents to lower motor neurons are extremely important, as shown by the effect of section of dorsal spinal roots. Following deafferentation of lower cervical segments, for example, there is severe impairment of the motor functions of the upper limb, even to the point of uselessness.

PYRAMIDAL VERSUS EXTRAPYRAMIDAL SYSTEMS

An understanding of the specific contributions of the pyramidal and extrapyramidal systems to motor functions has gradually evolved during the present century and continues to be a subject of investigation. One difficulty stems from differences between experimental results in animals, including subhuman primates, and the traditional clinical interpretation of motor deficits resulting from lesions that involve the pyramidal system. The problem can probably be appreciated to best advantage by considering the historical development of the concepts of these motor systems.

THE PYRAMIDAL SYSTEM

By the beginning of the present century, cortical stimulation studies on experimental animals were fairly well advanced. A motor area from which movements could be elicited on weak stimulation had been delineated in the cortex of the frontal lobe. At this stage of investigation the assumption was made that the pyramidal tract consisted of fibers that originated primarily, if not exclusively, from the motor cortex of the precentral gyrus. It was known that the pyramidal tract was a relatively recent phylogenetic acquisition, achieving its greatest development in man. It was natural, therefore, that the impairment of voluntary motor function consequent to ablation of the motor cortex in animals or its pathologic involvement in humans led to the concept that the pyramidal system represented the great descending pathway for all voluntary motor activity.

With the greater degree of sophistication in both anatomic and physiologic experimentation, certain presumptions leading to the concept of a strict association between the pyramidal system and voluntary motor function had to be revised. Anatomic studies showed, as noted above, that fibers from the primary motor area constituted about 40 percent of the fibers of the pyramidal tract, the remainder originating in other areas of frontal lobe cortex and in cortex of the parietal lobe. Physiologic studies on both lower mammals and subhuman primates disclosed that the effects of pyramidal tract section were less devastating than one might expect on the basis of traditional views. In addition, it was shown that ablation of the motor cortex added a more severe and complex deficit in motor function to that already present in an animal whose pyramidal tract had been sectioned previously. Thus by 1940 anatomists and physiologists were becoming aware of the shortcomings of equating the pyramidal system strictly with the primary motor cortex (Brodmann's area 4) or of the strict equation of the pyramidal system and voluntary motor function.

THE EXTRAPYRAMIDAL SYSTEM

Many reports appeared in the literature correlating involuntary movement disorders with degenerative changes in various subcortical nuclei. By definition these nuclei are included in the extrapyramidal system. These involuntary movement disorders, now collectively referred to as the dyskinesias, therefore became known as extrapyramidal syndromes, of which the following are the most important. The variable tremors and rigidity of Wilson's disease are associated with a special type of degenerative change in the lenticular nucleus resulting from a disorder of copper metabolism. Degenerative changes of various kinds in the corpus striatum are associated with involuntary movements of choreiform or athetoid type. Choreiform

movements are jerky, rapid, and purposeless, involving particularly the axial and proximal limb musculature. Athetoid movements are slow, sinuous, and aimless, most frequently involving the distal musculature of the extremities. Degenerative changes in these conditions may not be limited to the corpus striatum, but they are less widespread than those seen in dystonia musculorum deformans, the most grotesque of the dyskinesias which also is associated with striatal pathology. This disorder consists of slow, writhing movements of various parts of the axial and limb musculature. The involuntary movements are more sustained than those of chorea and athetosis, thus accounting in part for its more grotesque nature and the tendency to development of contractures of various parts of the body musculature.

The best pathologic correlation within the class of dyskinesias is that of hemiballismus, which is nearly always associated with pathologic changes in the contralateral subthalamic nucleus. Hemiballismus consists of sudden, flailing, gross movements of the proximal musculature of the limbs. The commonest dyskinesia, paralysis agitans or Parkinson's disease, is caused by neuronal degeneration in the substantia nigra and is characterized by muscular rigidity, a fine tremor, and poverty of movement (bradykinesia). Finally, lesions of the cerebellum lead to a variety of motor disturbances including a specific type of ataxia, hypotonia, and a characterstic intention tremor. Cerebellar lesions may be said in general to lead to errors in the rate, range, force, and direction of willed movements.

The clinical and pathologic observations summarized above lent support to the concept that the extrapyramidal system was concerned with involuntary and stereotyped movements without being involved directly with voluntary motor functions.

THE PRESENT POSITION

Naturally occurring lesions in man rarely, if ever, interrupt the pyramidal pathway without simultaneous involvement of extrapyramidal connections. The effects of a pure pyramidal lesion (careful sectioning of the pyramid in the medulla for example) can only be studied in experimental animals. Even when subhuman primates are studied in this way caution must be exercised in transferring information thus obtained to the human situation. The possibility that the normally functioning pyramidal tract may be responsible for more activities than those that disappear when the tract is sectioned must also be considered. Recognizing the above problems, more recent, well performed studies seem to have made untenable the hypothesis that all voluntary, nonstereotyped movement is mediated by way of the pyramidal system. Many observers now believe that the pyramidal system confers speed and agility on voluntary motor behavior, with the important specific contribution of enabling primates to use the individual digits in an independent and nonstereotyped manner. It follows that much of voluntary movement is mediated by the extrapyramidal motor system. It should also be noted that there is no increase in muscle tonus following a pure pyramidal lesion in the experimental animal, and that spasticity is a typical feature of experimental lesions within the extrapyramidal pathways.

The admixture of involvement of pyramidal and extrapyramidal pathways is best illustrated by the so-called "upper motor neuron lesion," which occurs most frequently in the cortex, medullary center, or internal capsule. In addition to affecting neurons of the pyramidal system such a lesion also affects large numbers of extrapyramidal fibers connecting the cortex with motor centers, including the corpus striatum, substantia nigra, red nucleus, and the reticular formation. Similarly, a lesion in the brain stem or spinal cord is most unlikely to interrupt the pyramidal tract without the simultaneous involvement of one or more extrapyramidal pathways. For example, a lesion in the lateral white column of the cord will involve not only the lateral corticospinal tract but also reticulospinal fibers and the rubrospinal tract.

After the effects of the acute lesion wear off the characeristic signs of an upper motor neuron lesion include varying degrees of voluntary paralysis, spasticity with exaggerated tendon reflexes, and the sign of Babinski. According to the concept summarized here the impairment of voluntary movement is partly pyramidal and partly extrapyramidal in origin. The pyramidal deficit is most evident in the voluntary paralysis of the muscles of the arm, in particular the muscles that normally allow for individual movements of the digits, and perhaps in voluntary paralysis of the muscles of facial expression. The sign of Babinski is also considered to be a pyramidal sign. Interruption of extrapyramidal pathways appears to be responsible for the muscle spasticity and hyperactive deep reflexes, although they are still clinically referred to as "pyramidal signs." The term "upper motor neuron" remains useful in order to distinguish the signs noted above from those of a "lower motor neuron" lesion. In the latter, interruption of the final common pathway results in flaccid paralysis and absence of stretch reflexes.

In view of the overlapping nature of the pyramidal and extrapyramidal motor systems anatomically and functionally, several neuroscientists have strongly advocated that the terms "pyramidal" and "extrapyramidal" be discarded. However, these terms are so firmly entrenched, especially in clinical usage, that their discontinuance could only take place over many years.

SUGGESTIONS FOR ADDITIONAL READING

Bertrand G: Stimulation during stereotactic operations for dyskinesias. J Neurosurg 24:419–423, 1966

Bertrand G, Blundell J, Musella R: Electrical exploration of the internal capsule and neighbouring structures during stereotaxic procedures. J Neurosurg 22:333–343, 1965

Brodal A: Some data and perspectives on the anatomy of the so-called "extrapyramidal system." Acta Neurol Scand 39 (suppl 4):17–38, 1963

Brooks VB, Stoney SD: Motor mechanisms: The role of the pyramidal system in motor control. Ann Rev Physiol 33: 337–392, 1971

Bucy PC: Is there a pyramidal tract? Brain 80:376–392, 1957

Coxe WS, Landau WM: Patterns of Marchi degeneration in the monkey pyramidal tract following small discrete cortical lesions. Neurology (Minneap) 20:89–100, 1970

Denny–Brown D: The Basal Ganglia and Their Relation to Disorders of Movement. London, Oxford University Press, 1962

Denny–Brown D: The Cerebral Control of Movement. Liverpool, Liverpool University Press, 1966

Felix D, Wiesendanger M: Pyramidal and non-pyramidal motor cortical effects on distal forelimb muscles of monkeys. Exp Brain Res 12:81–91, 1971

Koella WP: Organizational aspects of some subcortical motor areas. Int Rev Neurobiol 4:71–116, 1962

Lassek AM: The Pyramidal Tract. Springfield, Ill., Thomas, 1954

Lawrence DG, Kuypers HGJM: The functional organization of the motor system in the monkey. I. The effects of bilateral pyramidal lesions. Brain 91:1–14, 1968

Lawrence DG, Kuypers HGJM: The functional organization of the motor system in the monkey. II. The effects of lesions of the descending brain–stem pathways. Brain 91:15–36, 1968

Martin JP: The Basal Ganglia and Posture. Philadelphia, Lippincott, 1967

Walshe FMR: Critical Studies in Neurology. Edinburgh, Livingstone, 1948

24

Visceral Afferents and the Autonomic Nervous System

The primary role of both afferent and efferent visceral nerves is to maintain a state of homeostasis in the internal environment (the "milieu interieur" of Claude Bernard) for optimal bodily efficiency. This end is attained through regulation of the organs and structures concerned with digestion, circulation, respiration, excretion, and maintenance of normal body temperature. In addition to the regulating role of the visceral reflexes the activity of smooth muscles, glandular elements, and cardiac muscle is altered by influences from the highest levels of the brain, especially in response to emotional reactions to the external environment.

Afferent impulses of visceral origin reach the central nervous system through primary sensory neurons that do not differ significantly from those supplying general sensory endings for the somatic senses. Under normal conditions visceral afferent impulses elicit subconscious reflex responses and a feeling of fullness of hollow organs such as the stomach, rectum, and bladder. Impulses originating in the viscera also contribute to feelings of well-being or malaise. In the presence of abnormal function and disease, visceral afferents carry impulses for pain. The painful sensation is characteristically referred to that part of the body wall which is supplied by the same spinal nerves as those supplying the affected viscus.

The motor or efferent supply of smooth muscle, cardiac muscle, and gland cells differs from that of voluntary muscles in that the connection between the central nervous system and the viscus consists of a succession of two neurons rather than a single motor neuron. The cell body of the first neuron is situated in the brain stem or spinal cord; its axon terminates on a neuron in an autonomic ganglion and the axon of the latter neuron ends on effector cells. The two neurons are called preganglionic and postganglionic neurons, respectively. Because of the foregoing special feature of the visceral efferent system and because of its involuntary nature, Langley (1898) assigned the term "autonomic nervous system" to the visceral efferents exclusively. Although separate consideration of visceral efferents as the autonomic system continues to be the usual practice, this is to some extent unfortunate because the role of visceral reflexes tends to be obscured.

VISCERAL AFFERENTS

The senses of smell and taste, which are special senses eliciting visceral responses, come under the heading of *special visceral afferents*. The remaining central input from the viscera consists of *general visceral afferents*, some features of which will now be considered.

The cell bodies of visceral afferent neurons are located in the ganglia of those cranial and spinal nerves that include the autonomic outflow. The oculomotor and facial nerves are exceptions; they include visceral efferent neurons but not general visceral afferents. As described in more detail below, the autonomic system consists of a sympathetic division or system (thoracolumbar) and a parasympathetic division or system (bulbosacral). The sympathetic division is included in T1 through L2 or L3 spinal nerves; the parasympathetic division is included in the oculomotor, facial, glossopharyngeal, and vagus nerves, together with the second, third, and fourth sacral nerves. The dendrites of visceral afferent neurons traverse autonomic ganglia and plexuses without interruption to reach the viscera. For example, visceral afferent fibers associated with the sympathetic outflow traverse the paravertebral ganglia constituting the sympathetic trunk or chain, and the prevertebral or collateral sympathetic plexuses. The latter plexuses, in which irregular groups of sympathetic

nerve cells are located, surround the abdominal aorta and its major branches, especially the celiac, superior mesenteric, and inferior mesenteric arteries. The detailed anatomy of autonomic ganglia and plexuses is included in textbooks of gross anatomy.

Sensory neurons conducting impulses from the viscera can be classed in two categories: 1) afferents that elicit autonomic reflex responses (physiologic afferents), and 2) afferents that are stimulated in the presence of disturbed function and disease (pain afferents). Physiologic afferents accompany both the sympathetic and parasympathetic outflow (especially the latter), while pain afferents correspond to the region of sympathetic outflow almost exclusively.

PHYSIOLOGIC AFFERENTS

As noted above, the cell bodies of primary sensory neurons in the region of the sympathetic division are located in the dorsal root ganglia of T1 through L2 or L3 spinal nerves. The dendrites of these cells enter the sympathetic trunk by way of white communicating rami (Fig. 3-1). The fibers then traverse the cardiac, pulmonary, and splanchnic nerves, which arise from the sympathetic trunk, for distribution to the organs of the thorax and abdomen. Except for fibers ending in pacinian corpuscles, the visceral afferent fibers terminate as nonencapsulated branches, often in the form of quite complex branching of the end of the dendrite. Axons of visceral afferent neurons enter the spinal cord by T1 through L2 or L3 dorsal roots and terminate in the spinal gray matter. Impulses conveyed by some of these axons impinge on neurons of the intermediolateral cell column either directly or through intercalated neurons in the dorsal gray horn, including cells of the visceral afferent nucleus. The sympathetic outflow to thoracic and abdominal viscera completes spinal reflex arcs for the viscera.

In addition to the reflexes noted above, an ascending visceral system of fibers constitutes a poorly defined pathway originating in the visceral afferent nucleus and probably other cells of the dorsal horn. The fibers run in the deeper part of the lateral white column; rostral transmission also includes spinospinalis relays. The impulses reach the reticular formation of the brain stem and, through further relays in the reticular formation, impinge on the thalamus and hypothalamus.

Visceral afferents of special physiologic importance are associated with the parasympathetic or bulbosacral division of the autonomic system. The following examples will serve to illustrate the role of these afferents in homeostasis and the reflex arcs of which they form the afferent limb.

Cardiovascular System

Terminal dendritic branches in the aortic arch and the carotid sinus at the bifurcation of the common carotid artery serve as baroreceptors, signaling changes in arterial blood pressure. The cell bodies of neurons supplying the aortic arch are situated in the inferior ganglion of the vagus nerve, while those for the carotid sinuses are in the inferior ganglion of the glossopharyngeal nerve. The central processes terminate in the nucleus of the solitary tract in the medulla, from where fibers pass to cardiovascular centers in the reticular formation. These centers are in turn connected with the dorsal motor nucleus of the vagus nerve and with the intermediolateral cell column of the cord by means of reticulospinal fibers. Through the reflex pathways thus established, a rapid increase in arterial pressure causes a decrease in heart rate (vagus nerve) and vasodilation through inhibition of the vasoconstrictor action of the sympa-

thetic outflow. A fall in arterial pressure, such as occurs following hemorrhage, initiates reflex responses which are the reverse of those caused by a rise in arterial pressure. Visceral afferents in the glossopharyngeal and vagus nerves are therefore important in the maintenance of normal arterial blood pressure.

Another reflex, the details of which are not fully understood, serves to regulate venous pressure. As described originally by Bainbridge, nerve endings in the wall of the right atrium and adjacent large veins are stimulated by a rise in venous pressure. The impulses are conducted centrally by visceral afferents in the vagus nerve. The response is cardiac acceleration, with lowering of venous pressure, by inhibition of vagal efferents and excitation of sympathetic efferents to the heart. Among other modifications of the concept of the Bainbridge reflex (or effect) that may be necessary, there is the possibility that afferent impulses initiating cardiac acceleration may originate in some part of the pulmonary vascular bed.

Respiratory System

There are respiratory centers in the brain stem for automatic control of respiratory movements. The centers are located in the reticular formation of the medulla where they consist of an inspiratory center medially and a more laterally placed expiratory center. In addition, a pneumotaxic center in the pontine reticular formation regulates the rhythmicity of inspiration and expiration. Inspiration is initiated by stimulation of neurons in the inspiratory center by carbon dioxide of the circulating blood, the impulses reaching lower motor neurons supplying the diaphragm and intercostal muscles by means of reticulospinal connections.

Visceral afferents in the vagus nerve constitute the afferent limb of the Hering-Breuer reflex, through which expiration is initiated. Nerve terminals in the bronchial tree, especially the smaller branches, discharge at an increasing rate as the lungs are inflated. Impulses reach the expiratory center through a relay in the nucleus of the solitary tract; neurons supplying the respiratory muscles are inhibited by means of reticulospinal fibers.

Respiratory movements are also influenced by stimuli arising from the carotid bodies which lie near the bifurcation of the common carotid arteries, and from small aortic bodies adjacent to the aortic arch. Nerve terminals in these bodies function as chemoreceptors that are sensitive to a decrease in oxygen tension in the circulating blood. The resulting impulses reach the nucleus of the solitary tract through neurons with cell bodies in the inferior ganglia of the glossopharyngeal and vagus nerves. Further connections with respiratory centers in the brain stem bring about an increase in the rate and depth of respiratory movements. This reflex is especially important in vigorous exercise, when a person is exposed to a lowered oxygen tension such as at high altitudes, or in any circumstances that produce asphyxia.

Other Systems

Sensory fibers in the vagus nerve are distributed to the digestive tract as far caudally as the junction of the transverse and descending colon (splenic flexure). The endings are stimulated by stretch (distention) or active contraction of the smooth musculature, or by irritation of the mucosa. Although motility and secretion in the gastrointestinal tract occur in the absence of an extrinsic nerve supply, they are modified by reflexes consisting of vagal afferents and efferents. Vagal afferent impulses also contribute to the feeling of fullness when the stomach is distended and that of hunger when the stomach is empty. Excessive stimulation may result in nausea.

The distal colon and rectum are supplied by afferent fibers in the second, third, and fourth sacral nerves and their splanchnic branches (nervi erigentes). Reflexes through the corresponding sacral segments —the sacral portion of the parasympathetic system providing the efferent limb of the reflex arc—function in emptying of the large bowel. The feeling of fullness of the lower colon and rectum results from transmission of data to the brain through the ascending visceral system of fibers. Similarly, the sensation of fullness of the urinary bladder leads to emptying of the bladder, subject to voluntary control.

PAIN AFFERENTS

The sensory neurons for pain of visceral origin are associated with the sympathetic division of the autonomic nervous system. The cell bodies of primary sensory neurons are therefore in the dorsal root ganglia of the thoracic and upper two or three lumbar nerves. The dendrites of these neurons reach the sympathetic trunk by way of white communicating rami; they run in the trunk for variable distances and then continue to the viscera by way of cardiac, pulmonary, and splanchnic branches of the sympathetic trunk. The termination of the corresponding dorsal root axons in the spinal gray matter is not known precisely; however, the majority probably enter the dorsolateral fasciculus along with somatic pain fibers and end in the substantia gelatinosa. Synaptic contacts are made in the substantia gelatinosa with dendrites of cells that transmit impulses for visceral pain to the brain. The ascending pathway for visceral pain may coincide, in part, with the pathway for somatic pain, i.e., through crossed fibers in the lateral spinothalamic tract. There also appears to be crossed and uncrossed conduction by means of fibers deep in the lateral white column. The impulses reach the thalamus through the spinal lemniscus and extralemniscal relays in the reticular formation, along with impulses for pain from somatic structures.

The viscera are themselves insensitive to touch, cutting, cold and heat; operations on visceral structures may therefore be carried out under local anesthesia. The pain endings are stimulated in various ways in the presence of abnormal function or disease. Most commonly the pain is caused by distention of hollow viscera, which in turn may result from forcible contractions of smooth muscles at certain sites in the viscus. Such a mechanism probably operates when there is obstruction of the bile ducts or ureter, causing biliary or renal colic. Visceral pain also results from rapid stretching of the capsule of a solid organ, such as the liver and spleen. Peritoneal irritation contributes to the pain of inflammatory disease. In the case of anginal pain and the pain of coronary thrombosis, the effective stimulus is produced by anoxemia of the cardiac muscle. The stimulus is probably chemical in nature, perhaps a lowering of pH because of accumulation of acid metabolites.

Referred Pain

Visceral pain has certain characteristics that distinguish it from pain originating in somatic structures, notably diffuse localization and radiation to cutaneous areas. The latter characteristic is called "referred pain." The cutaneous zone of reference for a viscus coincides with the segmental distribution of the somatic sensory fibers that enter the same spinal segments as the fibers coming from the viscus in question. The principle of referred pain is illustrated by the following examples.

The heart is supplied with pain afferents

which course centrally in the middle and inferior cervical branches and thoracic cardiac branches of the sympathetic trunk. Axons of the primary sensory neurons enter spinal segments T1 through T4 or T5 on the left side; pain of cardiac origin is therefore referred to the left side of the chest and the inner aspect of the left arm.

In the case of pain arising from distention of the gallbladder or bile ducts the impulses pass centrally in the greater splanchnic nerve on the right side, entering the cord through the seventh and eighth thoracic dorsal roots. The painful sensation is referred to the upper quadrant of the abdomen and the infrascapular region on the right side. Disease of the liver or gallbladder may irritate the peritoneum covering the diaphragm. The resulting pain is felt in the lower chest wall if it originates in the periphery of the diaphragm, which is supplied by the lower intercostal nerves. However, the pain is referred to the region of the shoulder when the central area of the diaphragm is affected because this area is supplied with sensory fibers by the phrenic nerve, which originates from the third, fourth, and fifth cervical segments.

To cite a few additional examples, pain of gastric origin is referred to the epigastrium because the stomach is supplied with pain afferents that reach the seventh and eighth thoracic segments by way of the greater splanchnic branch of the sympathetic trunk. Pain of duodenal origin, as in duodenal ulcer, is referred to the anterior abdominal wall just above the umbilicus, both this cutaneous area and the duodenum being supplied by the ninth and tenth thoracic nerves. Afferent fibers from the appendix are included in the lesser splanchnic nerve and impulses enter the tenth thoracic segment of the cord. The pain of appendicitis is referred initially to the region of the umbilicus, shifting to the lower right quadrant of the abdomen if the parietal peritoneum becomes involved in the inflammatory process. Pain afferents supplying the renal pelvis and ureter are included in the least splanchnic nerve; impulses enter the first and second lumbar segments and the pain is felt in the loin and inguinal region.

There is still no entirely satisfactory explanation for the referral of pain of visceral origin to the surface of the body. One postulate implicates spinal reflexes consisting of visceral afferent neurons, intercalated cells in the spinal gray matter, and cells of the intermediolateral or sympathetic column. Such a reflex could cause tonic vasoconstriction in a cutaneous area supplied by those segments receiving afferents from the affected viscus. A further assumption is made to the effect that metabolic products in the area of vasoconstriction may not be carried away and that these substances stimulate peripheral pain endings. According to another suggestion, visceral and somatic pain afferents synapse with common tract cells in the spinal gray matter, the latter cells being then excited by subliminal cutaneous stimuli when played upon by impulses of visceral origin.

The explanation in favor at present is based on a projection of impulses related to visceral and somatic pain from a specific cord segment to the same group of cells in the ventral posterior thalamic nucleus. Since discrete or topographic projections of sensory pathways on the thalamus are the basis of cortical interpretation of the source of stimuli, and since pain of cutaneous origin is a common experience compared with pain of visceral origin, the source of the stimuli may be wrongly interpreted as cutaneous. It is of interest to recall in the present context that John Hunter, a pioneer anatomist and surgeon, called referred pain "a delusion of the mind." Even if the last hypothesis mentioned proves to be correct, spinal reflexes remain the explanation for

muscle spasm in response to visceral pain. Such a response is commonly seen as rigidity of abdominal muscles when there is inflammatory disease of a viscus. The reflex arc consists of visceral pain afferents, intercalated neurons, and ventral horn motor cells. This is one of several examples in which there is a connection between visceral and somatic innervation.

VISCERAL EFFERENT OR AUTONOMIC SYSTEM

By definition "viscera" refers to the organs of the thoracic and abdominal cavities. The smooth muscle and secretory cells of the viscera and cardiac muscle come under the dual influence of the sympathetic and parasympathetic divisions of the autonomic system. They are functionally antagonistic to one another, and a delicate balance between them maintains a more or less constant level of visceral activity (homeostasis) under conditions that usually prevail. Structures elsewhere which consist of smooth muscles or exocrine gland cells also have an autonomic innervation; for the most part this is by either sympathetic or parasympathetic fibers rather than fibers of both autonomic divisions. Such structures include the muscles of the iris and ciliary body of the eye, smooth muscles in the orbit, the lacrimal and salivary glands, sweat glands, arrector pili muscles attached to hair follicles, and many blood vessels.

With the exception of the adrenal medulla and the pineal gland, autonomic influence on the endocrine glands is mainly through changes in the blood flow through the glands. However, the level of activity of the endocrine glands is determined most importantly by pituitary hormones, and the pituitary gland is controlled by the hypothalamus. Conversely, hormones have an important influence on the nervous system; the two systems, nervous and endocrine, function in close collaboration.

PARASYMPATHETIC DIVISION

Preganglionic parasympathetic neurons, which have long axons, are located in nuclei of the brain stem and in the sacral cord. Postganglionic neurons with short axons are located in peripheral or terminal ganglia near or within the structure being innervated. Examples of peripheral ganglia are the ciliary, pterygopalatine, submandibular, and otic ganglia of the head, together with the diffusely arranged peripheral neurons in the heart, in the pulmonary plexus, and in the myenteric and submucosal plexuses of the gastrointestinal tract.

The role of the parasympathetic system is to bring about changes that are designed to conserve and restore the energy sources of the body. The responses include a decrease in the rate and force of the heart beat, lowering of the blood pressure, and augmentation of the activity of the digestive system. Acetylcholine is the chemical mediator at the synapses between preganglionic and postganglionic neurons and also at the contacts between postganglionic terminals and effector cells. The parasympathetic system is therefore said to be "cholinergic." The system acts in localized and discrete regions rather than causing a mass reaction throughout the body. The discrete nature of the response is a result of two factors: 1) each preganglionic neuron synapses with a limited number of postganglionic neurons, and the latter end on a limited number of effector cells; and 2) acetylcholine is rapidly inactivated by cholinesterase, hence each parasympathetic discharge is of short duration.

The preganglionic parasympathetic nuclei and the sites of the corresponding postganglionic cells are as follows: 1) *Edinger–Westphal nucleus* of the oculo-

motor complex and ciliary ganglion; 2) *superior salivatory nucleus* of the facial nerve and submandibular ganglion; 3) *lacrimal nucleus* of the facial nerve and pterygopalatine ganglion; 4) *inferior salivatory nucleus* of the glossopharyngeal nerve and otic ganglion; 5) *dorsal motor nucleus* of the vagus nerve and cardiac ganglia, ganglia in the pulmonary plexus, cells in the myenteric and submucosal plexuses of the gastrointestinal tract, and postganglionic neurons at other sites; and 6) *sacral parasympathetic nucleus* and postganglionic neurons scattered in the walls of pelvic viscera.

SYMPATHETIC DIVISION

As noted above, the sympathetic outflow originates in the intermediolateral cell column of all thoracic spinal segments and the upper two or three lumbar segments. (In some individuals, the column extends into the eighth cervical segment.) The axons of preganglionic neurons reach the sympathetic trunk by way of the corresponding ventral roots and white communicating rami. With respect to the sympathetic supply of structures in the head and thorax, the preganglionic fibers terminate in ganglia of the sympathetic chain. For smooth muscles and glands of the head, the synapses between pre- and postganglionic neurons are mainly in the superior cervical ganglion of the sympathetic trunk. In the case of thoracic viscera, the synapses are in the three cervical sympathetic ganglia (superior, middle, and inferior) and the upper five ganglia of the thoracic part of the chain.

Preganglionic fibers for abdominal and pelvic viscera continue through the sympathetic trunk and the splanchnic branches of the trunk. The fibers terminate on postganglionic neurons located in plexuses surrounding the main branches of the abdominal aorta, notably the celiac plexus and the superior and inferior mesenteric plexuses. The sympathetic supply to the adrenal medulla is exceptional. The secretory cells of the medulla, like postganglionic sympathetic neurons, are derived from the neural crest of the embryo. The adrenal medulla is consequently supplied directly by preganglionic sympathetic neurons.

For the body wall, preganglionic fibers terminate in all ganglia of the sympathetic trunk, from which postganglionic fibers are distributed by way of gray communicating rami and spinal nerves to blood vessels, arrector pili muscles, and sweat glands.

The sympathetic system stimulates activities that are accompanied by an expenditure of energy stores. These include acceleration of the heart rate and increase in force of the heart beat, rise of arterial pressure, elevation of the blood sugar level, and direction of blood flow to skeletal muscles at the expense of visceral and cutaneous circulation. Sympathetic responses are most dramatically expressed during stress and emergency situations. However, the "flight or fight" responses to strong sympathetic stimulation are only extreme examples of processes that are going on all the time. One can lead a normal existence in a sheltered environment in the absence of sympathetic function, but reactions to stress are lacking. The neurotransmitter between pre- and postganglionic neurons is acetylcholine, as in the parasympathetic system. However, in the case of the sympathetic system, norepinephrine (noradrenaline) is the transmitter substance between postganglionic terminals and effector cells. The sympathetic system is therefore said to be "adrenergic." The sympathetic supply to sweat glands is cholinergic, constituting an exception to the general rule. Cutaneous areas, in general, lack parasympathetic fibers; this may be related to the fact that sudomotor fibers are anatomically sympathetic but functionally parasympathetic.

Unlike the discrete functioning of the parasympathetic system, the sympathetic system tends to operate as a total unit throughout the body. This diffuse effect results from two factors which are the converse of those present in the parasympathetic system. 1) Each sympathetic preganglionic neuron synapses with as many as 30 or more postganglionic neurons and each of the latter ends on numerous effector cells. Hence, there is much divergence of stimuli. 2) Norepinephrine liberated at postganglionic terminals, and epinephrine (adrenaline) and norepinephrine secreted by the adrenal medulla on sympathetic stimulation, are deactivated slowly. As expressed by Cannon, "the sympathetics are like the loud and soft pedals, modulating all the tones together, while the parasympathetics are like the separate keys."

EXAMPLES OF AUTONOMIC INNERVATION

The autonomic innervation of certain structures may now be summarized. Descriptive details are omitted; autonomic nuclei within the central nervous system have been referred to in earlier chapters and detailed accounts of peripheral portions of the autonomic system are included in textbooks of gross anatomy.

SMOOTH MUSCLES OF THE EYE AND ORBITAL CAVITY

Parasympathetic

Preganglionic fibers from the Edinger–Westphal nucleus are carried by the oculomotor nerve to the orbit, where they terminate in the ciliary ganglion. Postganglionic fibers are distributed to the constrictor pupillae and ciliary muscles of the eye through short ciliary nerves. *Function:* pupillary constriction (miosis); thickening of the lens by contraction of the ciliary muscle, which reduces tension on the supporting ligament of the lens (the ciliary zonule).

Sympathetic

Preganglionic neurons are located in the upper two thoracic spinal segments, from where axons travel to the superior cervical ganglion of the sympathetic trunk. Postganglionic fibers reach the orbit by way of the internal carotid plexus and that of the ophthalmic artery, traverse the ciliary ganglion, and continue to the dilator pupillae muscle through short ciliary nerves. Other sympathetic fibers supply the smooth muscle component (tarsal muscle) of the levator palpabrae superioris muscle and Müller's orbital muscle (the latter being rudimentary in man). *Function:* pupillary dilation (mydriasis); retraction of the upper eyelid; exophthalmos (insignificant in man).

GLANDS IN THE HEAD
Parasympathetic

Submandibular and Sublingual Salivary Glands. The preganglionic neurons make up the superior salivatory nucleus, which is represented by an ill-defined cluster of cells in the pontine tegmentum medial to the motor nucleus of the facial nerve. Fibers from the superior salivatory nucleus end in the submandibular ganglion, which they reach by traversing the sensory root of the facial nerve (nervus intermedius), the facial nerve and its chorda tympani branch, and finally the lingual branch of the mandibular nerve. Short postganglionic fibers then proceed to the submandibular and sublingual glands. *Function:* stimulation of salivary secretion and vasodilation.

Lacrimal Gland and Mucosal Glands of the Nose and Palate. The preganglionic cells are in the pontine tegmentum (lacrimal nucleus), in the same region as the superior salivatory nucleus. Preganglionic fibers traverse the nervus intermedius and facial nerve proper, enter its greater petrosal branch, and terminate in the pterygopalatine ganglion. Postganglionic fibers

reach the lacrimal gland through the zygomatic branch of the maxillary nerve; other fibers are distributed to the mucosa of the nose and palate through nasopalatine and palatine branches of the maxillary nerve. *Function:* stimulation of secretion and vasodilation.

Parotid Gland. The inferior salivatory nucleus, which is situated just caudal to its superior counterpart, contains the cell bodies of preganglionic neurons. The axons leave the brain stem in the glossopharyngeal nerve, then traverse its tympanic branch and the tympanic plexus in the wall of the middle ear, from which they constitute the lesser petrosal nerve and terminate in the otic ganglion. Postganglionic fibers reach the parotid gland by way of the auriculotemporal branch of the mandibular nerve. *Function:* stimulation of salivary secretion and vasodilation.

Sympathetic

The preganglionic neurons are similar to those described above for innervation of smooth muscles in the eye and orbital cavity. Postganglionic fibers are distributed to the glands through the nerve plexuses surrounding the internal and external carotid arteries. *Function:* vasoconstriction, which decreases secretion.

HEART
Parasympathetic

Preganglionic fibers from the dorsal motor nucleus of the vagus nerve enter the cardiac branches of the vagus, synapsing with postganglionic neurons in the cardiac plexuses and in scattered cell clusters in the walls of the atria of the heart. Postganglionic fibers supply the sinoatrial and atrioventricular nodes, muscle fibers of the atria and ventricles, and the coronary arteries. *Function:* cardiac inhibition, i.e., reduction of the rate and force of the heart beat; vasoconstriction of the coronary arteries.

Sympathetic

Preganglionic fibers originate in the upper five or six thoracic spinal segments; they terminate in the corresponding ganglia of the sympathetic chain and in the three cervical ganglia. Postganglionic fibers reach the heart by way of the superior, middle, and inferior cardiac branches of the cervical portion of the sympathetic trunk, and through varying numbers of thoracic cardiac nerves. The fibers terminate in the nodes, on cardiac muscle fibers, and in coronary vessels. *Function:* cardiac acceleration and dilation of the coronary arteries.

LUNGS
Parasympathetic

Preganglionic fibers from the dorsal motor nucleus of the vagus nerve reach the pulmonary plexus through pulmonary branches of the nerve and end in tracheal and bronchial ganglia embedded in the plexus. Postganglionic fibers supply the smooth muscle and mucosal glands of the trachea and bronchial tree, and also blood vessels of the lung. *Function:* bronchoconstriction and stimulation of secretion.

Sympathetic

Preganglionic fibers from spinal segments T3 through T5 synapse in the inferior cervical ganglion of the sympathetic chain and the upper four or five thoracic ganglia. Postganglionic fibers traverse pulmonary branches of the sympathetic trunk and the pulmonary plexus to supply the smooth muscle and glands of the trachea and bronchial tree, together with blood vessels. *Function:* bronchodilation and inhibition of secretion. (Although autonomic fibers have been shown to supply pulmonary and bronchial blood vessels, the functional significance of such innervation is debated.)

STOMACH AND INTESTINE
Parasympathetic

Vagal preganglionic fibers traverse the esophageal plexus and enter the abdomen in the anterior and posterior vagal trunks. The fibers achieve a wide distribution to abdominal viscera, including the stomach and the intestine as far as the splenic flexure of the colon. Those

fibers supplying the gastrointestinal tract terminate on postganglionic neurons in the myenteric (Auerbach's) and submucosal (Meissner's) plexuses. The short postganglionic fibers end on smooth muscle and gland cells. *Function:* increase in peristaltic rate and tonus of smooth muscle; relaxation of sphincters; stimulation of secretion.

Sympathetic

Preganglionic fibers from spinal segments T5 through T12 traverse the sympathetic trunk and its greater and lesser splanchnic branches, terminating on postganglionic neurons in the celiac and superior mesenteric ganglia. Axons of the latter cells are distributed to the stomach with the celiac artery, and to the intestine as far as the splenic flexure with the superior mesenteric artery. Blood vessels for the stomach and intestine are also supplied with sympathetic fibers. *Function:* inhibition of peristalsis and contraction of sphincters; inhibition of secretion; vasoconstriction.

DESCENDING COLON AND PELVIC VISCERA
Parasympathetic

Preganglionic fibers originate in the parasympathetic nucleus in the ventral gray horn of spinal segments S2 through S4. The fibers traverse the pelvic splanchnic branches (nervi erigentes) of the corresponding spinal nerves and terminate on postganglionic neurons in the walls of organs innervated. These visceral structures include the descending colon, sigmoid colon, rectum, bladder, prostate, seminal vesicle, testis, uterus and tubes, ovaries, erectile tissue, and blood vessels supplying pelvic organs. *Function:* contraction of the smooth muscle of the lower bowel and the detrusor muscle of the bladder; stimulation of glands; vasodilation; erection.

Sympathetic

Preganglionic fibers originate in spinal segments T12 through L2 or L3, traverse the lumbar splanchnic branches of the sympathetic trunk, and synapse with postganglionic neurons in the inferior mesenteric plexus. From the latter site, fibers are distributed to the pelvic organs noted above. *Function:* inhibition of peristalsis in the lower bowel; contraction of muscles in the trigone of the bladder; ejaculation of semen; vasoconstriction.

KIDNEY

Nerve fibers assumed to be efferent have been described ending in relation to renal tubules and glomeruli. However, true secretory fibers appear to be of little importance because the denervated kidney can carry on approximately normal function.

The activity of the renal tubules is influenced by vasomotor fibers. The vasodilator supply is parasympathetic and consists of preganglionic vagal fibers and postganglionic cells in the renal plexus surrounding the renal artery and vein. The sympathetic is vasoconstrictor to renal vessels. Preganglionic sympathetic fibers from segments T11 through L1 synapse in the celiac ganglion, and postganglionic fibers are distributed through the renal plexus to branches of the renal artery within the kidney.

ADRENAL GLAND

The adrenal medulla is supplied by preganglionic sympathetic neurons directly, postganglionic sympathetic fibers as well as a parasympathetic supply being lacking. The fibers come from spinal cord segments T8 through T11 and reach the gland by way of the lesser splanchnic branch of the sympathetic trunk. As mentioned above, the absence of postganglionic sympathetic neurons stems from the fact that the secretory cells of the medulla arise from neural crest cells and are comparable in their origin to postganglionic neurons. The transmitter substance between the nerve terminals and the secretory cells is acetylcholine, as at synapses between pre- and postganglionic neurons. Sympathetic stimulation of the medulla increases the output of epinephrine and norepinephrine.

Convincing evidence of innervation of secretory cells of the adrenal cortex is lacking. However, the blood vessels of both parts of the gland are supplied by postganglionic sympathetic fibers. The preganglionic neurons correspond to those ending on parenchymatous cells of the medulla. The postganglionic neurons are mainly in the aorticorenal plexus, which is an extension of the celiac plexus.

PERIPHERAL BLOOD VESSELS

Preganglionic cells for blood vessels in the body wall and extremities are located throughout the intermediolateral cell column; their axons reach the sympathetic trunk through the ventral roots and white communicating rami from T1 through L2 or L3 segments. Many of the fibers run rostrally and caudally to synapse with postganglionic neurons in all chain ganglia. Postganglionic fibers enter all spinal nerves through the gray communicating rami and are distributed to blood vessels of the skin and deep structures, especially the muscles. While vessels supplying some visceral structures (e.g., salivary glands, heart, and kidney) receive parasympathetic as well as sympathetic efferents, peripheral blood vessels have only a sympathetic supply. Sympathetic stimulation causes vasoconstriction of cutaneous vessels and vasodilation of blood vessels in skeletal muscle.

BLOOD VESSELS OF THE HEAD

In addition to having a sympathetic innervation for vasoconstriction, a parasympathetic supply which is vasodilator in function has been demonstrated for arteries supplying some structures in the head. The preganglionic sympathetic fibers are from T1 and T2 spinal segments, and most of them synapse with postganglionic cells in the superior cervical ganglion. Fibers from the latter ganglion are distributed along the various branches of the internal and external carotid artery systems. In addition, postganglionic fibers from the inferior cervical ganglion accompany the vertebral and basilar arteries and their branches. With respect to cerebral arteries, sympathetic fibers supplying the branches on the surface of the brain and arterioles in the pia mater are more numerous than fibers supplying blood vessels in the brain substance.

Most of the preganglionic parasympathetic fibers are included in the facial nerve; those supplying the arterial branches to the lacrimal, submandibular, and sublingual glands have already been noted. Other preganglionic fibers in the facial nerve enter the greater petrosal nerve and join the internal carotid plexus in the region of the middle cranial fossa. Parasympathetic vasodilator fibers to the parotid gland are included in the glossopharyngeal nerve and accompany the secretomotor fibers. In all cases, the postganglionic neurons are in small clusters of cells in the periarterial plexuses.

ARRECTOR PILI MUSCLES AND SWEAT GLANDS

The sympathetic supply of both the smooth muscles attached to hair follicles (for piloerection) and the sweat glands corresponds to that of cutaneous blood vessels. The postganglionic terminals in sweat glands are cholinergic; they are therefore parasympathetic with respect to the chemical transmitter, although sympathetic anatomically.

CENTRAL CONTROL OF THE AUTONOMIC SYSTEM

The cells of origin of the autonomic outflow come under the influence of centers situated at various levels of the nervous system. The major controlling and integrating center is the hypothalamus, but centers in the reticular formation and visceral afferent nuclei are also very important. Impulses from the brain stem reach the intermediolateral cell column of the cord and the sacral parasympathetic nucleus by way of reticulospinal connections (descending autonomic fibers).

As described in the early part of the chapter, most of the general visceral afferent neurons of physiologic importance are associated with the parasympathetic system; vagal afferents are especially important. The impulses thus conveyed centrally are relayed to autonomic efferent nuclei through the nucleus of the solitary tract and the reticular formation. The special visceral sense of taste has similar connections. Fibers from the olfactory and limbic systems reach brain stem nuclei of autonomic significance through the olfactotegmental component of the medial forebrain bundle. These systems also project to the brain stem through a complex pathway that includes the habenular nucleus, midbrain nuclei, and the dorsal longitudinal fasciculus. Through the foregoing connections and also through projections of the olfactory and limbic systems to the hypothalamus, visceral functions are influenced by the sense of smell (a special visceral sense) and by the emotions. Visceral centers in the reticular formation of the brain stem include the cardiovascular centers, excitatory and inhibitory, which send fibers principally to the dorsal motor nucleus of the vagus nerve and the intermediolateral cell column of the cord.

Impulses from the hypothalamus reach autonomic efferent neurons through the dorsal longitudinal fasciculus and the mammillotegmental tract, with relays in the reticular formation. The hypothalamus also has an important controlling influence on the endocrine system. The supraopticohypophyseal system of the hypothalamus and neural lobe of the pituitary gland is in itself an endocrine organ. The hypothalamus controls hormone production in the anterior lobe of the pituitary by means of releasing factors, which reach the anterior lobe through the pituitary portal system of blood vessels.

The hypothalamus, in turn, receives afferents from several sources. These include visceral afferent impulses, both general and for taste, by way of ascending fibers in the brain stem, and impulses from olfactory cortex and the limbic system through the medial forebrain bundle. Other important afferents to the hypothalamus come from the medial and anterior thalamic nuclei, the amygdala, and the hippocampus; these parts of the brain are of special significance with respect to the emotions. Corticohypothalamic fibers, most of them originating in the orbital cortex of the frontal lobe, bring the hypothalamus under the influence of the neocortex. Hypothalamic neurons are also sensitive to slight changes in the temperature, the osmolarity, and the level of various chemical substances (including hormones) in the circulating blood. By the various means outlined above, the autonomic system comes under a wide range of influences, extending from primitive visceral afferents to psychic processes at the cortical level.

SUGGESTIONS FOR ADDITIONAL READING

Appenzeller O: The Autonomic Nervous System: An Introduction to Basic and Clinical Concepts. New York, American Elsevier, 1970

Crosby EC, Humphrey T, Lauer EW: Correlative Anatomy of the Nervous System. New York, Macmillan, 1962

Kuntz A: The Autonomic Nervous System, 4th ed. Philadelphia, Lea & Febiger, 1953

Pick J: The Autonomic Nervous System: Morphological, Comparative, Clinical and Surgical Aspects. Philadelphia, Lippincott, 1970

Romanes GJ (ed.): Cunningham's Textbook of Anatomy, 10th ed. London, Oxford University Press, 1964

Blood Supply
and Meninges

25

Blood Supply of the Central Nervous System

Vascular lesions are responsible for more neurologic disorders than any other category of disease process. Arterial occlusion by a thrombus, which is usually followed by infarction of a portion of the region supplied by the affected artery, is the most common type of cerebral vascular accident. Since the thrombus usually develops where there is intimal damage from atheromatous changes in the vessel wall, this type of arterial occlusion occurs mainly in those past middle life. It should be pointed out that arterial occlusion may be intracranial or extracranial. A large proportion of occlusive problems result from impairment of cerebral circulation because of stenosis in the extracranial portion of a carotid or vetebral artery. Occlusion of an artery by an embolus occurs most often in young people.

The slender, thin-walled arteries that penetrate the base of the brain to supply the internal capsule and basal ganglia are especially prone to rupture. Hypertension and degenerative changes of the vessels are important factors leading to cerebral hemorrhage. Aneurysms usually occur at the site of branching of one of the larger arteries at the base of the brain. An aneurysm may rupture, in which case the bleeding is typically into the subarachnoid space; however, the hemorrhage may be intracerebral.

There are anastomotic channels between branches of the major arteries on the surface of the brain. There are also communications at the arteriolar level, and the capillary bed is continuous throughout the brain. These anastomoses, however, are usually inadequate to sustain the circulation in the region supplied by a particular blood vessel when that vessel is occluded. The neurologic consequences of arterial occlusion depend on several factors which include the caliber of the occluded vessel, the collateral blood flow that is available, and the time elapsing to complete occlusion

349

(these factors determine the size of the infarcted area). The location of the damage
is of special importance because this determines the particular gray areas and fiber
connections that are rendered nonfunc-
tional. Because of the practical importance
of cerebral vascular disease and because
the neurologic signs depend on the site of
the lesion, an understanding of the distribution of the arteries supplying the brain
becomes a matter of necessity.

The blood supply of the brain (and the
spinal cord) has a special interest because
of the metabolic demands of nervous tissue. The brain depends on aerobic metabolism of glucose and is one of the most
metabolically active organs of the body.
Although composing only 2 percent of the
body weight, the brain receives approximately 17 percent of the cardiac output
and consumes about 20 percent of the
oxygen utilized by the whole body. Unconsciousness follows cessation of cerebral
circulation in about 10 seconds.

ARTERIAL SUPPLY OF THE BRAIN

The brain is supplied by the paired internal
carotid and vertebral arteries through an
extensive system of branches.

INTERNAL CAROTID ARTERY SYSTEM

The *internal carotid artery*, which is a
terminal branch of the common carotid
artery, traverses the carotid canal in the
base of the skull and enters the middle
cranial fossa beside the dorsum sellae of
the sphenoid bone. Beyond this point the
artery undergoes the following sequence of
bends which constitute the "carotid siphon"
in a cerebral angiogram. The internal
carotid artery first runs forward horizontally within the cavernous venous sinus,
then turns upward on the inner side of the

anterior clinoid process. At this point, the
artery enters the subarachnoid space by
piercing the dura mater and arachnoid,
courses backward below the optic nerve,
and finally turns upward immediately lateral to the optic chiasma. This brings the
artery under the anterior perforated substance where it divides into two terminal
branches, the middle and anterior cerebral
arteries (Fig. 25–1).

Collateral Branches

The following branches arise from the
internal carotid artery before the terminal
bifurcation.

Hypophyseal Arteries. These vessels originate from the cavernous and postclinoid
portions of the internal carotid artery. In
addition to supplying the neural lobe of the
pituitary gland (hypophysis), hypophyseal
arteries enter the median eminence of the
hypothalamus. The latter vessels break up
into capillary loops, into which hypothalamic releasing factors gain access, and the
capillary loops drain through small veins
into the sinusoids of the anterior lobe of the
pituitary gland. This constitutes the important pituitary portal system through which
the hypothalamus influences the output of
pituitary hormones.

Ophthalmic Artery. This branch comes off
immediately after the internal carotid
artery enters the subarachnoid space. The
ophthalmic artery passes forward into the
orbit, supplying the eye and other orbital
contents, the frontal area of the scalp, the
frontal and ethmoid air sinuses, and parts
of the nose.

Posterior Communicating Artery. This
slender vessel arises from the internal
carotid artery close to the terminal bifurcation. The posterior communicating artery
runs backward to join the proximal part of

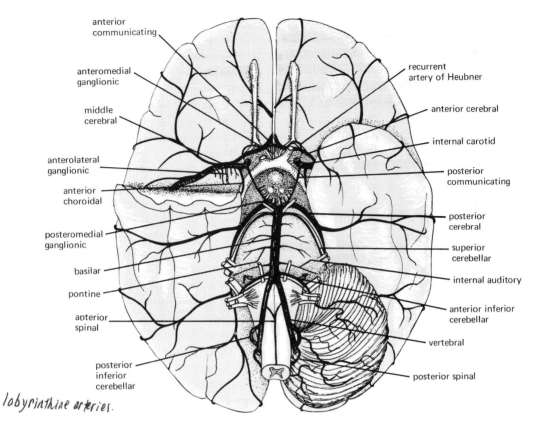

labyrinthine arteries.

FIG. 25–1. The blood supply of the brain as seen on the basal surface.

the posterior cerebral artery, thereby forming part of the arterial circle of Willis (see below).

Anterior Choroidal Artery. This branch, which comes off the distal part of the internal carotid artery or the beginning of the middle cerebral artery, has a wider distribution than the name suggests. The artery passes back along the optic tract and choroid fissure at the medial edge of the temporal lobe. In addition to supplying the choroid plexus in the inferior horn of the lateral ventricle, the anterior choroidal artery gives off branches to the optic tract, uncus, amygdala, hippocampus, globus pallidus, lateral geniculate nucleus, and the ventral part of the internal capsule. The further distribution of this artery varies

considerably, but additional branches have been traced into the subthalamus, the ventral portion of the thalamus, and the rostral part of the midbrain (including the red nucleus). The anterior choroidal artery is said to be prone to thrombosis because of its small caliber and rather long subarachnoid course. The globus pallidus and hippocampus, both of which are supplied in part by the anterior choroidal artery, are said to be favored sites of neuronal degeneration as a result of circulatory deficiency.

Middle Cerebral Artery

Of the terminal branches of the internal carotid artery, the middle cerebral artery is the larger and the direct continuation of the parent vessel (Fig. 25–1). This artery runs deep in the lateral fissure between the frontal and temporal lobes. *Frontal, parietal,* and *temporal branches* emerge from the lateral fissure and ramify over the dorsolateral surface of the hemisphere (Fig. 25–2).

The area of distribution of the middle cerebral artery includes the sensorimotor strip surrounding the rolandic sulcus, except for the dorsal part of the strip for the lower extremity. Occlusion of the artery therefore results in contralateral paralysis most noticeable in the lower part of the face and the arm, together with general sensory deficits of the cortical type. The auditory cortex is also included in the area of distribution; however, a unilateral lesion causes little impairment of hearing because of the bilateral cortical projection from the organ of Corti. Occlusion of a branch of the middle cerebral artery in the dominant hemisphere is the principal cause of aphasia (Chapter 15). The cortical areas concerned are the sensory language area in the temporal and parietal lobes, especially Wernicke's area in the temporal lobe, and Broca's area in the inferior frontal gyrus (Fig. 25–2).

Anterior Cerebral Artery

The smaller terminal branch of the internal carotid artery is the anterior cerebral artery, which is first directed medially above the optic nerve (Fig. 25–1). The two anterior cerebral arteries almost meet at the midline where they are joined together by the *anterior communicating artery.* The anterior cerebral artery then ascends in the

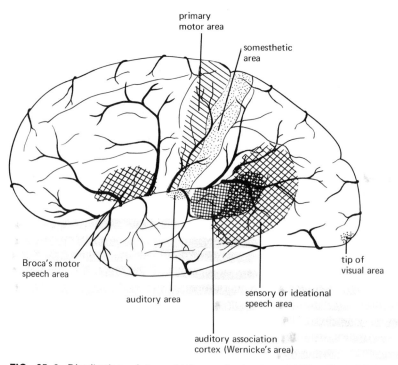

FIG. 25–2. Distribution of the middle cerebral artery on the dorsolateral surface of the cerebral hemisphere.

longitudinal fissure and bends backward around the genu of the corpus callosum (Fig. 25–3). Branches given off just distal to the anterior communicating artery supply the medial portion of the orbital surface of the frontal lobe, including the olfactory bulb and tract.

The artery continues along the upper surface of the corpus callosum as the *pericallosal artery*, and a large branch, the *callosomarginal artery*, follows the cingulate sulcus. The anterior cerebral artery supplies the medial portions of the frontal and parietal lobes and the corpus callosum. In addition, branches extend over the dorsomedial border of the hemisphere and supply a strip on the dorsolateral surface (Fig. 25–2). Since the dorsal part of the sensorimotor strip is included in the area of distribution of this artery, occlusion causes paralysis and sensory deficits in the contralateral leg.

A special branch of the anterior cerebral artery is given off just proximal to the anterior communicating artery. This is the *recurrent artery of Heubner*, which penetrates the anterior perforated substance to supply the ventral part of the head of the caudate nucleus, the adjacent portion of the putamen, and the anterior limb and genu of the internal capsule. The recurrent artery of Heubner is sometimes called the *medial striate artery* because of its contribution to the blood supply of the corpus striatum.

VERTEBRAL ARTERY SYSTEM

The *vertebral artery*, a branch of the subclavian artery, ascends in the foramina of

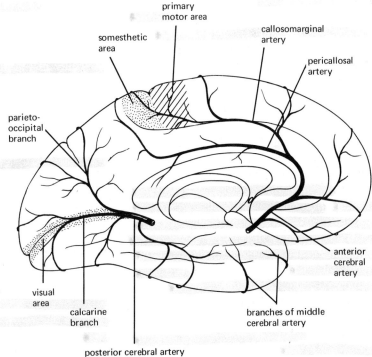

FIG. 25–3. Distribution of the anterior and posterior cerebral arteries on the medial surface of the cerebral hemisphere.

the transverse processes of the upper six cervical vertebrae. On reaching the base of the skull, the artery winds around the lateral mass of the atlas, pierces the posterior atlanto-occipital membrane, then enters the subarachnoid space at the level of the foramen magnum by piercing the dura mater and arachnoid. The vertebral artery runs forward with a medial inclination beneath the medulla oblongata, joining its fellow of the opposite side at the caudal border of the pons to form the *basilar artery*. The latter artery runs forward in the midline of the pons and divides into the *posterior cerebral arteries* (Fig. 25–1).

Branches of the Vertebral Artery

Spinal Arteries. The upper portion of the cervical cord receives blood through spinal branches of the vertebral arteries. A single *anterior spinal artery* is formed by a contribution from each vertebral artery. A *posterior spinal artery* arises on each side as a branch of either the vertebral or the posterior inferior cerebellar artery (Fig. 25–1). The spinal arteries continue the length of the cord, being reinforced at intervals by radicular arteries, as described below.

Posterior Inferior Cerebellar Artery. This vessel, which is the largest branch of the vertebral artery, pursues an irregular course between the medulla and the cerebellum. Branches are distributed to the posterior part of the cerebellar hemisphere, the inferior vermis, the central nuclei of the cerebellum, and the choroid plexus of the fourth ventricle. There are also medullary branches to the dorsolateral region of the medulla oblongata. Occlusion of the posterior inferior cerebellar artery therefore results in the lateral medullary or Wallenberg's syndrome (Chapter 7). In addition to branches from the posterior inferior cerebellar artery, many fine branches arising directly from the vertebral artery supply the medulla.

Branches of the Basilar Artery

In addition to terminal branches which will be considered separately, the basilar artery gives off the following branches to the pons, cerebellum, and inner ear.

Anterior Inferior Cerebellar Artery. Arising from the caudal end of the basilar artery, this vessel supplies the cortex of the inferior surface of the cerebellum anteriorly and the underlying white matter; it assists in the supply of the central cerebellar nuclei. In addition, slender twigs from the artery penetrate the upper medulla and lower pons.

Internal Auditory Artery. This vessel, also called the labyrinthine artery, is a branch of either the basilar or the anterior inferior cerebellar artery. The internal auditory artery ramifies throughout the membranous labyrinth of the inner ear, which it reaches by way of the internal auditory canal. Although of rare occurrence, occlusion of the artery results in the expected deafness in the corresponding ear.

Pontine Arteries. These are slender branches arising from the basilar artery along its length. They penetrate the pons and ramify in both the basal portion of the pons and the pontine tegmentum.

Superior Cerebellar Artery. This branch arises close to the terminal bifurcation of the basilar artery, ramifies over the dorsal surface of the cerebellum, and supplies the cortex, medullary center, and central nuclei. Branches from the proximal part of the superior cerebellar artery are distributed to the pons, the superior cerebellar peduncle, and the inferior colliculus of the midbrain.

Posterior Cerebral Artery

Each posterior cerebral artery, a terminal branch of the basilar artery, curves around the cerebral peduncle and reaches the medial surface of the hemisphere beneath the splenium of the corpus callosum (Fig. 25–3). The artery gives off *temporal branches,* which ramify over the inferior surface of the temporal lobe, and *calcarine* and *parieto-occipital branches,* which run along the corresponding sulci. All these arteries send branches around the border of the hemisphere to supply a peripheral strip on the dorsolateral surface (Fig. 25–2). The calcarine artery is of special significance as the main blood supply for the visual area of cortex. Occlusion of the vessel causes blindness in the contralateral field of vision. Central or macular vision is usually spared, perhaps because the large portion of the visual area at the occipital pole for macular vision is partially sustained by collateral circulation from the middle cerebral artery. However the possibility exists that "macular sparing" is an artifact of testing that results when the person being tested shifts his fixation point slightly during examination of the visual fields.

The *posterior choroidal artery* comes off the posterior cerebral artery in the region of the splenium and runs forward in the transverse fissure beneath the corpus callosum. The posterior choroidal artery supplies the choroid plexuses of the body of the lateral ventricle and the third ventricle, the posterior part of the thalamus, the fornix, and the tectum of the midbrain.

CORTICAL BRANCHES OF THE CEREBRAL ARTERIES

Anastomoses between branches of the anterior, middle, and posterior cerebral arteries are concealed in the sulci. The adequacy of these anastomoses is variable, but occasionally an anastomotic vessel is of sufficient caliber to sustain a portion of the territory of another artery if the latter is occluded. The cerebral arteries are interconnected through an arteriolar network in the pia mater. Short cortical branches from the pial plexus supply the rich capillary network of the cortex, while longer branches of arteries in the subarachnoid space penetrate into the white matter and form a more open capillary network.

Sympathetic fibers from cervical ganglia of the sympathetic chain form perivascular plexuses around the internal carotid and vertebral arteries. Some fibers can be followed to the finer ramifications of the blood vessels. Parasympathetic fibers, most of them coming from the facial nerve, are also present in the perivascular plexuses. The functional significance of the autonomic supply of cerebral vessels is still obscure. The cerebral circulation changes according to fluctuations in local requirements; this is probably a response to alterations in carbon dioxide and hydrogen ion concentrations. Circulatory changes of autonomic origin are probably superimposed on those caused by local chemical factors. Recent studies using histochemical stains for nerve fibers have shown that considerably more fibers are associated with blood vessels of various calibers than could be identified with the silver and methylene blue techniques used previously. The influence of autonomic innervation on cerebral blood flow may have more importance than is presently credited.

ARTERIAL CIRCLE (CIRCLE OF WILLIS)

The major arteries supplying the cerebrum are joined to one another at the base of the brain in the form of an *arterial circle* or *circle of Willis* (Fig. 25–1). Starting from the midline in front, the circle consists of the anterior communicating, anterior cerebral, internal carotid (a short segment), posterior communicating, and posterior cerebral arteries; then it continues to the starting point in reverse order. There is normally little exchange of blood between the main vessels through the slender communicating arteries. However, the arterial circle provides alternative routes when one of the major arteries leading into it is occluded. These anastomoses are frequently inadequate, especially in elderly persons in whom the lumina of the connecting arteries are often stenosed by vascular disease.

There are frequent variants of the conventional configuration of the arterial circle. The posterior cerebral artery is a branch of the internal carotid artery embryologically. In the course of development the posterior cerebral artery becomes a terminal branch of the basilar artery, the vestige of the embryologic condition being seen in the posterior communicating artery. The embryologic condition persists in about a third of all individuals, in whom one of the posterior cerebral arteries is a major branch of the internal carotid artery. The embryologic type of connection of the posterior cerebral artery occurs bilaterally very rarely. One of the anterior cerebral arteries may be unusually small in the first part of its course, in which case the anterior communicating artery has a larger than usual caliber.

GANGLIONIC ARTERIES

Numerous fine *ganglionic* or *perforating arteries* come off the circle of Willis and the proximal portions of the cerebral arteries (Fig. 25–1). Also known as central or nuclear branches of the arterial circle, these vessels supply the corpus striatum, internal capsule, diencephalon, and midbrain. The anterior and posterior choroidal arteries and the recurrent artery of Heubner may

also be considered as ganglionic arteries. The others constitute the following groups.

Anteromedial Group

These central branches arise from the first part of the anterior cerebral artery on both sides and from the anterior communicating artery. They penetrate the medial part of the anterior perforated substance and are distributed mainly to the preoptic and suprachiasmatic regions of the hypothalamus.

Anterolateral Group

This group of ganglionic arteries consists mainly of branches from the proximal portion of the middle cerebral artery. The vessels enter the anterior perforated substance and are also called *striate arteries* (or lateral striate arteries) because they supply a major portion of the corpus striatum. The region of distribution of the anterolateral ganglionic arteries includes the head of the caudate nucleus, putamen, lateral part of the globus pallidus, much of the internal capsule (anterior limb, genu, and dorsal portion of posterior limb), external capsule, and claustrum. Several of these vessels also send twigs into the lateral area of the hypothalamus.

Posteromedial Group

The posteromedial ganglionic arteries are branches of the initial portions of the posterior cerebral arteries and of the posterior communicating arteries. After penetrating the posterior perforated substance between the cerebral peduncles, the arteries are distributed to the anterior and medial portions of the thalamus, the subthalamus, the middle and posterior regions of the hypothalamus, and the medial parts of the cerebral peduncles of the midbrain.

Posterolateral Group

These ganglionic arteries come off the posterior cerebral artery as it curves around the cerebral peduncle. They are distributed to the posterior portion of the thalamus (including the geniculate bodies), the tectum of the midbrain, and the lateral part of the cerebral peduncle.

Distribution of Ganglionic Arteries

The following summary identifies the blood supply of structures situated within the region of the brain that is nourished by ganglionic or central arteries.

Head of caudate nucleus and putamen (*striatum*): anterolateral ganglionic arteries; recurrent artery of Heubner

Globus pallidus (*pallidum*): anterolateral ganglionic arteries; anterior choroidal artery

Thalamus: posteromedial and posterolateral ganglionic arteries; anterior and posterior choroidal arteries

Subthalamus: posteromedial ganglionic arteries; anterior choroidal artery

Hypothalamus: anteromedial, posteromedial, and anterolateral ganglionic arteries

Pineal gland: posterolateral ganglionic arteries

Internal capsule: anterolateral and posterolateral ganglionic arteries; anterior choroidal artery; recurrent artery of Heubner

Amygdala, uncus, and hippocampal formation: anterior choroidal artery; temporal branches of posterior cerebral artery

External capsule and claustrum: anterolateral ganglionic arteries

Tectum of midbrain: posterolateral ganglionic arteries; posterior choroidal artery; superior cerebellar artery

Cerebral peduncle: posteromedial and posterolateral ganglionic arteries; anterior choroidal artery

VENOUS DRAINAGE OF THE BRAIN

The capillary bed of the brain stem and cerebellum is drained by unnamed veins that empty into dural venous sinuses situated adjacent to the posterior cranial fossa. The cerebrum has an external and an internal venous system. The external cerebral veins lie in the subarachnoid space on all surfaces of the hemispheres, while the central core of the cerebrum is drained by internal cerebral veins situated beneath the corpus callosum in the transverse fissure. Both sets of cerebral veins empty into dural venous sinuses, which are identified in the following chapter.

EXTERNAL CEREBRAL VEINS

The *superior cerebral veins*, 8–12 in number, course upward over the dorsolateral surface of the hemisphere. On approaching the midsagittal line, these veins pierce the arachnoid, run between the arachnoid and the dura mater for 1–2 cm, and empty into the superior sagittal sinus or into venous lacunae adjacent to the sinus. The location of one of these veins may correspond with the central sulcus, in which case it is called the rolandic vein. Trauma to the head may tear a superior cerebral vein as it lies between the arachnoid and dura mater, resulting in subdural hemorrhage.

The *superficial middle cerebral vein* runs downward and forward along the sylvian fissure and empties into the cavernous sinus. However, anastomotic channels allow for drainage in other directions. These are the superior anastomotic vein (of Trolard), which opens into the superior sagittal sinus, and the inferior anastomotic vein (of Labbé), which opens into the transverse sinus.

The *deep middle cerebral vein* runs downward and forward in the depths of the sylvian fissure to the basal surface of the brain; the *anterior cerebral vein* corresponds with the anterior cerebral artery. These veins unite in the region of the anterior perforated substance to form the *basal vein* (of Rosenthal), which runs backward at the base of the brain, curves around the cerebral peduncle, and empties into the great cerebral vein (see below). The basal vein receives tributaries from the optic tract, tuber cinereum, mammillary bodies, uncus, and cerebral peduncles.

In addition to the named veins noted above, there are numerous small vessels that drain limited areas. These have no consistent pattern and empty into adjacent dural sinuses.

INTERNAL CEREBRAL VEINS

The internal venous system forms in the floor of the lateral ventricle and continues through the transverse cerebral fissure beneath the corpus callosum (Fig. 25–4). The *terminal vein,* known alternatively as the *thalamostriate vein,* begins in the region of the amygdaloid nucleus and follows the curve of the tail of the caudate nucleus on its medial side. The terminal vein receives tributaries from the corpus striatum, internal capsule, thalamus, fornix, and septum pellucidum. The *choroidal vein,* which is rather tortuous, runs along the choroid plexus of the lateral ventricle. In addition to draining the plexus, the choroidal vein receives tributaries from the hippocampus, fornix, and corpus callosum. The terminal and choroidal veins unite immediately behind the foramen of Monro to form the *internal cerebral vein.* The paired internal cerebral veins run posteriorly in the tela choroidea of the transverse fissure, uniting beneath the splenium of the corpus callosum to form the *great cerebral vein of Galen.* The latter vein, which is about 2 cm in length, receives the basal veins and tributaries from the cerebellum. The vein of Galen empties into the straight sinus, which is directed backward in the midline of the tentorium cerebelli.

BLOOD SUPPLY OF THE SPINAL CORD

SPINAL ARTERIES

Three arterial channels, the *anterior spinal artery* and the paired *posterior spinal arteries,* run longitudinally throughout the length of the cord. The anterior spinal artery originates in a Y-shaped configuration from the vertebral arteries, as described above, and runs caudally along the ventral median fissure. Each posterior spinal artery is a branch of either the vertebral or the posterior inferior cerebellar artery and consists of plexiform channels along the line of attachment of dorsal spinal roots.

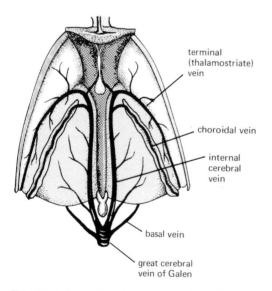

terminal (thalamostriate) vein

choroidal vein

internal cerebral vein

basal vein

great cerebral vein of Galen

FIG. 25–4. The internal cerebral system of veins.

The blood received by the spinal arteries from the vertebral arteries is sufficient for only the upper cervical segments of the spinal cord. The arteries are therefore reinforced at intervals in the following manner. The vertebral artery in the cervical region, the posterior intercostal branches of the thoracic aorta, and the lumbar branches of the abdominal aorta give off segmental *spinal arteries*, which enter the vertebral canal through the intervertebral foramina. The spinal arteries divide into branches that supply the vertebrae. In addition, some of the spinal arteries give rise to a special branch, usually referred to as a *radicular artery*, which courses along a spinal nerve root and joins either the anterior or the posterior spinal artery. There are approximately 12 anterior, and 14 posterior, radicular arteries, including both sides in each instance. The largest of these is an anterior radicular artery, known as the spinal artery of Adamkiewicz, which joins the anterior spinal artery in the upper lumbar region of the cord. The spinal cord is vulnerable to circulatory impairment if the important contribution by a radicular artery is shut off. This would occur, for example, following ligature of an intercostal artery that happens to contribute a radicular branch.

Sulcal branches arise in succession from the anterior spinal artery and enter the right and left sides of the cord alternately from the ventral median sulcus. The sulcal arteries are least frequent in the thoracic part of the cord. The anterior spinal artery supplies the ventral gray horns and the ventral and lateral white columns, including the lateral corticospinal tracts. Penetrating branches from the posterior spinal arteries supply the dorsal gray horns and the dorsal columns of white matter. A fine plexus (the vasocorona) derived from the spinal arteries is present on the lateral and ventral surfaces of the cord. Penetrating branches from the vasocorona supply a narrow zone of white matter beneath the pia mater.

SPINAL VEINS

The veins of the spinal cord have an irregular pattern; however, with this qualification six such veins are recognized. *Anterior spinal veins* run along the midline and each ventrolateral sulcus; *posterior spinal veins* are situated in the midline and along the dorsolateral sulci. The spinal veins are drained at intervals by up to 12 *anterior radicular veins* and a similar number of *posterior radicular veins*. The radicular veins empty into an epidural venous plexus, which in turn drains into an external vertebral plexus through channels in the intervertebral foramina. Blood from the external vertebral plexus empties into the vertebral, intercostal, and lumbar veins.

THE BLOOD–BRAIN BARRIER

Certain substances fail to pass from the capillary blood into the tissue of the central nervous system, although the same substances gain access to nonnervous tissues. This applies to some agents that would otherwise be useful therapeutically and to dye substances in experimental animals. The phenomenon is known as the "blood–brain barrier" and much research has been directed toward the identification of a barrier in an anatomic or physical sense.

The lumen of a capillary and the brain parenchyma are separated by the endothelial cell layer of the capillary, bounded by a basement membrane in which pericytes are embedded. It is currently thought that special properties of the endothelium, including an especially close approximation of endothelial cells in the form of tight junctions, make the chief contribution to

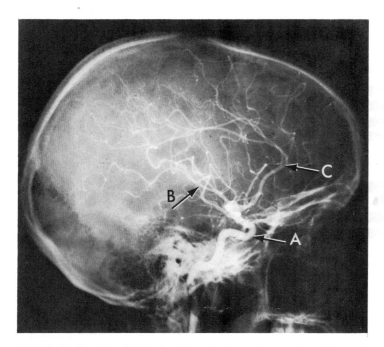

FIG. 25–5. Carotid angiogram, lateral view. *A.* carotid siphon; *B.* branches of middle cerebral artery; *C.* anterior cerebral artery. (Courtesy of Dr. J. M. Allcock)

the blood–brain barrier. Other possible factors include the perivascular foot-plates of astrocytic processes on the basement membranes of capillaries and the narrow intercellular spaces of nervous tissue, which are of the order of 200 Å in width. The blood–brain barrier in the anatomic sense is perhaps complex, with the principal barrier residing in special characteristics of the endothelium. The "barrier" is lacking or less evident in several components of the brain, notably in the area postrema in the medulla and in the neurohypophysis.

CEREBRAL ANGIOGRAPHY

In 1927, de Egas Moniz introduced the technique of cerebral angiography, which

has developed into a valuable diagnostic aid in the hands of the neuroradiologist. Briefly stated, the method consists of injecting a radiopaque solution into the artery, followed by serial X-ray photography at approximately 1 second intervals. The roentgenograms show the contrast medium in progressive stages of its passage through the arterial tree and the venous return. Injection into the common carotid artery or the internal carotid artery shows the distribution of the middle and anterior cerebral arteries (Figs. 25–5 and 25–6). Similarly, injection of the vertebral artery enables one to visualize the vertebral, basilar, and posterior cerebral arteries, together with their larger branches. The cerebral veins are seen in later roentgenograms of the series.

The technique of cerebral angiography is

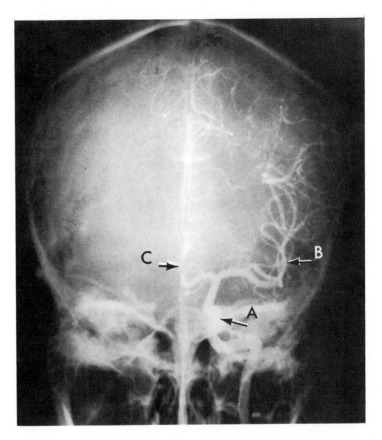

FIG. 25–6. Carotid angiogram, anteroposterior view. *A.* carotid siphon; *B.* branches of middle cerebral artery; *C.* anterior cerebral artery. (Courtesy of Dr. J. M. Allcock)

especially useful in localizing vascular malformations and aneurysms. The method often provides valuable information concerning occlusive vascular disease and space-occupying intracranial masses.

SUGGESTIONS FOR ADDITIONAL READING

Aird RB: Barriers in the brain. Sc Am 194/2:101–106, 1956

Bull JWD: Use and limitations of angiography in the diagnosis of vascular lesions of the brain. Neurology (Minneap) 11, Pt. 2:80–85, 1961

Gillilan LA: The arterial blood supply of the human spinal cord. J Comp Neurol 110:75–103, 1958

Harper AM, Deshmukh VD, Rowan JO, Jennett WB: The influence of sympathetic nervous activity on cerebral blood flow. Arch Neurol 27:1–6, 1972

Long DM: Capillary ultrastructure and the blood–brain barrier in human malignant brain tumors. J Neurosurg 32:127–144, 1970

Nelson E, Rennels M: Innervation of cranial arteries. Brain 93:475–490, 1970

Pappas GD: Some morphological considerations of the blood–brain barrier. J Neurol Sci 10:241–246, 1970

Shaw Dunn J, Wyburn GM: The anatomy of the blood brain barrier: A review. Scottish Med J 17:21–36, 1972

Stephens RB, Stilwell DL: Arteries and Veins of the Human Brain. Springfield, Ill., Thomas, 1969

Taveras JM: Angiographic observation in occlusive cerebrovascular disease. Neurology (Minneap) 11, Pt. 2:86–90, 1961

Truex RC, Carpenter MB: Human Neuroanatomy. Baltimore, Williams & Wilkins, 1969

26

Meninges and Cerebrospinal Fluid

The brain has a soft, gelatinous consistency, although the spinal cord is slightly firmer; without adequate protection the central nervous system would be especially vulnerable to trauma. The main function of the meninges is to provide support and protection for the brain and spinal cord, in addition to that offered by the skull and by the vertebral column and its ligaments.

The meninges consist of the thick dura mater externally, the delicate arachnoid lining the dura, and the thin pia mater which adheres to the brain and spinal cord. The latter two layers, which may be combined under the heading of the pia-arachnoid, bound the subarachnoid space filled with cerebrospinal fluid. The main support and protection provided by the meninges come from the dura mater and the cushion of cerebrospinal fluid in the subarachnoid space.

DURA MATER AND ASSOCIATED STRUCTURES

The inner surfaces of the bones enclosing the cranial cavity are clothed by periosteum, such as covers bones elsewhere. The inner periosteum is continuous with the periosteum on the outer surface of the cranium at the margins of the foramen magnum and smaller foramina for nerves and blood vessels. The cranial dura mater is attached intimately to the periosteum; the latter is often considered incorrectly as the outer layer of the dura.

PERIOSTEUM AND MENINGEAL BLOOD VESSELS

The *periosteum* consists of collagenous connective tissue and contains arteries, somewhat inappropriately called meningeal

363

arteries, that mainly supply the underlying bone. Of these vessels the largest is the middle meningeal artery, which is a branch of the maxillary artery entering the cranial cavity through the foramen spinosum in the floor of the middle cranial fossa. The artery divides into anterior and posterior branches soon after entering the middle fossa; these branches ramify over the lateral surface of the cranium, producing grooves on the underlying bones. A fracture in the temporal region of the skull may tear a branch of the middle meningeal artery. The extravasated blood accumulates between the bone and the periosteum, forming an epidural hematoma. As in the case of any space-occupying lesion in the nonexpansile cranial cavity, intracranial pressure rises and surgical intervention is usually necessary. Less extensive areas are supplied by several small arteries. These include meningeal branches of the ophthalmic artery, branches of the occipital artery traversing the jugular foramen and hypoglossal canal, and small twigs arising from the vertebral artery at the foramen magnum.

The meningeal arteries are accompanied by meningeal veins, which are also subject to tearing in fractures of the skull. The largest meningeal veins accompany the middle meningeal artery, leave the cranial cavity through the foramen spinosum or the foramen ovale, and drain into the pterygoid venous plexus.

DURA MATER

The *dura mater* or *pachymeninx* (thick membrane) is a dense, firm layer consisting of collagenous connective tissue. The *spinal dura* takes the form of a tube, pierced by the roots of spinal nerves, extending from the foramen magnum to the second sacral segment (Chapter 5). The spinal dura is separated from the wall of the spinal canal by an epidural space containing adipose

tissue and a venous plexus. The *cranial dura mater* is firmly attached to the periosteum, as described above, from which it receives small blood vessels. The smooth inner surface of the dura mater consists of simple squamous epithelium (mesenchymal epithelium). A thin film of fluid occupies the potential subdural space between the dura and arachnoid. The cranial dura mater has several features of importance, notably the dural reflexions or septa and the dural venous sinuses.

DURAL REFLEXIONS

The dura mater is reflected along certain lines to form the *dural reflexions* or *septa*. The intervals between the periosteum and the dura along the lines of attachment of the septa accommodate the dural venous sinuses (Fig. 26–1). Of the following dural septa, the largest ones partition the cranial cavity and provide support for parts of the brain (Fig. 26–2).

The *falx cerebri*, so named because of its sickle shape, is a vertical partition in the longitudinal fissure between the cerebral hemispheres. This dural septum is attached to the crista galli of the ethmoid bone in front, to the midline of the vault as far back as the internal occipital protuberance, and to the tentorium cerebelli. The free edge is close to the splenium, but some distance from the corpus callosum further forward. The anterior portion of the falx cerebri is often fenestrated.

The *tentorium cerebelli* intervenes between the occipital lobes of the cerebral hemispheres and the cerebellum. The attachment of the falx cerebri along the midline draws the tentorium upward, giving it a shallow tent-like configuration. The fixed border of the tentorium extends along the upper edges of the petrous temporal bones and is attached to the margins of the sulci on the occipital bone for the transverse

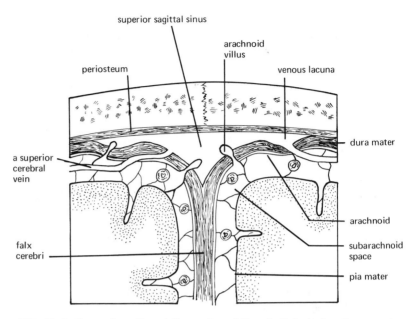

FIG. 26–1. Coronal section at the vertex of the skull, including the superior sagittal sinus and the attachment of the falx cerebri.

sinuses. The free border bounds the *tentorial notch,* also called the *incisura of the tentorium;* the incisura is completed by the sphenoid bone and accommodates the midbrain.

In the presence of certain pathologic conditions, neurologic signs may be produced by pressure of the firm edge of the tentorium on the midbrain. The narrow interval between the midbrain and the tentorial margin is the only communication between the subtentorial and supratentorial regions of the subarachnoid space. The cerebrospinal fluid produced in the ventricles enters the subarachnoid space of the posterior cranial fossa, then moves slowly upward around the midbrain to be absorbed into venous blood along the attached border of the falx cerebri. Obstruction of the subarachnoid space around the midbrain results in dilation of the ventricles and the subarachnoid space in the posterior

cranial fossa (communicating hydrocephalus).

The *falx cerebelli* is a small dural fold in the posterior fossa, extending vertically for a short distance between the cerebellar hemispheres. The *diaphragma sellae* roofs over the pituitary fossa or sella turcica of the sphenoid bone and has an opening for passage of the infundibular stalk of the pituitary gland.

NERVE SUPPLY OF THE DURA MATER

The cranial dura mater has a plentiful supply of sensory nerve fibers, mainly from the trigeminal nerve. The fibers terminate as unencapsulated endings, for the most part, and are of significance in certain types of headache.

The dura lining the anterior cranial fossa is supplied by ethmoid branches of the ophthalmic nerve. The mandibular nerve

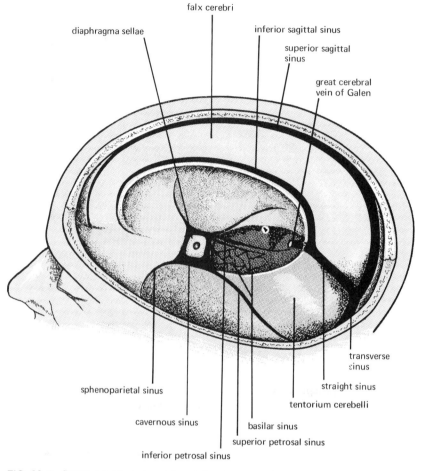

FIG. 26–2. Dural reflexions (septa) and dural venous sinuses.

supplies a large area through the nervus spinosum, which enters the middle cranial fossa with the middle meningeal artery and ramifies with the arterial branches. A meningeal branch comes off the maxillary nerve while still in the cranial cavity and joins those fibers of the nervus spinosum that accompany the anterior branch of the middle meningeal artery. The tentorium cerebelli and the dura lining the vault above it are supplied by several large branches coming off the first part of the ophthalamic nerve. These nerves run back-

ward in the tentorium, spreading out over the vault and in the falx cerebri. The dura lining the floor of the posterior cranial fossa is supplied by the vagus nerve and upper cervical nerves. The meningeal branch of the vagus nerve arises from the superior ganglion at the level of the jugular foramen, through which it enters the posterior fossa. Sensory twigs from the first three cervical spinal nerves enter the posterior fossa through the hypoglossal canal. (The first cervical nerve lacks a sensory component in about half of individuals.) Recurrent branches of all spinal nerves enter the vertebral canal through the intervertebral foramina and give off meningeal branches to the spinal dura mater.

DURAL VENOUS SINUSES

As described in the preceding chapter, the veins draining the brain empty into the venous sinuses of the dura mater, through which blood reaches the internal jugular veins. The sinuses are typically endothelium-lined spaces between the dura and the periosteum along lines of attachment of dural reflexions (Fig. 26-1). The location of most of the venous sinuses is indicated in Figure 26-2.

The *superior sagittal sinus* lies in the attached border of the falx cerebri. This sinus begins in front of the crista galli of the ethmoid bone, where there may be a narrow communication with nasal veins. Venous lacunae lie alongside the superior sagittal sinus and open into it. The superior cerebral veins drain into the sinus or into the lacunae. This sinus usually turns to the right at the internal occipital protuberance and continues as the transverse sinus on that side.

The *inferior sagittal sinus* is smaller than the one described above, runs along the free border of the falx cerebri, and receives veins from the medial aspects of the hemispheres. The inferior sagittal sinus opens into the *straight sinus, which lies in the attachment of the falx cerebri to the tentorium. The straight sinus receives the great cerebral vein of Galen* and therefore drains the system of internal cerebral veins. The straight sinus is usually continuous with the left transverse sinus. Venous channels connect the transverse sinuses across the midline and the configuration of dural sinuses at the internal occipital protuberance is known as the *confluence of the sinuses* or the *torcular Herophili*.

Each *transverse sinus* lies in a bony groove along the fixed margin of the tentorium cerebelli. On reaching the petrous temporal bone, the transverse sinus continues as the *sigmoid sinus*; the latter sinus follows a curved course in the posterior fossa on the mastoid portion of the petrous bone and becomes continuous with the internal jugular vein at the jugular foramen.

The *cavernous sinuses* are situated one on either side of the body of the sphenoid bone; each sinus receives the ophthalmic vein and the superficial middle cerebral vein. Venous channels in the anterior and posterior margins of the diaphragma sellae connect the cavernous sinuses and, with the latter, constitute the *circular sinus*. The cavernous sinus drains into the transverse sinus through the *superior petrosal sinus, running along the attachment of the tentorium to the petrous temporal bone.* The *inferior petrosal sinus* lies in the groove between the petrous bone and the clivus (basilar portion of the occipital bone), providing a communication between the cavernous sinus and the internal jugular vein. Small venous channels on the clivus constitute the *basilar sinus*, which is connected with the cavernous and inferior petrosal sinuses. Finally, the *sphenoparietal sinus* is a small venous channel under the lesser wing of the sphenoid bone draining into the cavernous sinus; the small *occipital sinus* in the falx cerebelli drains into the confluence of the sinuses. The sinuses at the base of the cranium receive veins from adjacent parts of the brain.

Emissary veins connect dural venous sinuses with veins outside the cranial cavity. Blood may flow in either direction in emissary veins, depending on venous pressure relationships. The parietal and mastoid vessels are the largest of the emissary veins. The parietal vein, one on either side, traverses the parietal foramen, joining the superior sagittal sinus with tributaries of the occipital veins. The mastoid emissary vein occupies the mastoid foramen and joins the sigmoid sinus with occipital and posterior auricular veins.

PIA–ARACHNOID

The *pia mater* and *arachnoid* develop initially as a single layer from the mesodermal tissue surrounding the embryonic brain and spinal cord. Fluid-filled spaces appear within the layer; these become the subarachnoid space, and the origin of the membranes from a single layer is reflected in the numerous trabeculae passing between them. Histologically, the pia and arachnoid consist of collagenous fibers and some elastic fibers. Both surfaces of the arachnoid and the outer surface of the pia mater are covered by mesenchymal epithelium of simple squamous type. The trabeculae crossing the subarachnoid space also consist of delicate strands of connective tissue with mesenchymal epithelial cells on their surfaces. The pia mater and arachnoid together constitute the leptomeninges (slender membranes).

The arachnoid is avascular and, as noted above, is separated from the dura by a film of fluid in the potential subdural space. The pia mater, which contains a network of fine blood vessels, adheres to the surface of the brain and spinal cord, following all their contours. The connective tissue fibers of the spinal pia mater tend to run in a longitudinal direction. This is accentuated along the ventromedian line of the cord, where a thickened strand of fibers superficial to the anterior spinal artery is known as the *linea splendens*. The *denticulate ligament*, described in Chapter 5, is derived from the pia mater.

The larger penetrating branches of blood vessels in the subarachnoid space are surrounded by a sleeve of pia mater. Within this sleeve the subarachnoid space extends into the *perivascular* or *Virchow–Robin spaces*, which continue in increasingly attenuated form to the level of the arteriolar bed.

SUBARACHNOID CISTERNS

The width of the subarachnoid space varies because the arachnoid rests on the dura mater, while the pia mater adheres to the irregular contours of the brain. The space is very narrow over the summits of gyri, relatively wide in the regions of cerebral fissures, and wider yet at the base of the brain and in the lumbar region of the spinal canal. Regions of the subarachnoid space containing more substantial amounts of fluid are called *subarachnoid cisterns* (Fig. 26–3). The cisterns are seen in pneumoencephalograms if the contained cerebrospinal fluid happens to be replaced with air.

The *cerebellomedullary cistern* (*cisterna magna*) occupies the interval between the cerebellum and the medulla oblongata, and receives cerebrospinal fluid through the foramen of Magendie. The basal cisterns beneath the brain stem and diencephalon include the *pontine* and *interpeduncular cisterns* and the *cistern of the optic chiasma.* The latter continues upward as the *cistern of the lamina terminalis*, which in turn continues into the *cistern of the corpus callosum* above this commissure. The subarachnoid space dorsal to the midbrain is called the *superior cistern* or, alternatively, the *cistern of the great vein of Galen.* The latter cistern, together with the subarachnoid space on the sides of the midbrain, are known as the *cisterna ambiens.* The *cistern of the lateral fissure* corresponds with the sylvian fissure. The *lumbar cistern* of the spinal subarachnoid space is especially large, extending from the second lumbar

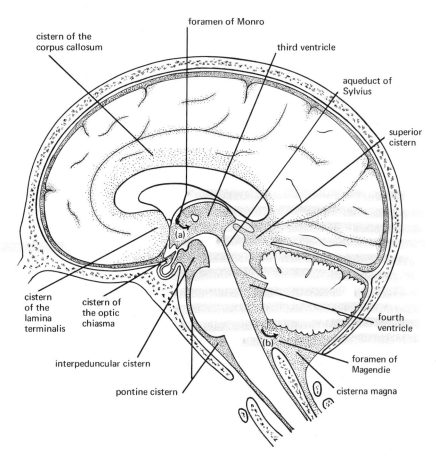

FIG. 26–3. Subarachnoid cisterns. (a) cerebrospinal fluid entering the third ventricle from the lateral ventricle through the foramen of Monro; (b) cerebrospinal fluid entering the cisterna magna from the fourth ventricle through the foramen of Magendie.

vertebra to the second segment of the sacrum. The lumbar cistern contains the cauda equina, formed by lumbosacral spinal nerve roots.

The meningeal layers and subarachnoid space extend around cranial nerves and spinal nerve roots for a short distance, approximately to the level of ganglia when these are present. For example, the semilunar ganglion of the trigeminal nerve is surrounded by extensions of the meninges; the dura-enclosed space occupied by the ganglion is known as Meckel's cavity or cave (cavum trigeminale). The most important meningeal extension clinically is that surrounding the optic nerve to its attachment to the eyeball. The central artery and vein of the retina run within the anterior part of the optic nerve and cross the extension of the subarachnoid space to join the ophthalmic artery and vein. An increase of cerebrospinal fluid pressure slows the return of venous blood, causing edema of the retina. This is most apparent on ophthalmoscopic examination as swelling of the optic papilla or disk (papilledema).

Inspection of the ocular fundi is an important part of the neurologic examination.

CEREBROSPINAL FLUID

The *cerebrospinal fluid* is produced mainly by the choroid plexuses of the lateral, third, and fourth ventricles, those in the lateral ventricles being the largest and most important.

The *choroid plexus* of the lateral ventricle is formed by an invagination of vascular pia mater (tela choroidea) on the medial surface of the cerebral hemisphere. The connective tissue picks up a covering layer of epithelium from the ependymal lining of the ventricle. The plexuses of the third and fourth ventricles are similarly formed by invaginations of the tela choroidea attached to the roofs of these ventricles. The choroid plexuses, which have a minutely folded surface, therefore consist of a core of connective tissue containing many wide capillaries and a surface layer of simple cuboidal or low columnar epithelium (the choroid epithelium) (Fig. 26–4). The surface area of the choroid plexuses of the two lateral ventricles combined is about 40 cm².

Several features of the choroid epithelium as seen in electron micrographs are of functional interest (Fig. 26–5). The large spherical nucleus, abundant cytoplasm, and numerous mitochondria indicate that the production of cerebrospinal fluid is at least partly an active process requiring expenditure of energy on the part of these cells. The plasma membrane at the free surface is greatly increased in area by irregular microvilli. The membranes of adjoining cells are thrown into complicated folds at the base of the cells. The choroid

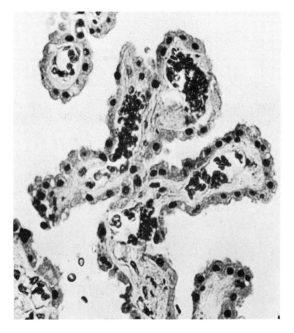

FIG. 26–4. A fragment of choroid plexus showing the large capillaries and choroid epithelium. Hematoxylin and eosin stain. ×400

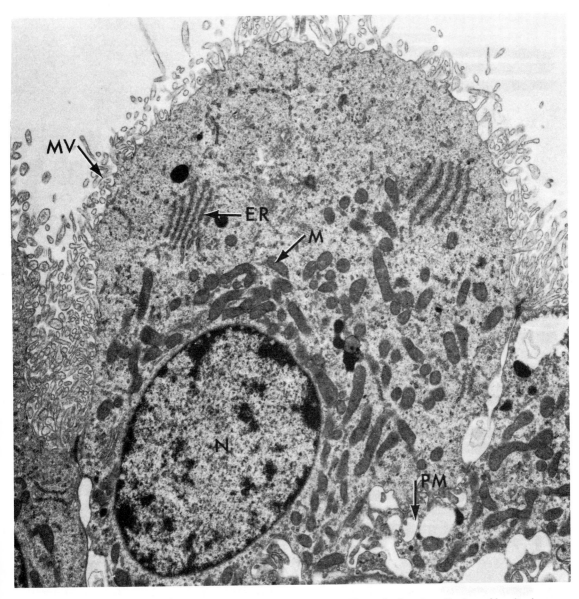

FIG. 26–5. Electron micrograph of a choroid epithelial cell. *ER*, endoplasmic reticulum; *M*, mitochondria; *MV*, microvilli; *N*, nucleus; *PM*, folds of plasma membrane. (Courtesy of Dr. D. H. Dickson) ×8,800

epithelial cells bear motile cilia in the embryo, and patches of ciliated epithelium persist for varying periods postnatally. A basement membrane separates the epithelium from the subjacent stroma with its rich vascular network. The capillaries are unlike those supplying nervous tissue generally in that the junctions between endothelial cells appear to be more permeable and the cells have fenestrations or pores closed by thin diaphragms.

Production of cerebrospinal fluid is a

complex process, the details of which are still being studied. The capillary blood is separated from the ventricular lumen by endothelium, a basement membrane, and the choroid epithelium. Some components of the plasma negotiate these layers with difficulty, others enter the cerebrospinal fluid readily by diffusion, and still others reach the fluid with the assistance of metabolic activity on the part of choroid epithelial cells. An important factor appears to be active transport of certain ions (notably sodium ions) through the epithelial cells, followed by passive movement of water to maintain the osmotic equilibrium between cerebrospinal fluid and blood plasma.

The flow of cerebrospinal fluid is from the lateral ventricles into the third ventricle through the foramina of Monro, and then into the fourth ventricle by way of the aqueduct of Sylvius. Cerebrospinal fluid leaves the ventricular system through the foramen of Magendie and the foramina of Luschka, the former opening into the cisterna magna and the latter into the pontine cistern. From these sites there is a sluggish movement of fluid through the spinal subarachnoid space, determined in part by movements of the vertebral column. More importantly, the cerebrospinal fluid flows slowly forward through the basal cisterns and then upward over the medial and dorsolateral surfaces of the cerebral hemispheres.

The main site of absorption of the cerebrospinal fluid into venous blood is through the *arachnoid villi* projecting into dural venous sinuses, especially the superior sagittal sinus and adjacent venous lucunae (Fig. 26–1). The arachnoid villi consist of a thin cellular layer, derived from the mesenchymal epithelium of the arachnoid and the endothelium of the sinus, which encloses an extension of the subarachnoid space containing trabeculae. The absorptive mechanism depends on the higher hydrostatic

pressure of the cerebrospinal fluid compared with venous blood in the dural sinuses, the difference of colloidal osmotic pressure between the virtually protein-free cerebrospinal fluid and the blood, and possibly active transport by cells forming the walls of the arachnoid villi. The arachnoid villi become hypertrophied with age, when they are called *arachnoid granulations* or *pacchionian bodies;* these may be sufficiently large to produce erosion or pitting of the cranial bones.

While the choroid plexuses are the main source of cerebrospinal fluid and the arachnoid villi of its absorption, there are exchanges between blood plasma and cerebrospinal fluid elsewhere. Studies using radioactive isotopes in experimental animals show that the chemical composition of cerebrospinal fluid is determined in part by passive, two-way transfer of solutes across the ependymal lining of the ventricles and the walls of small blood vessels in the pia mater. Some cerebrospinal fluid is probably absorbed into lymphatic vessels adjacent to the extensions of the subarachnoid space around cerebrospinal nerves.

The cerebrospinal fluid volume varies from 80 to 200 ml, with an average of about 130 ml; these figures include the fluid in both the ventricles and the subarachnoid space. The ventricular system alone contains from 15 to 40 ml of fluid. The rate of production of fluid is thought to be sufficient to effect a total replacement in 24 hours. The pressure of cerebrospinal fluid is from 80 to 180 ml of water when a person is recumbent; the pressure in the lumbar cistern is approximately twice the above values when measured in a sitting position. Venous congestion in the closed space of the cranial cavity and spinal canal, as produced by straining or coughing, is reflected in a prompt rise of cerebrospinal fluid pressure.

Cerebrospinal fluid is clear and colorless,

with a specific gravity of 1.003–1.008. The few cells present are mainly lymphocytes. These vary in number from one to eight in each cubic millimeter; a count of over ten cells is indicative of disease. The glucose level is about half that of blood, and the protein content is very low (15–45 mg per 100 ml).

When there is an excess of cerebrospinal fluid, the condition is known as *hydrocephalus,* of which there are several types. *External hydrocephalus,* in which the excess fluid is mainly in the subarchnoid space, is found in senile atrophy of the brain. *Internal hydrocephalus* refers to dilation of the ventricles. All the ventricles are enlarged if the foramina of Magendie and Luschka are occluded, the third and lateral ventricles if the obstruction is in the aqueduct of Sylvius, and one lateral ventricle only in the rare occurrence of occlusion of the foramen of Monro on one side. The term *communicating hydrocephalus* refers to a combination of internal hydrocephalus and subtentorial external hydrocephalus. In this instance, the flow of cerebrospinal fluid through the tentorial incisure around the midbrain is obstructed.

SUGGESTIONS FOR ADDITIONAL READING

Alksne, JF, Lovings ET: Functional ultrastructure of the arachnoid villus. Arch Neurol 27:371–377, 1972

Bowsher D: Cerebrospinal Fluid Dynamics in Health and Disease. Springfield, Ill., Thomas, 1960

Bull JWD: The volume of the cerebral ventricles. Neurology (Minneap) 11:1–9, 1961

Crosby EC, Humphrey T, Lauer EN: Correlative Anatomy of the Nervous System. New York, Macmillan, 1962

Davson, H: Physiology of the Cerebrospinal Fluid. London, Churchill, 1967

Davson H, Hollingsworth G, Segal MB: The mechanism of drainage of the cerebrospinal fluid. Brain 93:665–678, 1970

Dohrmann, GJ: The choroid plexus: A historical review. Brain Res 18:197–218, 1970

Dohrmann GJ, Bucy PC: Human choroid plexus: A light and electron microscopic study. J. Neurosurg 33:506–516, 1970

Jones EG: On the mode of entry of blood vessels into the cerebral cortex. J Anat 106:507–520, 1970

Kimmel DL: Innervation of spinal dura mater and dura mater of the posterior cranial fossa. Neurology (Minneap) 11:800–809, 1961

Millen JW, Woollam DHM: On the nature of the pia mater. Brain 84:514–520, 1961

Millen JW, Woollam DHM: The Anatomy of the Cerebrospinal Fluid. London, Oxford University Press, 1962

Penfield W, McNaughton F: Dural headache and innervation of the dura mater. Arch Neurol Psychiatry 44:43–75, 1940

Wolstenholme GEW, O'Connor CM (eds.): Ciba Foundation Symposium on the Cerebrospinal Fluid: Production, Circulation and Absorption. London, Churchill, 1958

Woollam DHM, Millen JW: The perivascular spaces of the mammalian central nervous system and their relation to the perineuronal and subarachnoid spaces. J Anat 89:193–200, 1955

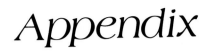

Appendix

Investigators Mentioned in the Text, Especially in Eponyms

ADAMKIEWICZ, ALBERT (1850–1921)

Polish pathologist. Described the blood supply of the spinal cord of man (an anterior radicular artery supplying the lumbar region of the cord is known as the artery of Adamkiewicz).

ANGSTRÖM, ANDERS JONAS (1814–1874)

Swedish physicist. Angström unit (Å) equals one-ten-thousandth of a micron.

ARGYLL ROBERTSON, DOUGLAS MORAY COOPER LAMB (1837–1909)

Scottish ophthalmologist. The Argyll Robertson pupil includes, among other signs, pupillary constriction with accommodation, but not in response to light.

AUERBACH, LEOPOLD (1828–1897)

German anatomist. Auerbach's plexus (myenteric plexus) in the gastrointestinal tract; end-bulbs of Held–Auerbach (synaptic end–bulbs or boutons terminaux).

BABINSKI, JOSEPH FRANÇOIS FÉLIX (1857–1932)

French neurologist of Polish origin. The Babinski sign, which consists of up-turning of the great toe and spreading of the toes on stroking the sole, is characteristic of an upper motor neuron lesion.

BAILLARGER, JULES GABRIEL FRANÇOIS (1806–1891)

French psychiatrist. The lines of Baillarger consist of two transverse strata of nerve fibers in the cerebral cortex.

BAINBRIDGE, FRANCIS ARTHUR (1874–1921)
British physiologist. Found that increase of pressure on the venous side of the heart accelerated the rate of beat.

BEEVOR, CHARLES EDWARD (1854–1908)
English neurologist. Contributed to knowledge of neurology, especially with respect to localization of function in the cerebral cortex.

BELL, SIR CHARLES (1774–1842)
Scottish anatomist, neurologist, and surgeon. Bell's palsy is a form of facial paralysis caused by interruption of conduction by the facial nerve. The Bell–Magendie law states that dorsal spinal roots are sensory, while ventral roots are motor.

BERNARD, CLAUDE (1813–1878)
French physiologist and one of the great investigators of the nineteenth century. One of his outstanding contributions was the demonstration of vasomotor mechanisms.

BIELSCHOWSKY, MAX (1869–1940)
German neuropathologist and neurologist. Bielschowsky's silver staining method for nerve cells and fibers.

BODIAN, DAVID
Contemporary American anatomist who has made important contributions to neurology. Bodian's stain for nerve cells and fibers, using the organic silver compound protargol.

BOWMAN, SIR WILLIAM (1816–1892)
English anatomist and ophthalmologist. His name is attached to glands in the olfactory mucosa, the capsule of the renal glomerulus, and a membranous layer of the cornea.

BREUER, JOSEF (1842–1925)
Austrian physician and psychologist. Contributed to our knowledge of reflexes controlling respiratory movements.

BROCA, PIERRE PAUL (1824–1880)
French pathologist and anthropologist. Localized the cortical motor speech area in the inferior frontal gyrus; also described a band of nerve fibers (the diagonal band of Broca) in the anterior perforated substance on the basal surface of the cerebral hemisphere.

BRODMANN, KORBINIAN (1868–1918)
German neuropsychiatrist. Brodmann's cytoarchitectural map of the cerebral cortex, although contested, is used frequently when referring to specific regions of the cortex.

BROWN–SÉQUARD, CHARLES EDOUARD (1817–1894)
British physiologist and neurologist. The Brown–Séquard syndrome consists of the sensory and motor abnormalities that follow hemisection of the spinal cord.

BRUCH, KARL WILHELM LUDWIG (1819–1884)
German anatomist. Bruch's membrane is the innermost layer of the choroid coat of the eye, separating the capillary layer of the choroid from the retina.

BUCY, PAUL C.
Contemporary American neurosurgeon. The Klüver–Bucy syndrome is caused by extensive bilateral lesions of the temporal lobes.

BÜNGNER, OTTO VON (1858–1905)
German neurologist. Described the endoneurial tubes containing modified Schwann cells in the distal portion of a sectioned peripheral nerve (bands of von Büngner).

CAJAL, See Ramón y Cajal.

CANNON, WALTER BRADFORD (1871–1945)
Outstanding American physiologist who contributed much to our understanding of autonomic regulation of visceral functions. Among other contributions, he developed the concept of homeostasis of the internal environment and demonstrated the "fight or flight" reactions of the body to stress.

CLARKE, JACOB AUGUSTUS LOCKHARD (1817–1880)
English anatomist and neurologist. Among numerous contributions, described the nucleus dorsalis of the spinal cord, which is also known as Clarke's column.

CORTI, MARCHESE ALFONSO (1822–1888)
Italian histologist. Described the sensory epithelium of the cochlea (organ of Corti).

CUSHING, HARVEY (1869–1939)
Pioneer American neurosurgeon. Contributed to many basic aspects of neurology, including the function of the pituitary gland, pituitary tumors, tumors of the eighth cranial nerve, and classification of brain tumors.

DARKSCHEWITSCH, LIVERIJ OSIPOVICH (1858–1925)
Russian neurologist. Nucleus of Darkschewitsch in central gray matter of the midbrain.

DE EGAS MONIZ, ANTÔNIO CAETANO DE ABREAU FRIERE (1874–1955)
Portuguese physician. Awarded Nobel Prize in 1949 for demonstration of therapeutic value of prefrontal leukotomy; introduced the technique of cerebral angiography in 1927.

DEITERS, OTTO FRIEDRICH KARL (1834–1863)
German anatomist. The lateral vestibular nucleus, which is the origin of the vestibulospinal tract, is known as Deiters' nucleus.

DUSSER DE BARENNE, JOHANNES GREGORIUS (1885–1940)
Dutch neurophysiologist. Studied cortical function and introduced the technique of physiologic neuronography.

EDINGER, LUDWIG (1855–1918)
German neuroanatomist and neurologist. An outstanding teacher of functional neuroanatomy and a pioneer in comparative neuroanatomy. The Edinger–Westphal nucleus is the parasympathetic component of the oculomotor nucleus.

FERRIER, SIR DAVID (1843–1928)
Scottish neuropathologist, neurophysiologist, and neurologist. Best known for his studies of the motor and sensory areas of the cerebral cortex.

FLECHSIG, PAUL EMIL (1847–1929)
German psychiatrist and neurologist. Flechsig's method of tracing fiber tracts in the immature brain and spinal cord is based on differing times of myelination for different tracts.

FOERSTER, OTFRID (1873–1941)
German neurologist and neurosurgeon. Made important contributions to the study of epilepsy, pain, the distribution of dermatomes, brain tumors, and the cytoarchitecture and functional localization of the cerebral cortex; introduced the chordotomy operation for intractable pain.

FOREL, AUGUSTE H. (1848–1931)
Swiss neuropsychiatrist. Described certain fiber bundles in the subthalamus, which are known as the fields of Forel. The ventral tegmental decussation of Forel in the midbrain consists of crossing rubrospinal and rubroreticular fibers. Forel also proposed the Neuron Theory on the basis of the response of nerve cells to injury.

FRIEDREICH, NIKOLAUS (1826–1882)
German physician. Best known for his studies of neuromuscular disorders; hereditary spinal ataxia is known as Friedreich's ataxia.

FRITSCH, GUSTAV THEODOR (1838–1927)
German anthropologist and anatomist. With Hitzig, he studied localization of motor function in the dog's cerebral cortex by electrical stimulation.

FRÖLICH, ALFRED (1871–1953)
Austrian pharmacologist and neurologist. Described the adiposogenital syndrome, which is caused by a lesion involving the hypothalamus.

GALEN, CLAUDIUS (131–201)
Roman physician. Galen was the leading medical authority of the Christian world for 1400 years. His name is attached to the great cerebral vein.

GASSER, JOHANN LAURENTIUS
Eighteenth century Austrian anatomist. The sensory (semilunar) ganglion of the trigeminal nerve was named for him by one of his students, A.B.R. Hirsch, in 1765.

GENNARI, FRANCESCO (1750–1796?)
Italian physician. Described the white line in the visual cortex, now known as the line of Gennari, while still a medical student in Parma, Italy.

GOLGI, CAMILLO (1843–1926)
Italian histologist. Introduced a silver staining method which provided the basis of numerous advances in neurohistology. Awarded the Nobel Prize in Physiology and Medicine in 1905 (with Santiago Ramón y Cajal). Golgi staining method, type I and type II neurons, tendon spindles, etc.

GRÜNBAUM, ALBERT S.F. (later Leyton, A.S.F.) (1869–1921)
British bacteriologist and physiologist. Worked with Sir Charles Sherrington on functional localization of the cerebral cortex.

GUDDEN, BERNHARD ALOYS VON (1824–1886)

German neuropsychiatrist. Described the partial crossing of optic nerve fibers in the optic chiasma together with certain small commissural bundles adjacent to the chiasma. Gudden also studied connections in the brain by observing changes subsequent to lesions made in the brains of young animals.

HEAD, SIR HENRY (1861–1940)

English neurologist. Studied the dermatomes, cutaneous sensory physiology, and especially sensory disturbances and aphasia following cerebral lesions.

HELD, HANS (1866–1942)

German anatomist. Made extensive studies of interneuronal relationships (axonal synaptic terminals or end-bulbs of Held–Auerbach).

HENLE, FRIEDRICH GUSTAV JACOB (1809–1885)

German anatomist and a pioneer in histology. The endoneurial sheath surrounding individual fibers of a peripheral nerve is known as the sheath of Henle.

HENSEN, VICTOR (1835–1924)

German embryologist and physiologist. Studied the anatomy and physiology of the sense organs (cells of Hensen in the organ of Corti).

HERING, HEINRICH EWALD (1866–1948)

German physiologist. Best known for his study of the reflex that initiates expiration.

HEROPHILUS (ca. 300–250 B.C.)

Greek physician in Alexandria. Made early observations on the anatomy of the brain and other organs. The confluence of the dural venous sinuses at the internal occipital protuberance is known as the torcular Herophili.

HESCHL, RICHARD (1824–1881)

Austrian anatomist and pathologist. Described the anterior transverse temporal gyri (Heschl's convolutions), which serve as a landmark for the auditory area of the cerebral cortex.

HEUBNER, JOHANN OTTO LEONHARD (1843–1926)

German pediatrician. Described the recurrent branch of the anterior cerebral artery.

HIS, WILHELM (1831–1904)

Swiss anatomist and a founder of human embryology. Proposed the Neuron Theory on the basis of his embryologic studies of the development of nerve cells.

HITZIG, EDUARD (1838–1907)

German physiologist and neurologist. Studied localization of motor function in the cerebral cortex of dogs and monkeys by electrical stimulation.

HORNER, JOHANN FRIEDRICH (1831–1886)

Swiss ophthalmologist. Horner's syndrome, caused by interruption of sympathetic innervation of the eye, includes pupillary constriction and ptosis of the upper eyelid.

HORSLEY, SIR VICTOR ALEXANDER HADEN (1857–1916)

A founder of neurosurgery in England. Studied the motor cortex and other parts of the brain by electrical stimulation; introduced the Horsley–Clarke stereotaxic apparatus.

HUNTER, JOHN (1728–1793)

Outstanding British anatomist and pioneer surgeon of the eighteenth century. His collection of anatomic and pathologic specimens formed the basis of the Hunterian Museum of the Royal College of Surgeons.

HUNTINGTON, GEORGE SUMNER (1850–1916)

American general medical practitioner. Described a hereditary form of chorea resulting from neuronal degeneration in the corpus striatum and cerebral cortex.

JACKSON, JOHN HUGHLINGS (1835–1911)

English neurologist and pioneer of modern neurology. Gave a thorough description of focal epilepsy (jacksonian seizures) resulting from local irritation of the motor cortex.

KLÜVER, HEINRICH

Contemporary American psychologist. The Klüver–Bucy syndrome is caused by bilateral lesions of the temporal lobes.

KORSAKOFF, SERGEI SERGEIEVICH (1854–1900)

Russian psychiatrist. Korsakoff's psychosis or syndrome, which is usually a sequel of chronic alcoholism, includes a memory defect, fabrication of ideas, and polyneuritis.

KRAUSE, WILHELM JOHANN FRIEDRICH (1833–1910)

German anatomist. Described sensory endings in the skin, including the end-bulbs of Krause.

LABBÉ, LÉON (1832–1916)

French surgeon. Studied the veins of the brain (lesser anastomotic vein of Labbé).

LANGLEY, JOHN NEWPORT (1852–1925)

English physiologist. Best known for his studies of the autonomic nervous system, a term which he introduced in 1898.

LANTERMAN, A.J.

Nineteenth century American anatomist. Described the incisures of Schmidt–Lanterman in myelin sheaths of peripheral nerve fibers.

LISSAUER, HEINRICH (1861–1891)

German neurologist. Described the dorsolateral fasciculus of the spinal cord (Lissauer's tract or zone).

LUSCHKA, HUBERT VON (1820–1875)

German anatomist. Among other contributions to anatomy, described the lateral apertures of the fourth ventricle (foramina of Luschka).

LUYS, JULES BERNARD (1828–1895)

French neurologist. Described the subthalamic nucleus (nucleus of Luys), whose degeneration causes hemiballismus.

MAGENDIE, FRANÇOIS (1783–1855)

French physiologist and pioneer of experimental physiology. The sensory function of dorsal spinal nerve roots and motor function of ventral roots constitutes the Bell–Magendie law. Also described the median aperture of the fourth ventricle (foramen of Magendie).

MARCHI, VITTORIO (1851–1908)

Italian physician and histologist. The Marchi staining method for tracing the course of degenerating myelinated fibers continues to be an invaluable neuroanatomic technique.

MARIE, PIERRE (1853–1940)

French neurologist. Described a number of disorders, including aphasia and hereditary cerebellar ataxia. The fasciculus sulcomarginalis of Marie is situated in the ventral white column of the spinal cord.

MARTINOTTI, GIOVANNI (1857–1928)

Italian physician and student of Golgi. Described a type of neuron known as the cell of Martinotti in the cerebral cortex.

MECKEL, JOHANN FRIEDRICH (1714–1774)

German anatomist. Especially known for his careful description of the trigeminal nerve. The semilunar ganglion is lodged in Meckel's cavity (or cave), which is bounded by dura mater.

MEISSNER, GEORG (1829–1905)

German anatomist and physiologist. His name is attached to touch corpuscles in the dermis and the submucous nerve plexus of the gastrointestinal tract.

MÉNIÈRE, PROSPER (1801–1862)

French otologist. Described the syndrome characterized by episodes of vertigo, nausea, and vomiting, occuring in some diseases of the inner ear.

MERKEL, FRIEDRICH SIEGMUND (1845–1919)

German anatomist. Described tactile endings in the epidermis, known as Merkel's disks.

MEYER, ADOLPH (1866–1950)

A prominent American psychiatrist. Those fibers of the geniculocalcarine tract that loop far forward in the temporal lobe constitute Meyer's loop.

MEYNERT, THEODOR HERMANN (1833–1892)

Austrian neuropsychiatrist and neurologist. The habenulointerpeduncular fasciculus is also called the fasciculus retroflexus of Meynert. The dorsal tegmental decussation of Meynert in the midbrain consists of crossing tectobulbar and tectospinal fibers.

MONAKOW, CONSTATIN VON (1853–1930)

Neurologist of Russian birth who lived in Switzerland. Made fundamental contributions to knowledge of the thalamus, red nucleus, rubrospinal tract, etc. The dorsolateral region of the medulla is known as Monakow's area.

MONIZ, See de Egas Moniz.

MONRO, ALEXANDER (1733–1817)

Scottish anatomist, also known as Alexander Monro (Secundus). Including tenure by his father (Primus) and son (Tertius), the Chair of Anatomy in the University of Edinburgh was occupied by Alexander Monros for over a century. The interventricular foramen between the lateral and third ventricles is known as the foramen of Monro.

MÜLLER, HEINRICH (1820–1864)

German anatomist. Müller's orbital muscle and cells of Müller in the retina.

NAUTA, WALLE JETZE HARINX

Contemporary American neuroanatomist. Has made numerous contributions to knowledge of the functional anatomy of the central nervous system. The Nauta silver staining method is used widely for tracing the course of nerve fibers.

NISSL, FRANZ (1860–1919)

German neuropsychiatrist. Made important contributions to neurohistology and neuropathology. Introduced a method of staining gray matter with basic aniline dyes to show the basophil material (Nissl bodies) of nerve cells.

PACCHIONI, ANTONIO (1665–1726)

Italian anatomist. The arachnoid villi become hypertrophied with age and are then known as arachnoid granulations or pacchionian bodies.

PACINI, FILIPPO (1812–1883)

Italian anatomist and histologist. Described the sensory endings known as the corpuscles of Vater–Pacini.

PARKINSON, JAMES (1775–1824)

English physician, surgeon, and paleontologist. Described "shaking palsy" or paralysis agitans, which is frequently referred to as Parkinson's disease.

PENFIELD, WILDER GRAVES

Contemporary Canadian neurosurgeon. Has made fundamental contributions to neurocytology and neurophysiology; including functions of the cerebral cortex, speech mechanisms, and factors underlying epilepsy.

PERLIA, RICHARD

Nineteenth century German ophthalmologist. Described a region of the oculomotor nucleus as a center for ocular convergence (nucleus of Perlia).

PERRONCITO, A. (1882–1929)

Italian histologist. Described the whorls of regenerating fibers (spirals of Perroncito) in the central stump of a sectioned peripheral nerve.

PURKINJE, JOHANNES (JAN) EVANGELISTA (1787–1869)

Bohemian physiologist, pioneer in histologic techniques, and accomplished histologist. Described the Purkinje cells of the cerebellar cortex, Purkinje fibers in the heart, etc.

RAMÓN Y CAJAL, SANTIAGO (1852–1934)

Spanish histologist who is acknowledged as the foremost among neurohistologists. Awarded the Nobel Prize in Physiology and Medicine (with Camillo Golgi) in 1906. Among innumerable contributions, Cajal vigorously championed the Neuron Theory on the basis of his observations with silver staining methods.

RANVIER, LOUIS–ANTOINE (1835–1922)
French histologist and a founder of experimental histology. Described the nodes of Ranvier in the myelin sheaths of nerve fibers.

RASMUSSEN, GRANT LITSTER
Contemporary American neuroanatomist. Has made numerous contributions to neuro-anatomy, including a description of the olivocochlear bundle.

REIL, JOHANN CHRISTIAN (1759–1813)
German physician. The insula, lying in the depths of the lateral fissure of the cerebral hemisphere, is known as the island of Reil.

REISSNER, ERNST (1824–1878)
German anatomist. The vestibular membrane of the cochlea is known as Reissner's membrane.

RENSHAW, BIRDSEY (1911–1948)
American neurophysiologist. Certain intercalated neurons in the ventral gray horn of the spinal cord are called Renshaw cells.

REXED, BROR
Contemporary Swedish neuroanatomist. Divided the gray matter of the spinal cord into regions (laminae of Rexed) on the basis of differences in cytoarchitecture.

RIO HORTEGA, PIO DEL (1882–1945)
Spanish histologist, who worked in his later years in England and Argentina. Best known for his studies of neuroglial cells, especially the microglia.

ROBIN, CHARLES PHILIPPE (1821–1885)
French anatomist. The perivascular spaces of the brain are known as Virchow–Robin spaces.

ROLANDO, LUIGI (1773–1831)
Italian anatomist. Among various contributions to neurology, described the central sulcus of the cerebral hemisphere and the substantia gelatinosa of the spinal cord.

ROMBERG, MORITZ HEINRICH (1795–1873)
German neurologist. Romberg's sign consists of unsteadiness or swaying of the body when standing with the feet close together and the eyes closed (present in tabes dorsalis).

ROSENTHAL, FRIEDRICH CHRISTIAN (1779–1829)
German anatomist. Studied the veins of the brain (basal vein of Rosenthal).

RUFFINI, ANGELO (1864–1929)
Italian anatomist. Described sensory endings, especially those known as the end-bulbs of Ruffini.

RUSSELL, JAMES SAMUEL RISIEN (1863–1939)
British physician and neurologist. Published on diseases of the nervous system and described the uncinate fasciculus of efferent cerebellar fibers.

SCARPA, ANTONIO (1747–1832)

Italian anatomist and surgeon. Made numerous contributions to anatomy, including a description of the vestibular ganglion.

SCHMIDT, HENRY D. (1823–1888)

American anatomist and pathologist. Described the incisures of Schmidt–Lanterman in myelin sheaths of peripheral nerve fibers.

SCHÜTZ, H.

German anatomist. Described the dorsal longitudinal fasciculus of the brain stem in 1891.

SCHWANN, THEODOR (1810–1882)

German anatomist. Formulated the Cell Theory (with M. J. Schleiden) and described the neurolemmal cells (Schwann cells) of peripheral nerve fibers.

SHERRINGTON, SIR CHARLES SCOTT (1856–1952)

English neurophysiologist. A foremost contributor to basic knowledge of the function of the nervous system. His researches included studies of reflexes, decerebrate rigidity, reciprocal innervation, the synapse, and the concept of the integrative action of the nervous system.

SYDENHAM, THOMAS (1624–1689)

English physician, known as the English Hippocrates. Described the form of chorea to which his name is attached.

SYLVIUS, FRANCIS DE LA BOE (1614–1672)

French anatomist. Gave the first description of the lateral fissure of the cerebral hemisphere.

SYLVIUS, JACOBUS (also known as Jacques Dubois) (1478–1555)

French anatomist. Described the cerebral aqueduct of the midbrain.

TROLARD, PAULIN (1842–1910)

French anatomist. Described the venous drainage of the brain (greater anastomotic vein of Trolard).

VATER, ABRAHAM (1684–1751)

German anatomist. Among other contributions to anatomy, described the sensory endings known as the corpuscles of Vater–Pacini.

VICQ D'AZYR, FELIX (1748–1794)

French anatomist and a leading comparative anatomist. The mammillothalamic tract bears his name.

VIRCHOW, RUDOLPH LUDWIG KARL (1821–1902)

German pathologist. Founder of cellular pathology, or modern pathology. The perivascular spaces of the brain are known as Virchow–Robin spaces.

WALDEYER, HEINRICH WILHELM GOTTFRIED (1836–1921)
German anatomist. Popularized the Neuron Theory on the basis of studies by Cajal, Forel, His, and others.

WALLENBERG, ADOLF (1862–1949)
German physician. Described the lateral medullary syndrome.

WALLER, AUGUSTUS VOLNEY (1816–1870)
English physician and physiologist. Described the degenerative changes in the distal portion of a sectioned peripheral nerve, now known as wallerian degeneration.

WARWICK, ROGER
Contemporary British anatomist. Among other contributions, described the organization of the oculomotor nucleus with respect to the ocular muscles which it supplies.

WEBER, SIR HERMANN DAVID (1823–1918)
English physician. Described the midbrain lesion causing hemiparesis and ocular paralysis.

WEIGERT, KARL (1843–1905)
German pathologist. Introduced several staining methods, including a stain for myelin and therefore for white matter in sections of nervous tissue.

WERNICKE, CARL (1848–1905)
German neuropsychiatrist. Made a special study of disorders in the use of language. Wernicke's sensory language area, Wernicke's aphasia.

WESTPHAL, KARL FRIEDRICH OTTO (1883–1890)
German neurologist. Among other contributions to neurology, described the Edinger–Westphal nucleus in the oculomotor complex.

WILLIS, THOMAS (1621–1675)
English physician. One of the dominating figures in English medicine of the seventeenth century and one of the founders of the Royal Society. Among numerous contributions to the anatomy of the brain, described the arterial circle that bears his name.

WILSON, SAMUEL ALEXANDER KINNIER (1878–1937)
British neurologist. Described hepatolenticular degeneration, now known as Wilson's disease.

WRISBERG, HEINRICH AUGUST (1739–1808)
German anatomist. Among other contributions to anatomy, described the sensory root of the facial nerve (nervus intermedius of Wrisberg).

Glossary of Neuroanatomic Terms

Adiadochokinesia. *a,* neg. + Gr. *diadochos,* succeeding + *kinesis,* movement. Inability to perform rapidly alternating movements. Also called dysdiadochokinesia.

Agnosia. *a,* neg. + Gr. *gnōsis,* knowledge. Lack of ability to recognize the significance of sensory stimuli (auditory, visual, tactile, etc., agnosia).

Agraphia. *a,* neg. + Gr. *graphō,* to write. Inability to express thoughts in writing, due to a central lesion.

Ala cinerea. L. wing + *cinereus,* ashen-hued. Vagal triangle in floor of fourth ventricle.

Alexia. *a,* neg. + Gr. *lexis,* word. Loss of the power to grasp the meaning of written or printed words and sentences.

Allocortex. Gr. *allos,* other + L. *cortex,* bark. The phylogenetically older cerebral cortex, consisting of three layers. Includes paleocortex and archicortex.

Alveus. L. trough. The thin layer of white matter covering the ventricular surface of the hippocampus.

Amacrine. *a,* neg. + Gr. *makros,* long + *is, inos,* fiber. Amacrine nerve cell of the retina.

Ammon's horn. The hippocampus, which has an outline in cross-section suggestive of a ram's horn. Also known as the cornu Ammonis. Ammon: an Egyption diety with a ram's head.

Amygdala. L. from Gr. *amygdalē,* almond. Amygdala or amygdaloid nucleus in the temporal lobe of the cerebral hemisphere.

Anopsia. *an,* neg. + Gr. *opsis,* vision. A defect of vision.

Aphasia. *a,* neg. + Gr. *phasis,* speech. A defect of the power of expression by speech or of comprehending spoken or written language.

Apraxia. *a,* neg. + Gr. *prattō,* to do. Inability to carry out purposeful movements in the absence of paralysis.

Arachnoid. Gr. *arachnē,* spider's web + *eidos,* resemblance. The delicate meningeal layer forming the outer boundary of the subarachnoid space.

Archicerebellum. Gr. *archē,* beginning + diminutive of cerebrum. A phylogenetically old part of the cerebellum, functioning in the maintenance of equilibrium.

Archicortex. Gr. *archē,* beginning + L. *cortex,* bark. Three-layered cortex included in the limbic system; located mainly in the hippocampus and dentate gyrus of the temporal lobe.

Astereognosis. *a,* neg. + *stereos,* solid + *gnōsis,* knowledge. Loss of ability to recognize objects or to appreciate their form by touching or feeling them.

Astrocyte. Gr. *astron,* star + *kytos,* hollow (cell). A type of neuroglial cell of ectodermal origin.

Asynergy. *a,* neg. + Gr. *syn,* with + *ergon,* work. Disturbance of that proper association in the contraction of muscles which assures that the different components of an act follow in proper sequence, at the proper moment, and of the proper degree, so that the act is executed accurately.

Ataxia. *a,* neg. + Gr. *taxis,* order. A loss of power of muscle coordination, with irregularity of muscle action.

Athetosis. Gr. *athetos,* without position or place. An affection of the nervous system, caused by degenerative changes in the corpus striatum and cerebral cortex, and characterized by bizarre, writhing movements of the fingers and toes, especially.

Autonomic. Gr. *autos,* self + *nomos,* law. Autonomic system: the efferent or motor innervation of viscera.

Autoradiography. Gr. *autos,* self + L. *radius,* ray + Gr. *graphō,* to write. A technique that uses a photographic emulsion to detect the location of radioactive isotopes in tissue sections. Also called radioautography.

Axolemma. Gr. *axōn,* axis + *lemma,* husk. The plasma membrane of an axon.

Axon. Gr. *axōn,* axis. Efferent process of a neuron conducting impulses to other neurons or to muscle fibers (striated and smooth) and gland cells.

Axon hillock. The region of the nerve cell body from which the axon arises; it contains no Nissl material.

Axon reaction. Changes in the cell body of a neuron following damage to its axon.

Axoplasm. Gr. *axōn,* axis + *plasm,* anything formed or molded. The cytoplasm of the axon.

Baroreceptor. Gr. *baros,* weight + *receptor,* receiver. A sensory nerve terminal that is stimulated by changes in pressure.

Brachium. L. from Gr. *brachiōn,* arm. As used in the central nervous system, denotes a large bundle of fibers connecting one part with another (e.g., brachia associated with the cerebellum and the colliculi of the midbrain).

Bradykinesia. Gr. *brady,* slow + *kinesis,* movement. Abnormal slowness of movements.

Brain stem. In the mature human brain, usually denotes the medulla, pons, and midbrain. In descriptions of the embryonic brain the diencephalon is included as well.

Bulb. The medulla oblongata; but in the context of "corticobulbar tract," refers to the brain stem, in which motor nuclei of cranial nerves are located.

Calamus scriptorius. L. *calamus,* a reed, therefore a reed pen. Refers to an area in the caudal part of the floor of the fourth ventricle, which is shaped somewhat like a pen point.

Calcar. L. spur, used to denote any spur-shaped structure. Calcar avis, an elevation on the medial aspect of the lateral ventricles at the junction of posterior and inferior horns. Also calcarine sulcus of occipital lobe, which is responsible for the calcar avis.

Cauda equina. L. horse's tail. The lumbar and sacral spinal nerve roots in the lower part of the spinal canal.

Caudate nucleus. Part of the corpus striatum, so-named because it has a long extension or tail.

Cerebellum. L. diminutive of *cerebrum,* brain. A large part of the brain with motor functions, situated in the posterior cranial fossa.

Cerebrum. L. brain. The principal portion of the brain, including the diencephalon and cerebral hemispheres, but not the brain stem and cerebellum.

Chordotomy. Gr. *chordē,* cord + *tomē,* a cutting. Division of the lateral spinothalamic tract for intractable pain. Also spelled "cordotomy."

Chorea. L. from Gr. *choros,* a dance. A disorder characterized by irregular, spasmodic, involuntary movements of the limbs or facial muscles. Attributed to degenerative changes in the neostriatum.

Choroid. Gr. *chorion*, a delicate membrane + *eidos*, form. Choroid or vascular coat of the eye; choroid plexuses in the ventricles of the brain. Also spelled "chorioid."

Chromatolysis. Gr. *chrōma*, color + *lysis*, dissolution. Dispersal of the Nissl material of neurons following axon section or in viral infections of the nervous system.

Cinerea. L. *cinereus*, ashen–hued, from *cinis*, ashes. Refers to gray matter, but limited in usage. Tuber cinereum (basal portion of the hypothalamus, from which the pituitary stalk arises); tuberculum cinereum (slight elevation on medulla formed by spinal tract and nucleus of trigeminal nerve); ala cinerea (vagal triangle in floor of fourth ventricle).

Cingulum. L. girdle. A bundle of association fibers in the white matter of the cingulate gyrus on the medial surface of the cerebral hemisphere.

Claustrum. L. a barrier. A thin sheet of gray matter, of unknown function, situated between the lenticular nucleus and the insula.

Clava. L. club. A slight swelling on the dorsal surface of the medulla, produced by the nucleus gracilis.

Corona. L. from Gr. *korōnē*, a crown. Corona radiata (fibers radiating from the internal capsule to various parts of the cerebral cortex).

Corpus callosum. L. body + *callosus*, hard. The main neocortical commissure of the cerebral hemispheres.

Corpus striatum. L. body + *striatus*, furrowed or striped. A mass of gray matter, with motor functions, at the base of the cerebral hemisphere.

Cortex. L. bark. Outer layer of gray matter of the cerebral hemispheres and cerebellum.

Cuneus. L. wedge. A gyrus on the medial surface of the cerebral hemisphere. Fasciculus cuneatus in the spinal cord and medulla; nucleus cuneatus in the medulla.

Dendrite. Gr. *dendritēs*, related to a tree. A process of a nerve cell, on which axons of other

neurons terminate. Also peripheral process of a primary sensory neuron.

Dentate. L. *dentatus*, toothed. Dentate nucleus of the cerebellum; dentate gyrus in the temporal lobe.

Diencephalon. Gr. *dia*, through + *enkephalos*, brain. Part of the cerebrum, consisting of the thalamus, epithalamus, subthalamus, and hypothalamus. The posterior of the two brain vesicles formed from the prosencephalon of the developing embryo.

Dura. L. *durus*, hard. Dura mater (the thick external layer of the meninges).

Dysmetria. Gr. *dys*, difficult or disordered + *metron*, measure. Disturbance of the power to control the range of movement in muscular action.

Emboliform. Gr. *embolos*, plug + L. *forma*, form. Eboliform nucleus of the cerebellum.

Endoneurium. Gr. *endon*, within + *neuron*, nerve. The delicate connective tissue sheath surrounding an individual nerve fiber of a peripheral nerve. Also called the sheath of Henle.

Engram. Gr. *en*, in + *gramma*, mark. Used in psychology to mean the lasting trace left in the psyche by previous experience; a latent memory picture.

Entorhinal. Gr. *entos*, within + *rhis* (rhin-), nose. The entorhinal area is the anterior part of the parahippocampal gyrus of the temporal lobe adjacent to the uncus. Functions as olfactory association cortex.

Ependyma. Gr. *ependyma*, an upper garment. Lining epithelium of the ventricles of the brain and central canal of the spinal cord.

Epineurium. Gr. *epi*, upon + *neuron*, nerve. The connective tissue sheath surrounding a peripheral nerve.

Epithalamus. Gr. *epi*, upon + *thalamos*, inner chamber. A region of the diencephalon above the thalamus; includes the pineal gland.

Exteroceptor. L. *exterus*, external + *receptor*, receiver. A sensory receptor which serves to acquaint the individual with his environment (exteroception).

Extrapyramidal system. In broadest terms, consists of all motor parts of the central nervous system except the pyramidal motor system. "Extrapyramidal system" is subject to various interpretations.

Falx. L. sickle. Two of the dural partitions in the cranial cavity are the falx cerebri and the small falx cerebelli.

Fasciculus. L. diminutive of *fascis*, bundle. A bundle of nerve fibers.

Fastigial. L. *fastigium*, the top of a gabled roof. Fastigial nucleus of the cerebellum.

Fimbria. L. *fimbriae*, fringe. A band of nerve fibers along the medial edge of the hippocampus, continuing as the fornix.

Forceps. L. a pair of tongs. Used in neurologic anatomy for the U-shaped configuration of fibers constituting the anterior and posterior portions of the corpus callosum (forceps minor and forceps major).

Fornix. L. arch. The efferent tract of the hippocampus, arching over the thalamus and terminating mainly in the mammillary body of the hypothalamus.

Fovea. L. a pit or depression. Fovea centralis (the depression in the center of the macula lutea of the retina).

Funiculus. L. diminutive of *funis*, cord. An area of white matter which may consist of several functionally different fasciculi, as in lateral funiculus (column) of white matter of the spinal cord.

Ganglion. Gr. knot or subcutaneous tumor. A swelling composed of nerve cells, as in cerebrospinal and sympathetic ganglia.

Gemmule. L. *gemmula*, diminutive of *gemma*, bud. Minute projections on dendrites of certain neurons, especially pyramidal cells and Purkinje cells, for synaptic contact with other neurons.

Genu. L. *genus*, knee. Anterior end of corpus callosum; genu of facial nerve. Also geniculate ganglion of facial nerve and geniculate nuclei of thalamus.

Glia. Gr. glue. Neuroglia, the interstitial or accessory cells of the central nervous system.

Gliosome. Gr. *glia*, glue + *soma*, body. Granules in neuroglial cells, in particular astrocytes.

Globus pallidus. L. a ball + pale. Medial part of lenticular nucleus of corpus striatum. Also globose nuclei of cerebellum.

Gracilis. L. slender. Fasciculus gracilis of the spinal cord and medulla; nucleus gracilis of the medulla.

Granule. L. *granulum*, diminutive of *granum*, grain. Used to denote small neurons, such as granule cells of cerebellar cortex and stellate cells of cerebral cortex. Hence, granular cell layers of both cortices.

Habenula. L. diminutive of *habena*, strap or rein. A small swelling in the epithalamus, adjacent to the posterior end of the roof of the third ventricle.

Hemiballismus. Gr. *hēmi*, half + *ballismos*, jumping. A violent form of motor restlessness involving one side of the body, caused by a destructive lesion involving the subthalamic nucleus.

Hemiplegia. Gr. *hēmi*, half + *plēgē*, a stroke. Paralysis of one side of the body.

Hippocampus. Gr. *hippocampus*, sea horse. A gyrus which constitutes an important part of the limbic system; produces an elevation on the floor of the inferior (temporal) horn of the lateral ventricle.

Homeostasis. Gr. *homois*, like + *stasis*, standing. A tendency toward stability in the internal environment of the organism.

Hydrocephalus. Gr. *hydrōr*, water + *kephalē*, head. Excessive accumulation of cerebrospinal fluid in the ventricles.

Hypothalamus. Gr. *hypo*, under + *thalamos*, inner chamber. A region of the diencephalon which serves as the main controlling center of the autonomic nervous system.

Indusium. L. a garment, from *induo*, to put on. Indusium griseum, a thin layer of gray matter on the upper surface of the corpus callosum (gray tunic).

Infundibulum. L. funnel. The funnel-shaped stalk connecting the hypothalamus with the neural lobe of the pituitary gland.

Insula. L. island. Cerebral cortex concealed from surface view and lying at the bottom of the lateral fissure. Also called the island of Reil.

Interoceptor. L. *inter*, between + *receptor*, receiver. One of the sensory end-organs within viscera.

Isocortex. Gr. *isos*, equal + L. *cortex*, bark. Cerebral cortex having six layers (neocortex).

Kinesthesia. Gr. *kinēsis*, movement + *aisthēsis*, sensation. The sense of perception of movement.

Konicortex. Gr. *konis*, dust + L. *cortex*, bark. Areas of cerebral cortex containing large numbers of small neurons; typical of sensory areas.

Lemniscus. Gr. *lēmniskos*, fillet (a ribbon or band). Used to designate a bundle of nerve fibers in the central nervous system, e.g., medial lemniscus and lateral lemniscus.

Lenticular. L. *lenticula*, a lentil (of the shape of a lentil or a lens). Lenticular nucleus, a component of the corpus striatum. Also called lentiform nucleus.

Leptomeninges. Gr. *leptos*, slender + *mēninx*, membrane. The arachnoid and pia mater.

Limbus. L. a border. Limbic lobe: a C-shaped configuration of cortex on the medial surface of the cerebral hemisphere, consisting of the cingulate and parahippocampal gyri. Limbic system: Limbic lobe, hippocampal formation, and portions of the diencephalon, especially the mammillary body and anterior thalamic nucleus.

Limen. L. threshold. Limen insulae: the basal part of the insula (island of Reil); included in the lateral olfactory area.

Locus ceruleus. L. place + *caeruleus*, dark blue. A small dark spot on either side of the floor of the fourth ventricle; marks the position of a group of nerve cells that contain melanin pigment.

Macroglia. Gr. *makros*, large + *glia*, glue. The larger types of neuroglial cells, namely, astro-

cytes, oligodendrocytes, and ependymal cells; of ectodermal origin.

Macrosmatic. Gr. *makros*, large + *osmē*, smell. Having the sense of smell strongly or acutely developed.

Macula. L. a spot. Macula lutea: a spot at the posterior pole of the eye, having a yellow color when viewed with red-free light. Maculae sacculi and utriculi: sensory areas in the vestibular portion of the membraneous labyrinth.

Mammillary. L. *mamilla*, diminutive of *mamma*, breast (shaped like a nipple). Mammillary bodies: small swellings on the basal surface of the hypothalamus.

Massa intermedia. A bridge of gray matter connecting the thalami of the two sides across the third ventricle; present in 70 percent of brains.

Medulla. L. marrow, from *medius*, middle. Medulla spinalis: spinal cord. Medulla oblongata: caudal portion of the brain stem. In current usage, "medulla" refers to the medulla oblongata.

Mesencephalon. Gr. *mesos*, middle + *enkephalos*, brain. The midbrain; the second of the three primary brain vesicles.

Mesocortex. Gr. *mesos*, middle + L. *cortex*, bark. Cerebral cortex that is intermediate between three-layered and six-layered cortex (present in the cingulate gyrus).

Mesoglia. Gr. *mesos*, middle + *glia*, glue. Microglial cells, of mesodermal origin.

Metathalamus. Gr. *meta*, after + *thalamos*, inner chamber. The medial and lateral geniculate bodies (nuclei).

Metencephalon. Gr. *meta*, after + *enkephalos*, brain. Pons and cerebellum; the anterior of the two divisions of the rhombencephalon or posterior primary brain vesicle.

Microglia. Gr. *mikros*, small + *glia*, glue. Neuroglial cells of mesodermal origin, belonging to the reticuloendothelial system of cells of the body.

Microsmatic. Gr. *mikros*, small + *osmē*, smell. Having a sense of smell, but of relatively poor development.

Mitral. L. *mitra*, a coif or turban (bishop's miter). Mitral cell of the olfactory bulb.

Mnenomic. Gr. *mnēmē*, memory. Pertaining to memory.

Molecular. L. *molecula*, diminutive of *moles*, mass. Used in neurohistology to denote tissue containing large numbers of fine nerve fibers, and which therefore has a punctate appearance in silver-stained sections. Molecular layers of cerebral and cerebellar cortices.

Myelencephalon. Gr. *myelos*, marrow + *enkephalos*, brain. Medulla oblongata; the posterior of the two divisions of the rhombencephalon or posterior primary brain vesicle.

Neocerebellum. Gr. *neos*, new + diminutive of cerebrum. The phylogenetically newest part of the cerebellum, present in mammals and especially well developed in man. Ensures smooth muscle action in the finer voluntary movements.

Neocortex. Gr. *neos*, new + L. *cortex*, bark. Six-layered cortex, characteristic of mammals and constituting most of the cerebral cortex in man.

Neostriatum. Gr. *neos*, new + L. *striatus*, striped or grooved. The phylogenetically newer part of the corpus striatum consisting of the caudate nucleus and putamen; the striatum.

Neuraxis. Gr. *neuron*, nerve + L. *axis*, axle (axis). Used as a short form when referring to the brain and spinal cord. Occasionally refers to an axon.

Neurobiotaxis. Gr. *neuron*, nerve + *bios*, life + *taxis*, arrangement. The tendency of nerve cells to move during embryologic development toward the area from which they receive the most stimuli.

Neurofibril. Gr. *neuron*, nerve + L. *fibrilla*, diminutive of *fibra*, a fiber. Delicate filaments in the cytoplasm of neurons.

Neuroglia. Gr. *neuron*, nerve + *glia*, glue. Accessory or interstitial cells of the central nervous system; includes astrocytes, oligodendrocytes, microglial cells, and ependymal cells.

Neurolemma. Gr. *neuron*, nerve + *lemma*, husk. The delicate sheath surrounding a peripheral nerve fiber consisting of a series of neurolemma cells or Schwann cells.

Neuron. Gr. a nerve. The morphologic unit of the nervous system consisting of the nerve cell body and its processes (dendrites and axon).

Neuropil. Gr. *neuron*, nerve + *pilos*, felt. A complex net of nerve cell processes occupying the intervals between cell bodies in gray matter.

Nociceptive. L. *noceo*, to injure + *capio*, to take. Responsive to injurious stimuli.

Nystagmus. Gr. *nystagmos*, a nodding, from *nystazō*, to be sleepy. An involuntary oscillation of the eyes.

Obex. L. barrier. A small transverse fold overhanging the opening of the fourth ventricle into the central canal of the closed portion of the medulla.

Oligodendrocyte. Gr. *oligos*, few + *dendron*, tree + *kytos*, hollow (cell). A neuroglial cell of ectodermal origin; forms the myelin sheath in the central nervous system in the same manner as the Schwann cell in peripheral nerves.

Operculum. L. a cover or lid, from *opertus*, to cover. Frontal, parietal, and temporal opercula bound the lateral fissure of the cerebral hemisphere and conceal the insula.

Pachymeninx. Gr. *pachys*, thick + *mēninx*, membrane. The dura mater.

Paleocerebellum. Gr. *palaios*, ancient + diminutive of cerebrum. A phylogenetically old part of the cerebellum functioning in postural changes and locomotion.

Paleocortex. Gr. *palaios*, ancient + L. *cortex*, bark. Three-layered olfactory cortex.

Paleostriatum. Gr. *palaios*, ancient + L. *striatus*, striped or grooved. The phylogenetically older and efferent part of the corpus striatum; the globus pallidus or pallidum.

Pallidum. L. *pallidus*, pale. The globus pallidus of the corpus striatum; medial portion of the lenticular nucleus comprising the paleostriatum.

Pallium. L. cloak. The cerebral cortex with subjacent white matter, but sometimes used synonymously with cortex.

Paraplegia. Gr. *para*, beside + *plēgē*, a stroke. Paralysis of both legs and lower part of trunk.

Perikaryon. Gr. *peri*, around + *karyon*, nut, kernel. The cytoplasm surrounding the nucleus. Sometimes refers to the cell body of a neuron.

Perineurium. Gr. *peri*, around + *neuron*, nerve. The connective tissue sheath surrounding a bundle of nerve fibers in a peripheral nerve.

Pia mater. L. tender mother. The thin innermost layer of the meninges, attached to the surface of the brain and spinal cord; forms the inner boundary of the subarachnoid space.

Pineal. L. *pineus,* relating to the pine. Shaped like a pine cone (pertaining to the pineal gland).

Pneumoencephalography. Gr. *pneuma,* air + *enkephalos,* brain + *graphō,* to write. The replacement of cerebrospinal fluid by air, followed by x-ray examination (pneumoencephalogram); permits visualization of the ventricles and subarachnoid space.

Pons. L. bridge. That part of the brain stem which lies between the medulla and the midbrain; appears to constitute a bridge between the right and left halves of the cerebellum.

Proprioceptor. L. *proprius,* one's own + *receptor,* receiver. One of the sensory endings in muscles, tendons, and joints; provides information concerning movement and position of body parts (proprioception).

Prosencephalon. Gr. *pros,* before + *enkephalos,* brain. The forebrain, consisting of the telencephalon (cerebral hemispheres) and diencephalon; the anterior primary brain vesicle.

Pulvinar. L. a cushioned seat. The posterior projection of the thalamus beneath which the medial and lateral geniculate bodies are situated.

Putamen. L. shell. The larger and lateral part of the lenticular nucleus of the corpus striatum.

Pyramidal system. Corticospinal and corticobulbar tracts. So called because the corticospinal tracts occupy pyramid-shaped areas on the basal aspect of the medulla. The term pyramidal tract refers specifically to the corticospinal tract.

Pyriform. L. *pyrum,* pear + *forma,* form. Pyriform area is a region of olfactory cortex consisting of the uncus, limen insulae, and entorhinal area; has a pear-shaped outline in animals with a well-developed olfactory system.

Quadriplegia. L. *quadri,* four + Gr. *plēgē,* stroke. Paralysis affecting the four extremities. Also called tetraplegia.

Restiform. L. *restis,* rope + *forma,* form. Restiform body: the main mass of the inferior cerebellar peduncle, containing afferent fibers to the cerebellum.

Rhinal. Gr. *rhis,* nose, therefore related to the nose. Rhinal sulcus in the temporal lobe indicates the margin of the lateral olfactory area.

Rhinencephalon. Gr. *rhis* (rhin-), nose + *enkephalos,* brain. Refers, in man, to components of the olfactory system. In comparative neurology, structures incorporated in the limbic system (especially the hippocampus and dentate gyrus) are included.

Rhombencephalon. Gr. *rhombos,* a lozenge-shaped figure + *enkephalos,* brain. The pons and cerebellum (metencephalon) and medulla (myelencephalon); the posterior primary brain vesicle.

Rostrum. L. beak. Recurved portion of the corpus callosum, passing backward from the genu to the lamina terminalis.

Satellite. L. *satteles,* attendant. Satellite cells: flattened cells of ectodermal origin forming a capsule for nerve cell bodies in dorsal root ganglia and sympathetic ganglia. Also, satellite oligodendrocytes adjacent to nerve cell bodies in the central nervous system.

Septal area. Cortex and underlying septal nuclei, the latter extending into the septum pellucidum, beneath the genu and rostrum of the corpus callosum on the medial aspect of the frontal lobe. Also called the medial olfactory area.

Septum pellucidum. L. partition + transparent. A triangular double membrane separating the anterior horns of the lateral ventricles. Situated in the median plane, it fills in the interval between the corpus callosum and the fornix.

Somatic. Gr. *somatikos,* bodily, Used in neurology to denote the body, exclusive of the viscera (as in somatic efferent neurons supplying the skeletal musculature).

Somesthetic. Gr. *soma,* body + *aisthēsis,* perception. The consciousness of having a body. Somesthetic senses are the general senses of pain, temperature, touch, pressure, position, movement, and vibration. Also spelled "somatesthetic."

Splenium. Gr. *splēnion,* bandage. The thickened posterior extremity of the corpus callosum.

Stria terminalis. L. a furrow, groove + boundary, limit. A slender strand of fibers running along the medial side of the tail of the caudate nucleus. Originating in the amygdaloid nucleus, most of the fibers end in the septal area and hypothalamus.

Striatum. L. *striatus*, furrowed. The phylogenetically more recent part of the corpus striatum (neostriatum) consisting of the caudate nucleus and the putamen or lateral portion of the lenticular nucleus.

Subiculum. L. diminutive of *subex* (*subic-*), a layer. Transitional cortex between that of the parahippocampal gyrus and the hippocampus.

Substantia gelatinosa. A column of small neurons at the apex of the dorsal gray horn throughout the spinal cord.

Substantia nigra. A large nucleus with motor functions in the midbrain; many of the constituent cells contain dark melanin pigment.

Subthalamus. L. under + Gr. *thalamos,* inner chamber. Region of the diencephalon beneath the thalamus, containing fiber tracts and the subthalamic nucleus.

Synapse. Gr. *synaptō*, to join. The word was introduced by Sherrington in 1897 for the site of contact between neurons, at which site one neuron is excited or inhibited by another neuron.

Syringomyelia. Gr. *syrinx*, pipe, tube + *myelos,* marrow. A condition characterized by central cavitation of the spinal cord and gliosis around the cavity.

Tapetum. L. *tapete*, a carpet. Fibers of the corpus callosum sweeping over the lateral ventricle and forming the lateral wall of its posterior and inferior horns.

Tectum. L. roof. Roof of the midbrain consisting of the paired superior and inferior colliculi.

Tegmentum. L. cover, from *tego*, to cover. The dorsal portion of the pons; also the major portion of the cerebral peduncle of the midbrain, lying between the substantia nigra and the tectum of the midbrain.

Tela choroidea. L. a web + Gr. *chorioeidēs*, like a membrane. The vascular connective tissue continuous with that of the pia mater which continues into the core of the choroid plexuses.

Telencephalon. Gr. *telos,* end + *enkephalos,* brain. Cerebral hemispheres; the anterior of the two divisions of the prosencephalon or anterior primary brain vesicle.

Telodendria. Gr. *telos,* end + *dendrion,* tree. The terminal branches of axons.

Tentorium. L. tent. The tentorium cerebelli is a dural partition between the occipital lobes of the cerebral hemispheres and the cerebellum.

Thalamus. Gr. *thalamos,* inner chamber. A major portion of the diencephalon with sensory and integrative functions.

Torcular. L. wine press, from *torquere,* to twist. The confluence of the dural venous sinuses at the internal occipital protuberance was formerly known as the torcular Herophili.

Transducer. L. *transducere,* to lead across. A structure or mechanism for converting one form of energy into another; applied to sensory receptors.

Trapezoid body. Transverse fibers of the auditory pathway situated at the junction of the dorsal and basal portions of the pons.

Uncinate. L. hook-shaped. Uncinate fasciculus: association fibers connecting cortex of the basal surface of the frontal lobe with that of the temporal pole. Also a bundle of fastigiobulbar fibers (uncinate fasciculus of Russell) which curves over the superior cerebellar peduncle in its passage to the inferior cerebellar peduncle.

Uncus. L. a hook. The hooked-back portion of the rostral end of the parahippocampal gyrus of the temporal lobe, constituting a landmark for the lateral olfactory area.

Uvula. L. little grape. A portion of the inferior vermis of the cerebellum.

Vallecula. L. diminutive of *vallis*, valley. The midline depression on the inferior aspect of the cerebellum.

Vermis. L. worm. The midline portion of the cerebellum.

Zona incerta. Gray matter in the subthalamus representing a rostal extension of the reticular formation of the brain stem.

Index

Accessory body of Cajal, 14
Acetylcholine, 19, 37, 340
Action potential, 13
Adenohypophysis, 192
Adiodochokinesia, 166
Agnosia, 228, 229
Ala cinerea, 87
Alveus, 261, 262
Amnesia, 265–266
Ampulla of semicircular duct, 313
Amygdala, 256, 264–265
Amyotrophic lateral sclerosis, 80
Angiography, cerebral, 360
Ansa lenticularis, 183, 203, 325
Aphasia, 234–235
Apparatus, Golgi, 17
Apraxia, 233
Aqueduct, cerebral, of Sylvius, 106, 369
Alexia, 235
Allocortex, 216
Arachnoid, 368
  granulations, 372
  villi, 372
Archicerebellum, 153, 162, 314
Archicortex, 216, 220, 262
Area(s), of Broca, 235
  of Brodmann, 221–222
  entorhinal, 256
  intermediate olfactory, 257

Area(s) (*continued*)
  lateral olfactory, 256
  medial olfactory, 257
  of Monakow, 271
  postrema, 85, 149
  preoptic, of hypothalamus, 186
  prerubral, 183
  primary olfactory, 256
  pyriform, 257
  septal, 257
  striate, of cerebral cortex, 228
  vestibular, of rhomboid fossa, 87
  of Wernicke, 230, 235
Argyll Robertson pupil, 124, 297
Arterial circle of Willis, 355–356
Artery(-ies), anterior cerebral, 352–353
  anterior choroidal, 351
  anterior communicating, 352
  anterior inferior cerebellar, 354
  anterior spinal, 354, 358–359
  basilar, 354
  callosomarginal, 353
  central, of retina, 290, 292
  ganglionic (perforating), 356–357
  hypophyseal, 350
  internal auditory, 354
  internal carotid, 350
  meningeal, 363–364
  middle cerebral, 351–352

75 76 77 78 10 9 8 7 6 5 4 3